A MANUAL OF HUMAN

PHYSIOLOGY

A MANUAL OF HUMAN PHYSIOLOGY

BY

JOSEPH H. RAYMOND

GYAN

Published by

GYAN

Gyan Publishing House
5, Ansari Road
Daryaganj, New Delhi-110002
Phone: 011-47034999, 9811692060
E-mail: books@gyanbooks.com

Distribution Network
gyanbooks.com
India, USA, Canada, UK, Australia

ISBN: 978-93-6280-267-5 (HB)
First Published, 1894

2nd Impression 2024

Printed at: Gyan Press, Delhi.

A MANUAL OF HUMAN PHYSIOLOGY
Author: JOSEPH H. RAYMOND

PLATE I.

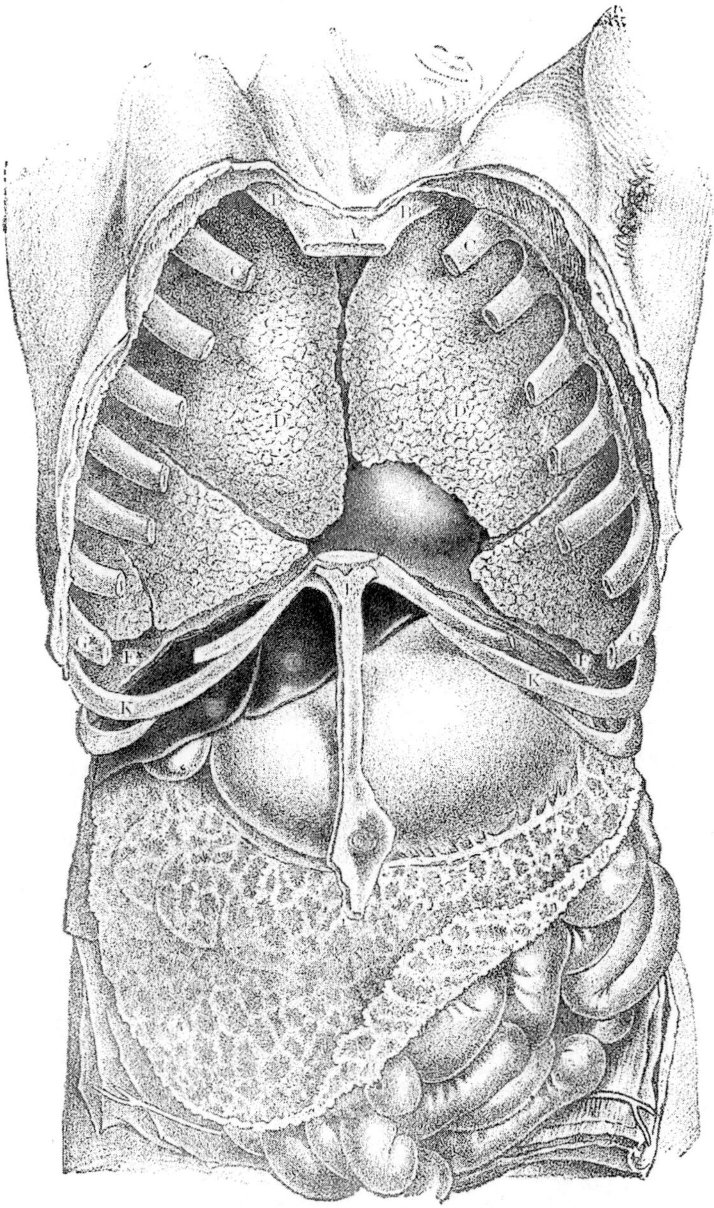

A, upper bone of sternum; *B*, *B*, two first ribs; *C*, *C*, second pair of ribs; *D*, *D*, right and left lungs; *E*, lower end of sternum: *F F*, right and left halves of the diaphragm in sections: the right half separating the right lung from the liver, the left half separating the left lung from the broad cardiac end of the stomach; *G*, *G*, eighth pair of ribs; *K*, *K*, ninth pair of ribs.

A MANUAL OF HUMAN PHYSIOLOGY

PREPARED WITH SPECIAL REFERENCE TO

STUDENTS OF MEDICINE

BY

JOSEPH H. RAYMOND, A. M., M. D.,

PROFESSOR OF PHYSIOLOGY AND HYGIENE IN THE LONG ISLAND COLLEGE HOSPITAL,
AND DIRECTOR OF PHYSIOLOGY IN THE HOAGLAND LABORATORY.

PHILADELPHIA
W. B. SAUNDERS
925 WALNUT STREET.
1894.

PREFACE.

THE author's experience of twenty years as a teacher of Physiology to medical students has brought him to the conclusion that in the short time allotted to the study of physiology in medical schools students can assimilate only the main facts and principles of this branch of medicine, which lies at the very foundation of a sound knowledge of the healing art; and that even if there were time to investigate the more recondite and abstruse parts of the subject, such an investigation would be profitless during this formative period. In his teaching the author has kept this thought constantly in mind, and in this manual has endeavored to put into a concrete and available form the results of his experience.

SEPTEMBER, 1894.

CONTENTS.

LIST OF ILLUSTRATIONS.

HUMAN PHYSIOLOGY.

INTRODUCTION.

Definitions.—Physiology is *the science which treats of functions.* By the term "function" is meant the characteristic work performed by an organ. An organ may be defined as a structure which performs a function. Lifeless things perform no functions, hence physiology has no dealings with inanimate things. Rocks, stones, and other members of the mineral kingdom at no time possess life; consequently they perform no functions, and with them physiology has no concern: we cannot speak of the physiology of minerals. Plants and animals are sometimes living and sometimes dead: when living they perform functions, when dead they perform no functions; in the latter condition they are like the rocks so far as function is concerned, and with them physiology has nothing whatever to do. It is only when they are living that they perform functions, and it is then and only then that with them physiology concerns itself.

Another definition which might be given of physiology is, that it is *the science which treats of vital phenomena.* A brief consideration of this definition will bring us to the same conclusion as did that of the above definition. Of life in its essence we know nothing. Metaphysicians have endeavored to explain life, and some have even ventured to point out its seat, but the fact remains that we are utterly ignorant of its nature. We only know that it exists by certain manifestations which it presents. When we see a growing plant or a moving animal, we say of each that it is alive. In the higher forms of animals and plants it is easy, under ordinary circumstances, to determine whether they are living or not, but in the lower forms this determination is sometimes a most difficult task. The evidences upon which reliance is placed to determine the presence or the absence of life are spoken of as "vital phenomena." Thus, if in examining an animal we find that its heart beats, we say that the animal is alive, but if the heart be motionless, we say that the animal is dead. This beating of the heart, therefore, is a vital phenomenon—that is, a manifestation of life. We speak also of this beating of the heart as its "function"; hence the first definition of physiology, that it is the science which treats of functions, and the second definition, that it is the science which treats of vital phenomena, amount to the same thing.

"Organ" Defined.—Let us for a moment consider what is meant by the term "organ." It has already been defined as a structure which performs a function. In speaking of the organs of an animal reference is usually had to such structures as the heart, the lungs, and the stomach, inasmuch as their size and the important work they perform force them upon our attention. These are indeed organs, for they perform functions; thus the function of the heart is to receive blood in one portion and to propel it from another portion, that of the lungs is to aërate the blood, and that of the stomach is to digest certain kinds of food; but the term *organ*, as used in physiology, has a much broader signification. A muscle, a nerve, and a blood-vessel are as truly organs as are the greater ones above spoken of, for each has its own function. Thus the function of a muscle is to contract, that of a nerve is to transfer nervous impulses, and that of a blood-vessel is to convey blood. At first sight it might seem that these functions were unimportant, and that the structures which performed them were hardly worthy of so dignified a name as organs; but a moment's reflection will show that without the contraction of muscles, the transference of nervous impulses, or the carrying of blood the life of an animal would as certainly cease as if it were deprived of its heart, of its lungs, or of its stomach.

Inasmuch as minerals, on the one hand, possess no organs, they perform no work—that is, they have no functions; therefore we do not speak of the physiology of a mineral. Plants and animals, on the other hand, possess organs, each of which performs its special function; and it is with them, as has been said, that physiology has to do. As we find organs in the animal, so do we find them in the plant; not the same organs, it is true, but as truly organs, for they respond to the same test. The roots of a plant absorb moisture and nourishment from the soil, this being their function; the green leaves take up from the air carbonic acid, with which and with water they form starch that is utilized by the plant, while oxygen is set free, this being the function of the leaves; the anthers and the ovaries of flowers are concerned in reproducing plants by forming new ones, this being their function. Thus we might continue to show that as in animals, so in plants, the different organs have their respective functions.

"Organic" and "Inorganic."—We can now understand the meaning of two very important terms—*organic* and *inorganic*. These terms are used in two senses: first, as to *structure*, and, second, as to *product*. When we say that a plant or an animal is "organic," we mean that it is made up of organs—that is, of structures which perform functions. The plant or the animal may be simple or may be complex, but, however simple or however complex, its parts do something, that something being the function of the part which acts. We say, therefore, that the plant or animal is organic, meaning that it is composed of organs—organic, then, as to structure. The rock has no organs, therefore it is *non-organic*, or is *inorganic*. These terms are used also in another sense. Thus we speak of honey as organic. Manifestly, we do not mean organic as to structure, for honey has no organs, but it is the product of the bee, which is an organic structure; hence honey is an organic product. The nectary of a flower is organic as to structure, and the nectar which it produces is organic in being the product of the nectary.

Branches of Physiology.—From these elementary considerations it is evident that physiology has to do with plants and animals only—that is, with organic structures and their products. That branch of the science which treats of the functions of plants is denominated Vegetable Physiology, and that which deals with the functions of animals is called Animal Physiology.

VEGETABLE PHYSIOLOGY.—We are concerned but indirectly with vegetable physiology, or so far only as its study helps us to understand some of the more obscure processes in animals. Some of these processes, being simpler in plants, are more easily studied in them, and what is there learned is of great assistance in understanding analogous processes in man. Thus a knowledge of fertilization as it occurs in the vegetable kingdom aids very much in elucidating the process of reproduction in the human species.

ANIMAL PHYSIOLOGY.—The same organs in different animals perform their functions in different ways. Thus the stomach of the cow and that of the dog act very dissimilarly, and a knowledge of the one would aid very little in acquiring a knowledge of the other. What is true of the stomach is true of other organs to a greater or lesser degree. Each class of animals has its own peculiarities as to functions—that is, has its own physiology. One who intends to devote his life to the treatment of the diseases of the lower animals must study the functions of those animals, while one who is preparing himself for the cure of human diseases must understand the functions of the organs of the human body, or Human Physiology.

Many hints, it is true, may be obtained by the student of human physiology from a study of the processes which take place in the lower animals, and many of the most valuable contributions made to physiological science have been based upon such a study; but it must ever be borne in mind that specific differences exist, and that we cannot infer too much from such observations. Thus one who studies the process of stomach digestion in a ruminant, such as the cow, will make a most serious blunder should he suppose that the process is the same in man. Errors of a similar character, though perhaps less glaring, have been made, notably in the process of reproduction. This process is so obscure that many opportunities which have presented themselves for investigation, both in the lower and in the higher animals, have been seized upon, but theories which have been accepted as proven, and which have largely depended on such observations, are now, in the light of more recent study, being questioned. Notwithstanding this disadvantage, had it not been for such studies many of the most important facts of medical science would have remained undiscovered. Inasmuch as functions cease with life, these observations can only be made upon living animals. *Vivisection*, therefore, has been of the greatest benefit to the human race, and those who decry it are daily reaping the results which it has attained, and which could never have been attained without it. Wanton and unnecessary experiments are to be condemned, but no terms of praise are too exalted to bestow upon those patient investigators who, through many long years, have laboriously and zealously pursued their studies and experiments, with no other end in view than to add to the sum of human knowledge and to contribute to the relief of human suffering.

Human Physiology Defined.—Human physiology is *the science which treats of the functions of the organs of the human body*. This science, together with *anatomy*, which treats of structure, and with *chemistry*, which treats of composition, lies at the foundation of rational medicine. No one can be a successful physician who does not understand at least the more important functions of the human body, and the greater the knowledge he possesses of physiology, the broader will be the scientific groundwork on which he has to build. Disease is a departure from the normal or physiological condition. A diseased organ performs its function in an abnormal manner, and to succeed in correcting the diseased condition we must first be able to recognize this abnormal action, which can only be done by knowing how the organ acts in health; that is, by understanding its physiology. Even with this knowledge we may be unable to accomplish the desired object, for the structure of the organ may be so changed that there can be applied no means which will restore it to its normal condition; but we are certainly more likely to succeed if possessed of a knowledge of its physiology than if ignorant of it. The study of human physiology is but the study of the human functions, and when we thoroughly understand these functions we have mastered the science.

Classification of Functions.—The functions of the body may be classified and defined as follows: 1. *Nutritive Functions*, which include those concerned directly with the maintenance of the individual, such as digestion, respiration, circulation, etc.; 2. *Nervous Functions*, which include those that bring the different organs of the body into harmonious relations with one another, and, in addition, bring the individual, through the special senses—sight, hearing, etc.—into relation with the world outside him; and 3. *Reproductive Functions*, which are concerned not with the individual, but with the *species*, which they perpetuate.

Physiological Chemistry.—Although physiology, strictly speaking, has nothing to do with composition, still, as a matter of necessity as well as of convenience, it is usual to preface the study of the functions of the human body with a greater or lesser consideration of its composition. This consideration is necessary, because, as a rule, medical students have an insufficient knowledge of this branch of chemistry—physiological chemistry—to take up at once the study of the functions with profit, and should the attempt be made confusion and loss of time would inevitably result. As an illustration we may refer to the function or series of functions by which the food is prepared for absorption—that is, digestion. Food is the material which is taken into the body to supply the waste of its tissues, and it must be of such a composition as will meet this want. To select the proper food-materials we must know of what the body is composed, and what are the changes which take place in its composition—what parts are wasted. For these reasons a study of *physiological chemistry* must precede a study of the functions of digestion. This is but one of many illustrations which might be given to show the importance of prefacing the study of physiology proper with a study of the chemistry of the body and of the food. We shall, therefore, arrange the topics to be discussed, and treat them, in the following order: I. Physiological Chemistry; II. Nutritive Functions; III. Nervous Functions; and IV. Reproductive Functions.

I. PHYSIOLOGICAL CHEMISTRY.

PHYSIOLOGICAL CHEMISTRY, as applied to the human body, may be defined as *the science which treats of the ingredients of the human body and of the human food.* These ingredients are spoken of by some writers as "proximate principles," by others as the "chemical basis," and by still others as "physiological ingredients." The latter term is the one which will be adopted, as it is the most expressive.

If the human body be analyzed into its ultimate chemical elements, it will be found that of the *sixty-nine* elements known to chemists no less than *fourteen* are found constantly present. These elements are oxygen, carbon, hydrogen, nitrogen, calcium, sodium, potassium, iron, phosphorus, sulphur, magnesium, chlorine, fluorine, and silicon. As fluorine and silicon occur in such small proportions, they may be omitted from consideration altogether.

To obtain most of these substances in their elementary form such processes must be adopted as will utterly destroy the tissues. In the body, in its living state, most of these substances do not exist in their elementary condition, and, however interesting it may be to know all the facts about them, still a knowledge of the properties of these elements does not help to an understanding of their offices in the human body. What is really desired to be known is, *under what forms* these elements exist in the body during life, and not what can be obtained by the analytical chemist.

Chemical elements and physiological ingredients are not interchangeable terms. A physiological ingredient may be defined as *a substance which exists in the body under its own form.* To determine, then, whether a given substance is or is not a physiological ingredient of the human body, it must be ascertained whether it does or does not exist there under its own form. For instance, if it is asked if carbon is a physiological ingredient, before the question could be answered we should have to determine whether carbon exists in the body under its own form; that is, as *carbon.*

Chemistry demonstrates that carbon, as an element, is found in nature in but three forms—namely, as coal, as the diamond, and as graphite or plumbago. In the human body none of these substances is found; therefore carbon does not exist under its own form, and consequently is not a physiological ingredient, although more than one-eighth of the body is made up of carbon, and this amount can be obtained from it. But this carbon does not exist under its own form—that is, free or uncombined—but it is all in a state of combination, as carbonates or in carbohydrates or other forms of combination, and when we obtain the carbon as an element these combinations are broken up and the carbon is set free. Water *is* a physiological ingredient, because it exists in the body under its own form, and can be obtained therefrom without the use of such violent means as are necessary to destroy chemical combinations.

It is exceedingly important to have a clear conception of what are and what are not physiological ingredients: all that can be learned of them and their properties will be of assistance, but a knowledge of the properties of their chemical elements will be of no assistance in our physiological studies, for the properties of a compound are not the sum of the properties of its component parts. One might be thoroughly conversant with the properties of oxygen and hydrogen, yet have no possible conception of the properties of water, which their combination forms.

Classification of Physiological Ingredients.—The physiological ingredients of the human body may be classified as follows: A. Inorganic Ingredients; B. Carbohydrates; C. Fatty Acids, Fats, and Allied Substances; D. Proteids; E. Albuminoids; F. Enzymes; G. Intermediate Products; H. Waste Products; and I. Coloring Matters.

A. Inorganic Ingredients.

1. Water.
2. Salts . . . . .
   - Sodium . . .
     - Chloride.
     - Phosphate.
     - Biphosphate.
     - Sulphate.
     - Carbonate.
     - Bicarbonate.
   - Potassium . .
     - Chloride.
     - Phosphate.
     - Sulphate.
     - Carbonate.
   - Calcium . . .
     - Phosphate.
     - Carbonate.
     - Fluoride.
   - Magnesium .
     - Phosphate.
     - Carbonate.
   - Ammonium . Chloride.
3. Iron } not free.
4. Silicon } not free.

5. Oxygen.
6. Hydrogen.
7. Nitrogen.
8. Marsh-gas.
9. Ammonia.
10. Sulphuretted Hydrogen.
11. Hydrochloric Acid.
12. Carbon Dioxide.

1. WATER (H_2O).—Water is one of the most important of the physiological ingredients. Its quantity is about 70 per cent. of the whole body, and it is found in all the tissues, both solid and fluid.

Quantity of Water in the Body.—The quantity (percentage) of water in the body is as follows:

Enamel of teeth	0.2
Bones	22.
Muscles	76.
Blood	78.
Milk	87.
Urine	93.
Gastric juice	97.
Saliva	99.

From this table it will be seen that while water makes up but a small part of the enamel of the teeth, it constitutes by far the greater part of the saliva. Between these two extremes it is present in different tissues in varying proportions. It should be said of these, and of most other quantities given in physiological tables, that they are not invariable, hence the analyses of different authorities will vary. The composition of the milk, for instance, is not always the same; therefore there will not invariably be 87 per cent. of water present, but the normal variations from this figure, either above or below, will not be very great, and these percentages may be regarded as averages.

Offices of Water.—We should naturally infer from the large quantity of water present in the body, and from its universal presence in all the solids and liquids, that its offices must be important; and a study of these demonstrates that this is a fact. It is the water which gives to *fluids* their fluidity. Without this property the blood could not circulate through the blood-vessels, nor dissolve and hold in solution the nutritive materials which it supplies to the tissues, nor carry the waste materials to the various organs whose duty it is to eliminate them. Without water the saliva would cease to be the important agent it is in softening the food in the mouth preparatory to its being swallowed. In short, without water as an integral part of the fluids of the body these fluids would cease to be fluids, and the many and varied offices which they subserve would at once be abolished, and life could no longer be maintained.

Equally important, though less apparent, are the various offices which are subserved by water in the *solids* of the body. From the above table it is seen that water exists in the muscles to the amount of 76 per cent. The striking property of muscles is their power of contractility, or ability to shorten. By the exercise of this property all the movements of the different parts of the body are accomplished: without this power locomotion would be impossible, the movements of the heart would cease, and death would quickly supervene. A muscle deprived of its water would cease to possess this contractile power—in other words, would lose its characteristic function.

As will be seen later, the skin possesses most important functions—those, for instance, of sensation, of excretion, and of protection. All these functions would be destroyed if the water in the skin were expelled. Perhaps this fact is nowhere more strikingly evident than in studying the functions of the skin of the palm of the hand. The pliability of this portion of the skin, by which objects are grasped, and the sense of touch, by which it can be determined whether they are hard or soft, whether rough or smooth, whether hot or cold, are both dependent on the presence of water in the skin, and the mere evaporation of the water would at once make the skin hard and rigid, its pliability would vanish, and its functions would cease.

Sources of Water.—The water which exists in the body is derived from two principal sources: first, from the food, and second, from its formation in the interior of the body, the former being the main source of supply. As water is a constituent part of every tissue of the human body, so it is of all the varieties of food, both solid and liquid, taken into the body.

The Quantity of Water in Food (percentage) is as follows:

Wheat bread (fresh)	33.
Mackerel	70.
Lean beef	70.
Potatoes	76.
Human milk	87.09
Cow's milk	87.41
Green vegetables	88.

From this table it will be seen that the greater part of potatoes and of green vegetables is water, and that even of bread, water constitutes at least a third. In some vegetables, such as the turnip, about 90 per cent. is water. In other words, three of every four pounds of potatoes and one of every three pounds of bread are water. In the liquid food, as milk, tea, and coffee, the proportion of water is, of course, still greater. The amount of water daily taken into the body in solid and liquid food aggregates 2000 c. c. In addition to this there is, as above stated, a small amount actually formed within the body.

One of the important ingredients of food is the class of carbohydrates. A study of their composition shows that hydrogen and oxygen exist in these substances in such proportion as to form water. In the various changes which these elements undergo in the body, water is formed. Besides this source there is reason to believe that a small quantity of water is formed by the action of free oxygen on some organic substances. The amount of water daily formed in these two ways is not far from 500 c.c., which makes, with the water taken in with the food, a total of 2500 c.c.

Avenues of Discharge from the Body.—The water which has been shown to form so essential a part of the body is not, however, a permanent ingredient; that is, while water is always present, it is not the same water: that which at one time exists in the tissues is soon replaced by other water. The amount daily discharged is equal to the amount taken in with the food and formed in the body—that is, about 2500 grammes. The avenues by which it passes out, and the proportion by each are as follows:

Large intestines, as fæces	4	per cent.
Lungs, as watery vapor	20	"
Skin, as perspiration	30	"
Kidneys, as urine	46	"

When discharged it is not pure water, but contains ingredients that vary according to the channel by which it is eliminated. The composition of these ingredients respectively will be studied in its appropriate place.

2. SALTS.—Sodium chloride, or common salt (NaCl), is present in all the solids and fluids. The *quantity* (percentage) in different solids and fluids is as follows:

Milk	0.03
Saliva	0.15
Gastric juice	0.17
Perspiration	0.22
Blood	0.33
Urine	0.55
Bones	0.70

The total quantity of common salt in the human body is 110 grammes.

Offices of Sodium Chloride.—The most important office which sodium chloride subserves is in connection with the process known as "osmosis," or the diffusion of liquids through animal membranes. A second office which it possesses is to hold in solution the globulins. These globulins are proteids which are not soluble in distilled water, as are the native albumins, but are soluble in dilute solutions of sodium chloride (1 per cent.). The importance of this office of common salt will be more fully appreciated in the study of the plasma of the blood, of which these globulins form an essential part. A third office which is attributable to it is to aid in the excretion of waste matter.

Source of Sodium Chloride.—The food taken into the body is the principal source of the sodium chloride which the body contains.

The quantity (percentage) *of this salt in some articles of food* is as follows:

Oats	0.01
Turnips	0.03
Potatoes	0.04
Cabbage	0.04
Beets	0.06

It has been the opinion of physiologists that sodium chloride is not present in sufficient amount in human food to satisfy the demands of the body; consequently, that an additional amount must be taken in as a condiment at the table or be added to the food during the process of cooking. But Dr. F. A. Cook, surgeon to the first Peary North-Greenland Expedition, states that the Eskimos who dwell between the seventy-sixth and seventy-ninth parallels use no salt or condiment of any kind in their food, which is entirely of meat and blubber only one-third cooked. This cooking is done in order that there may be obtained the blood of the meat, and this blood the Eskimos drink. However this may be with the Eskimos, it is the general experience that by the addition of salt the food is not only made more palatable, but the digestive juices are also increased and digestion improved. This insufficiency of salt in the food of man is seen also in that of some of the lower animals. While carnivora, or flesh-eating animals, find in their food all the salt they need, it is different with the herbivora, or vegetable-eaters. Especially noticeable is this fact in the ruminants. Boussingault many years ago demonstrated this by a series of experiments which he conducted. He selected two sets of bullocks as nearly as possible in the same condition of health, and to both sets he gave the same food, except that to one he gave salt, while to the other he gave none. Several months elapsed before any very marked difference could be detected, but at the end of a year, during which time the experiment continued, there were striking differences in the two sets. The bullocks that received the salt were in excellent physical condition, while those deprived of it were much inferior in every respect: their hide was rough, their hair tangled, and they were dull and apathetic.

Avenues of Discharge.—Sodium chloride is daily discharged from the body through the following channels and in the given amounts: urine, 13 grammes; perspiration, 2 grammes. There is a small amount also in mucous secretions.

Sodium Phosphate (Na_2HPO_4) *and Potassium Phosphate* (K_2HPO_4).—These salts are so intimately associated that they may be described together. They are frequently spoken of as the "alkaline phosphates," and they exist in all the solids and fluids of the body.

Offices of Alkaline Phosphates.—The most important office which these salts perform is to assist in giving alkalinity to the alkaline fluids—a property which, in the blood at least, is essential to life, and in some of the other fluids is necessary to the performance of their functions. The fluids of the body are, with but four exceptions, alkaline in reaction: these exceptions are gastric juice, perspiration, urine, and vaginal mucus. The following fluids are alkaline: plasma of the blood; lymph; aqueous humor; cephalo-rachidian fluid; pericardial fluid; synovia; mucus (except that of vagina); milk; spermatic fluid; tears; saliva; bile; pancreatic juice; and intestinal juice.

The alkalinity of the plasma of the blood is not an

accidental property. The fact that the blood of all animals hitherto examined has invariably been found alkaline would seem to indicate that this condition is an important one. Bernard has shown that if an acid be injected into the blood of an animal death will be produced, even though the amount injected is not enough to make the blood itself acid. One of the properties of the blood is to carry carbonic acid gas—one of the products of the waste of the tissues—to the lungs, where it is eliminated; and experiment has shown that the alkalescence of the blood enables it to carry more of this gas than it could were it neutral in reaction. In discussing the alkaline carbonates it will be seen that they take part in rendering alkaline the fluids in which they occur.

Source of Alkaline Phosphates.—The alkaline phosphates are taken into the body in the food, of which they form a constituent part.

Avenues of Discharge.—After fulfilling their offices in the body these alkaline salts are discharged in the perspiration, the mucus, and the urine. In the urine a portion of the sodium phosphate is converted into sodium biphosphate, or, as it is sometimes called, "acid sodium phosphate," which gives to the urine its acid reaction. In this fluid are discharged daily 4.5 grammes of the alkaline phosphates and the sodium biphosphate.

Sulphates.—Sodium sulphate (Na_2SO_4) and potassium sulphate (K_2SO_4) are found in the blood, lymph, aqueous humor, milk, saliva, mucus, perspiration, urine, and fæces. Their quantity is small, however, except in the urine, by which fluid they are discharged daily to the amount of 4 grammes.

Source of Sulphates.—These sulphates are taken in as

part of the solid food we eat and also in the water we drink. They are present in flesh, in eggs, in the cereals, and in other animal and vegetable foods. Drinking-water often contains these sulphates, and the sulphate of lime as well. Sulphates are undoubtedly formed to some extent within the body. In discussing the constitution of the albuminous ingredients of the food it will be seen that one of their elements is sulphur. Some of this sulphur becomes oxidized, forming sulphuric acid, which, being a stronger acid than carbonic, displaces it from the carbonates and unites with the alkaline bases, forming sulphates.

Carbonates.—Sodium carbonate (Na_2CO_3), sodium bicarbonate ($NaHCO_3$) and potassium carbonate (K_2CO_3) are salts which are known as the "alkaline carbonates," and are intimately associated with the alkaline phosphates.

Source of Carbonates.—These salts are, to some extent, introduced with the food, but are principally formed by the decomposition of the salts of the vegetable acids. In fruits, such as apples and cherries, and in vegetables, such as potatoes and carrots, are found malic, tartaric, and citric acids, united with sodium and potassium to form tartrates and citrates of sodium and potassium. When these fruits or vegetables are eaten, these salts are taken up by the blood, and while in the blood the organic acids are decomposed, and the bases uniting with carbonic acid, alkaline carbonates are formed, which are discharged in the urine. This accounts for the fact that after eating sufficient of such fruits or vegetables the urine becomes alkaline.

Office of Carbonates.—The alkalinity of the blood and of other alkaline fluids is, as has been stated, only partially due to the alkaline phosphates. In causing this reaction the alkaline carbonates have a share. In the blood of flesh-eating animals the phosphates are more abundant, this being due to the predominance of phosphates in muscular tissue, while in that of the herbivora the carbonates are in excess of the phosphates. Remembering, then, what has been said of the formation of the carbonates from the salts in fruits and vegetables, this difference in the blood is readily understood. In human blood there are both phosphates and carbonates to account for its alkalinity.

Potassium Chloride.—Potassium chloride (KCl) is found in many of the tissues, especially in the muscles, in blood-corpuscles, and in milk. This salt occurs also in gastric juice, in urine, and in perspiration. Like sodium chloride, it is neutral in reaction and is soluble in water.

Source of Potassium Chloride.—Potassium chloride is contained in both animal and vegetable foods.

Avenues of Discharge.—Potassium chloride is discharged in mucus, in urine, and in perspiration.

Calcium Salts.—Calcium phosphate, lime phosphate, or phosphate of lime ($Ca_3(PO_4)_2$).—Next to water, calcium phosphate is the most abundant physiological ingredient of the human body. Its total amount is 2400 grammes in a man weighing 65 kilogrammes.

The quantity (percentage) *of calcium phosphate* is as follows:

Blood	0.03
Urine	0.07
Milk	0.27
Bone	57.6
Enamel of teeth	88.5

The greater part of the calcium phosphate in the body

is in the bones. It is estimated that 6.4 per cent. of the body is bone, and in a man weighing 65 kilogrammes, an average weight, there would therefore be 2400 grammes of this salt Its presence in the fluids of the body is not in noteworthy amount, except in the milk.

Office of Calcium Phosphate.—The principal office of calcium phosphate is to give the bones their rigidity. During early life this salt is in small amount in the bones, and at this time the bones are soft and yielding. Later, as the phosphate is deposited in greater amount, these structures become more rigid and better adapted to sustain weight. In old age this salt is in excess of the organic ingredients of the bone, and at this period of life the bones are easily broken, much as a pipe-stem; while in infancy the bones bend, but do not break, or if they do break the fracture is not complete, but is similar to that which occurs in a green stick, commonly known as the "green-stick fracture" (Fig. 1). The flexible condition of the bones may be artificially produced by putting a long bone, like the fibula, into a jar containing dilute hydrochloric acid. The acid dissolves the calcium phosphate, and, although in appearance the bone is much the same as before, it will now be found so flexible as to permit its being tied in a knot (Fig. 2). In the blood, calcium phosphate, which is insoluble in alkaline fluids, is held in solution by the albuminous constituents. Were these withdrawn the calcium phosphate would at once be rendered insoluble, and would be precipitated.

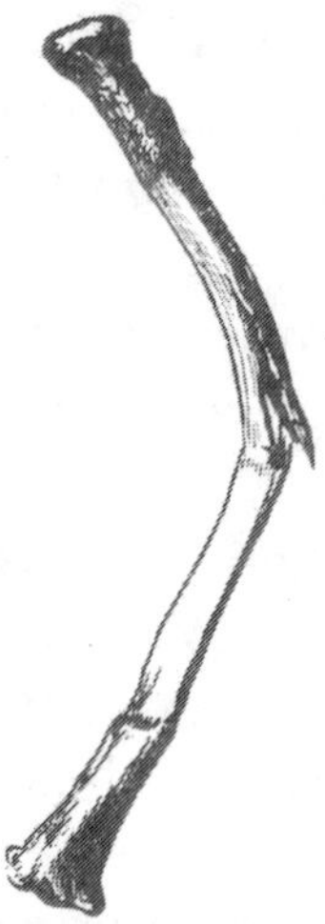

FIG. 1. Partial or "green-stick" fracture (Stimson).

Source of Calcium Phosphate.—Calcium phosphate is

an important ingredient of the animal and vegetable food of man. It is contained in flesh, in eggs, in milk, in wheat, in oats, in rice, in peas, in beans, in potatoes, in apples, in cherries, and in other alimentary substances. Its presence in milk needs especial comment. As has been stated, during early life calcium phosphate is in the bones in small amount. The milk, upon which the growing child relies for its nourishment, supplies the necessary amount of this salt to give the bones their firmness and rigidity. From this statement it will be seen that the adulteration of milk with water, even though the water is pure, may be of great injury to the child. To obtain the necessary amount of calcium phosphate a certain amount of milk must be taken. If half this amount be water, the quantity of the lime-salt present will be but one-half of what it should be, and the child is consequently defrauded. Of course, if impure water be used in the adulteration, there is the additional danger of introducing the germs of disease with the milk.

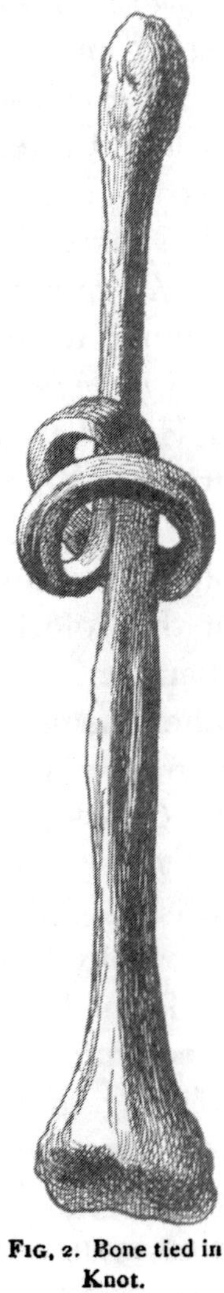

FIG. 2. Bone tied in Knot.

Avenues of Discharge.—A very small amount of calcium phosphate is discharged from the body—a fact which shows its permanent character. It is discharged in the urine, in the fæces, and in the perspiration.

Calcium Carbonate ($CaCO_3$).—This salt exists in the bones to the amount of about 300 grammes, in the teeth, in the blood, in lymph, in chyle, in the saliva, and sometimes in the urine. Like calcium phosphate, with which it is usually associated, it is insoluble in water; and when it exists in solution its solubility is due either to alkaline chlorides or to free carbonic acid.

Calcium Fluoride ($CaFl_2$) exists in bones and in the teeth, and is of little importance.

Magnesium Salts.—Magnesium phosphate (Mg_3PO_4) is found wherever calcium phosphate is found, and the two together are frequently spoken of as the "earthy phosphates." It is discharged by the urine.

Magnesium Carbonate ($MgCO_3$).—A trace of this salt is found in the blood.

Ammonium Salts.—Traces of ammonium chloride (NH_4Cl) are found in the gastric juice and in the urine.

3. IRON.—Iron is present in the hæmoglobin of the blood, in the hair, the bile, and the urine. Its presence in the coloring matter of the blood is its most striking characteristic. It exists in the blood combined with the other chemical elements, and not as an oxide. The total amount of iron in the blood of the body of a man weighing 65 kilogrammes is about 2.71 grammes.

Office of Iron.—The office of iron is not understood. It is regarded as a remarkable fact that without iron chlorophyll, the green coloring matter of plants, cannot be formed—in other words, that vegetable life is interfered with; and it is believed that its presence in the coloring matter of the blood of an animal is equally necessary for its nutrition.

Source of Iron.—All animal food containing blood contains iron. In addition, animal food is taken into the body in rye, barley, oats, wheat, peas, and strawberries.

Avenues of Discharge.—A small amount only of iron is discharged in the bile and the urine. After serving its purpose in the blood it is probably deposited in the hair.

4. SILICON (S).—It is not known in exactly what form silicon exists in the body, possibly as silicic acid.

5. OXYGEN (O).—This gas is absorbed from the air, and exists in the blood principally in loose combination with the hæmoglobin, though some of it is doubtless free.

6. HYDROGEN (H).—This gas is found in the alimentary canal and in the expired air, having been absorbed by the blood from the intestine.

7. NITROGEN (N).—Nitrogen is absorbed from the air by the blood, in which it exists in a dissolved state. Some nitrogen is formed also within the body.

8. MARSH GAS (CH_4).—This gas is found in the expired air, like hydrogen, having been absorbed from the intestines. Reiset found that 30 litres were expired in twenty-four hours.

9. AMMONIA (NH_3).—A small amount of ammonia is found in the expired air, probably derived from the blood.

10. SULPHURETTED HYDROGEN (H_2S).—This gas is found in the intestines.

11. HYDROCHLORIC ACID (HCl).—This acid exists in gastric juice.

12. CARBONIC DIOXIDE (CO_2).—This gas exists in many of the fluids, having been absorbed by them from the tissues. It is also present in blood and in expired air.

B. CARBOHYDRATES.

This class is so called because its members contain carbon united with hydrogen and oxygen in the proportion to form water. To be placed in this class a substance must have at least 6 atoms of carbon in its molecule. The carbohydrates either possess a sweet taste, as is the case with the sugars, or, if they do not, they are convertible into sugars. They also have the power of rotating a ray of polarized light.

The following table contains the groups which form this class, and the members of each group:

1. Starch Group	Starch. Soluble starch. Erythrodextrin. Achroödextrin. Maltodextrin. Glycogen. Cellulose.
2. Dextrose Group	Dextrose. Lævulose. Galactose. Inosit.
3. Cane-sugar Group	Saccharose. Maltose. Lactose.

1. Starch Group.

Starch $(C_6H_{10}O_5)_n$.—The exact formula for starch is not determined. Chemists agree that it is not $C_6H_{10}O_5$, but some multiple of this, as indicated by "*n*," and that "*n*" is not less than five. Starch is not found in the human body, except when it is taken in as food. It is very abundant in vegetable food. Indeed, it is said that starch exists in every chlorophyll-containing plant at some period of its existence. Starch is a substance of great interest, from the fact that it is the first organic substance produced by vegetables from inorganic matter. Animals have not the power to produce organic substances directly from members of the inorganic kingdom, but plants have, and they exercise this power, and from the organic materials thus produced animals are nourished. Plants may change the organic matter from one form to another, as starch to sugar, but were inorganic substances alone supplied to animals they would starve.

The inorganic substances out of which the plant forms the starch are carbonic acid and water, these being taken from the atmosphere and the soil. This process is represented by the following chemical formula:

$$\underset{\text{Carbonic acid.}}{(6CO_2} + \underset{\text{Water.}}{5H_2O)_n} = \underset{\text{Starch.}}{(C_6H_{10}O_5)_n} + \underset{\text{Oxygen.}}{O_n}$$

That is, the carbonic acid and the water are decomposed, the carbon and hydrogen, with some of the oxygen, unite and form starch, while the rest of the oxygen is set free. To bring about this change there must be present solar light and the green coloring matter, chlorophyll. If chlorophyll be absent, this change does not take place, nor does it when solar light is absent.

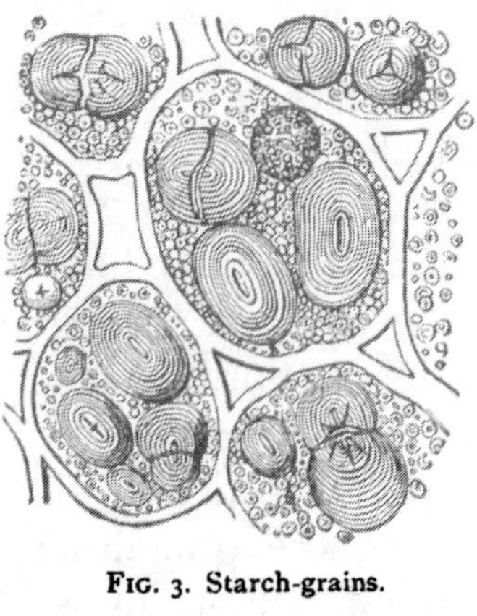
FIG. 3. Starch-grains.

Starch exists in plants in the form of grains, known as "starch-grains" or "starch-granules" (Fig. 3). They present a characteristic appearance under the microscope by which they may at once be recognized. Each granule presents a number of concentric markings and varies in size and shape in different plants; by these points of difference the plant from which the granules are derived may be identified. This fact is made use of in detecting adulterations, in which cheaper kinds of starch are mixed with more expensive kinds and sold for the latter at a higher price. The markings are caused by the arrangement of the material composing the granule in alternating layers of cellulose and granulose.

Quantity of Starch.—The quantity of starch (percentage) in the following food-plants is

Sweet potatoes	16.05
Potatoes	20.
Beans	33.
Peas	37.30
Wheat	57.88
Oats	60.59
Rye	64.65
Indian corn	67.55
Rice	88.65

The presence of starch is determined by the addition of a little tincture of iodine, which gives a blue color. This reaction is due to the granulose, and not to the cellulose. Starch cellulose differs in some respects from ordinary cellulose, as is demonstrated by its solubility in some reagents which do not dissolve the latter.

Starch is insoluble in cold water, but when boiling water is added to it in an amount twenty times its weight, the granules swell and burst and there is formed a gelatinous mass which is called "starch-paste." This paste will respond to the iodine test, showing it to be, principally at least, granulose. If the amount of water added should be one hundred times the weight of the starch, a solution of granulose is made, the insoluble cellulose falling to the bottom of the vessel. This starch solution will likewise respond to the iodine test.

Soluble Starch, or Amylodextrin $(C_6H_{10}O_5)_n$.—When starch-paste, produced in the manner above described, is heated to a temperature of 40° C. on a water-bath, and saliva is then added, the paste changes from a gelatinous to a watery condition, and in this fluid soluble starch now exists. This soluble starch gives also a blue color with iodine. It filters readily, whereas starch-paste, even in dilute solution, filters with difficulty. Soluble starch is dextro-rotatory; that is, it rotates the ray of polarized light to the right. This substance is the first product of the conversion of starch into sugar by saliva, and if the action be not stopped, as it may be by boiling, the stage of soluble starch is only a temporary one, it passing quickly into that of dextrin. As will be seen hereafter, the ingredient of the saliva that changes starch into soluble starch is a ferment—*ptyalin*—the action being one of hydrolysis. Pancreatic juice produces the same change as does saliva, and as the action of saliva is due to the ferment ptyalin, so is the action of pancreatic juice due to a ferment, *amylopsin*, both of which substances belong to the ferments or enzymes.

Erythrodextrin $(C_6H_{10}O_5)_n$.—If the action of either of these ferments upon starch be not arrested in the soluble-starch stage, erythrodextrin is formed. The blue color caused by the action of iodine on starch gradually changes into violet, reddish-violet, and then to reddish-brown as the starch gradually changes to erythrodextrin. This reddish-brown color produced by iodine is the test for erythrodextrin.

Achroödextrin $(C_6H_{10}O_5)_n$.—If the action of these ferments be continued, a still further change in the starch takes place. It passes into the condition of achroödextrin, and iodine fails to produce any color. A further change into maltose follows the formation of achroödextrin. In the action of these ferments upon starch outside the body the first product is a mixture of dextrin with the sugar, but within the body there is little doubt but that all the starch is converted into sugar, and as such is absorbed. If starch be treated with boiling dilute acids instead of with these enzymes, the changes just described take place with far greater rapidity, and dextrose results.

Maltodextrin $(C_6H_{10}O_5)_n$.—If diastase, the ferment contained in malt extract, be used instead of saliva or pancreatic juice, maltodextrin is formed; and indeed it is not certain that the latter substance is not formed in addition to the erythrodextrin and achroödextrin when saliva and pancreatic juice are employed. Maltodextrin differs from the dextrins already described in being more soluble in alcohol, in being diffusible, and in responding to Fehling's test. It also passes over into maltose by the continued action of the diastase.

Glycogen $(C_6H_{10}O_5)_n$.—The similarity between glycogen and starch has led to the term "animal starch" being applied to the former. Glycogen was first discovered in the liver, but has since been found to exist in the integument and the mucous membranes of the human embryo, in the placenta and the amnion, in white blood-corpuscles and in pus-corpuscles, in oysters and in other mollusca. For purposes of study it is usually obtained from the liver of an animal (a rabbit or a dog), in which it is stored up in amorphous granules around the nuclei of the liver-cells. Glycogen is soluble in water, and with iodine gives a port-wine color. This color does not distinguish it from erythrodextrin, but when it exists pure, as ordinarily it does not, it is precipitated by 60 per cent. alcohol, while the dextrins are not precipitated. Watery solutions are dextro-rotatory.

In general it may be said that the action of the enzymes and of boiling acids upon glycogen is the same as upon starch. The glycogen of the liver becomes converted, by physiological processes, into liver-sugar, which is regarded as identical with dextrose. In this process probably no maltose is formed, such as occurs in the artificial hydrolysis already described. This difference would seem to indicate that in the liver-cells there is no ferment to which this action can be attributed, for, so far as can be judged, most ferments produce maltose, and not dextrose, and up to the present time no dextrose-producing ferment has been obtained from the liver.

Cellulose $(C_6H_{10}O_5)_n$.—Nowhere in the animal body is cellulose found, but it exists in many of the vegetable alimentary principles upon which man relies for his nutrition. As has already been stated, it is a constituent of the starch-granule, and while in the raw state it is unaffected by the digestive fluids, yet when it is boiled it becomes converted into sugar as well as the granulose. While cellulose has not a marked nutritive value, still it is more than probable that the older view that it is of no value as a food-stuff is erroneous. It has recently been suggested that there is in the alimentary canal an undiscovered ferment which has the power of causing this conversion of the cellulose. This change takes place especially when those vegetables and fruits are eaten whose cell-walls are tender and have not yet become lignified or woody in character. The cellulose of some plants, such as the date, is regarded as a reserve material to be made use of in germination.

The presence of cellulose is recognized by the fact that when treated with strong sulphuric acid it becomes converted into a substance that is colored blue by iodine. Schulze's reagent is another test for its presence. This test consists in the production of a blue color when the substance is treated with iodine dissolved to saturation in a solution of chloride of zinc to which potassium iodide has been added.

2. Dextrose Group.

Dextrose (glucose, grape-sugar, diabetic sugar) ($C_6H_{12}O_6$) is normally found in the blood, chyle, lymph, and in very small amount in the urine. In the disease known as "diabetes mellitus" the quantity of dextrose in the blood and urine is very much increased. It is a substance of much interest, as it is in the form of dextrose that the carbohydrates of the food find their way into the blood. In its pure state dextrose is colorless and readily crystallizes; it is soluble in cold water, more so in hot water. It is dextro-rotatory, whence it derives its name. Dextrose reduces metallic oxides, a property which is made use of in determining its presence and in measuring its quantity. Tests based on this are Trommer's, Fehling's, Moore's, and others.

Fermentations of Dextrose.—Dextrose undergoes various fermentations: (1) Alcoholic; (2) Lactic; and (3) Butyric.

1. *Alcoholic Fermentation.*—In alcoholic fermentation, under the influence of yeast, the dextrose is decomposed and ethyl alcohol and carbonic anhydride are produced

($C_6H_{12}O_6 = 2C_2H_6O + 2CO_2$). This process is at the height of its activity when the temperature is 25° C.; when above 45° C. or below 5° C. it ceases. When sugar is present in the solution to the extent of more than 15 per cent., the process of fermentation will be arrested, by the alcohol produced, before all the sugar has been decomposed.

2. *Lactic Fermentation.*—When milk sours, the sugar which it contains is converted into lactic acid, constituting the lactic fermentation ($C_6H_{12}O_6 = 2C_3H_6O_3$). This fermentation is not confined to milk-sugar, but may occur also with dextrose. This change is brought about by the presence of specific micro-organisms. It is stated that there exists also in the mucous membrane of the stomach an enzyme which can change lactose, and possibly dextrose, into lactic acid.

3. *Butyric Fermentation.*—When the lactic fermentation is continued for some time, it is liable to pass into the butyric. This change is due to the action of a ferment (organized) upon the lactic acid. In the change hydrogen and carbonic anhydride are given off ($2C_3H_6O_3 = C_3H_7.COOH. + 2CO_2 + 2H_2$). The optimum (most favorable) temperature for the lactic and butyric fermentations is from 35° C. to 40° C. When the diet consists largely of carbohydrates, both these fermentations may occur in the alimentary canal.

Lævulose (left-rotating sugar, fruit-sugar, or mucin-sugar) ($C_6H_{12}O_6$) is found in many fruits and in honey, and is said to occur occasionally in urine. It is not crystallizable. When cane-sugar is treated with dilute mineral acids, it is decomposed into equal parts of dextrose and lævulose. Cane-sugar has a dextro-rotatory action on polarized light, but when changed by the acid the solution becomes lævo-rotatory, and the cane-sugar is said to be "inverted;" hence the mixture of dextrose and lævulose is sometimes spoken of as "invert-sugar." As will be seen in the consideration of cane-sugar, "inversion" takes place in the alimentary canal. Although in many respects lævulose is very similar to dextrose, still its action on polarized light serves to distinguish the two.

Galactose ($C_6H_{12}O_6$).—When lactose is boiled with dilute mineral acids it is changed into dextrose and galactose:

$$\underset{\text{Lactose.}}{C_{12}H_{22}O_{11}} + H_2O = \underset{\text{Dextrose.}}{C_6H_{12}O_6} + \underset{\text{Galactose.}}{C_6H_{12}O_6}$$

Inosit, or muscle-sugar ($C_6H_{12}O_6 + 2H_2O$), has been found in the muscles, lungs, liver, spleen, kidneys, and brain, and pathologically in urine. It occurs also in beans and grape-juice. Because of its sweet taste and its chemical composition it has been regarded as a carbohydrate, but as it has no rotatory action on polarized light, does not reduce metallic salts, and does not undergo the alcoholic fermentation, it is now regarded as belonging to the benzol series, and not as being a carbohydrate. Its ability to undergo lactic fermentation is very doubtful.

3. Cane-sugar Group.

Saccharose, or cane-sugar ($C_{12}H_{22}O_{11}$).—This sugar is not found in the human body, but it nevertheless plays an important part in the food of man. It occurs in the sugar-cane and in some other plants. It does not reduce metallic salts, it is soluble in water, it is dextro-rotatory, and it does not undergo alcoholic, but does readily undergo lactic, fermentation in presence of sour milk to which zinc oxide is added to fix the acid as formed. One of the interesting facts connected with saccharose is its property of "inversion," which, as we have seen, consists in its decomposition into equal parts of dextrose and lævulose, and to this mixture the name of "invert-sugar" has been given. This change is represented chemically as follows:

$$\underset{\text{Cane-sugar.}}{C_{12}H_{22}O_{11}} + \underset{\text{Water.}}{H_2O} = \underset{\text{Dextrose.}}{C_6H_{12}O_6} + \underset{\text{Lævulose.}}{C_6H_{12}O_6},$$

and may be produced by the action of acid, as has been described under "Lævulose." It takes place also in the small intestine under the influence of an enzyme of the intestinal juice—namely, *invertin.* This enzyme exists also in yeast, where it has the same power as in the intestinal juice.

Cane-sugar cannot be taken up as such by the blood, and when injected into an animal it is eliminated unaltered in the urine. When taken in as food it is absorbed, not as cane-sugar, but as invert-sugar, into which it has been changed. This inversion is most pronounced in the small intestine; it is claimed that it may take place also in the stomach, and that there exists in the gastric juice an enzyme which has this power.

Maltose ($C_{12}H_{22}O_{11} + H_2O$).—In considering maltodextrin it was stated that starch-paste, under the influence of diastase, passes into maltodextrin, and, if the action be continued, into maltose. When starch-paste or glycogen is treated with saliva, maltose is the principal sugar formed; prolonged treatment with pancreatic juice will produce, beside the maltose, some dextrose. Although pancreatic juice, on the one hand, acts in this manner, still the tissue of the small intestine or an extract of it has but slight action on the paste. On the other hand, the pancreatic juice rapidly changes maltose into dextrose. Maltose, like cane-sugar, injected into the blood is eliminated as maltose in the urine. From this fact it would appear that maltose is not absorbed as such in the intestine, but as dextrose; and it would further appear that, inasmuch as the tissue of the intestine has this converting power, the change from maltose into dextrose occurs while the process of absorption is actually taking place, and not before. The action of pancreatic juice on starch in the intestine will be further discussed in the consideration of the ferments of this fluid.

Maltose is soluble in water, but it is less soluble in alcohol than dextrose. It is crystallizable, dextro-rotatory, and reduces metallic salts. Maltose is distinguished from dextrose (1) by the difference in its rotatory power on polarized light, that of maltose being greater; (2) by maltose having a less reducing power, as when boiled with Fehling's solution only two-thirds as much cuprous oxide is separated out with maltose as with dextrose; (3) by Barfoed's reagent, which, consisting of a solution of cupric acetate in water to which acetic acid has been added, is reduced by dextrose, but not by maltose.

Lactose (milk-sugar, sugar of milk) ($C_{12}H_{22}O_{11}+H_2O$) is found only in milk, although it has been said to occur in the urine of lying-in women and in sucklings. It is crystallizable, less soluble in water than dextrose, and insoluble in alcohol. It is dextro-rotatory, its power in this respect being the same as that of dextrose. It does not reduce Barfoed's reagent. As above noted in speaking of galactose, lactose is changed into equal parts of sugar and dextrose by boiling it with dilute mineral acids.

Lactose by itself does not undergo alcoholic fermentation with yeast, but an alcoholic fermentation does take place in milk, as when mare's milk is used for the preparation of kumyss and kephir. This fermentation is due to special ferments, the nature of which is not fully understood. In Russia kephir ferment may be purchased. Lactose readily undergoes the lactic fermentation. It is this change which takes place in the souring of milk due to the action of a ferment. The character of the change in the case of lactose is the same as described in dextrose and saccharose. Lactose injected into the blood is eliminated by the urine, as are saccharose and maltose, and like them must therefore be changed in the alimentary canal during the process of absorption. This conversion, which is probably into dextrose and galactose, takes place, as in the case of maltose, while the sugar is passing through the walls of the intestines.

C. Fatty Acids, Fats, and Allied Substances.

Formic Acid.—This acid has been obtained from the spleen, thymus gland, pancreas, muscles, brain, blood, and urine.

Acetic Acid.—Fermentation of the food in the stomach may produce acetic acid. It has been found in normal and in diabetic urine.

Acetone.—Diabetic urine yields acetone on distillation; it is this substance which gives the ethereal odor to such urine. The blood of persons suffering from diabetes has also been found to contain it, and to its presence has been attributed the fatal coma which comes on in some cases of this disease. Acetone has been found also in the urine of healthy children, and it has been stated that it has been detected in their breath.

Propionic Acid.—This acid is found in perspiration, in fermenting diabetic urine, and it has been found also in the contents of the stomach and in normal urine.

Normal Butyric Acid is found in perspiration, in the contents of the large intestines, in the fæces, and in urine. It occurs also during lactic fermentation.

Isobutyric Acid occurs in fæces, and is one of the products of the putrefaction of proteids.

Caproic and *Caprylic Acids* are constituents of the perspiration, and, with *Capric Acid*, are found also in butter.

Neutral Fats are *palmitin*, *stearin*, and *olein*. They are regarded by chemists as compounds of glycerin and the respective fatty acid. Thus the acid of palmitin is *palmitic*; that of stearin, *stearic*; and that of olein, *oleic*. They are characterized by being insoluble in water, slightly soluble in alcohol, and very soluble in ether and chloroform. All fats are mixtures of the three varieties, the difference in the consistency of any given fat depending upon the proportion in which the neutral fats are present. Thus in the more solid fats, such as suet, stearin predominates, while in the fluid fats it is olein which is in excess. There is a difference also in the proportions of these substances in the fats of different animals. Human fat and that of carnivorous animals contain palmitin in excess over stearin and olein, while in that of the herbivora stearin predominates, and in that of fishes, olein.

Source of Fat in the Human Body.—Human fat is derived from the fats, the carbohydrates, and the proteids of the food. In fatty meats, nuts, eggs, milk, and other food more or less fat exists as a constituent, and undoubtedly contributes to the formation of the fat of the body. Food containing starch and sugar is also fattening in its nature, and persons who have an excess of fat are placed upon a diet containing a minimum of these ingredients. Herbivorous animals—the cow, for instance—rely entirely upon vegetable food for their support, and it is the carbohydrates which this contains that are converted into the fat of their milk or that which covers their muscles. That proteid food will also produce fat is shown by the amount of the latter which carnivorous animals put on.

Offices of Fat.—The offices which fat subserves in the human body are manifold: (1) It protects the underlying parts from injury, as in the palm of the hand and the sole of the foot; (2) it serves as a lubricator, as in the sebaceous matter poured out upon the skin, which keeps it soft and pliable; (3) it acts as a non-conductor of heat, aiding in the retention within the body of the vital heat, which would otherwise be lost so rapidly as to produce injurious results; (4) it serves as a reservoir when the supply of food is cut off or diminished; thus in wasting diseases the fat deposited in various parts of the body is absorbed and contributes to its nutrition; (5) it is a source of energy and of heat through its oxidation.

Important properties of fats, besides those already mentioned, which deserve special consideration, are two—that of forming a soap and that of forming an emulsion.

Saponification.—Fats are said to be saponifiable; that is, capable of being converted into a soap. If a fat be heated with a caustic alkali under pressure, it splits up into glycerin, and a fatty acid which unites with the alkali, the compound being a soap. Thus, if palmitin be the fat selected and the alkali be sodium, the palmitic acid, uniting with the sodium, would form sodium palmitate, a soap. If potassium were the alkali, the product would be potassium palmitate; similarly, stearin would form a stearate, and olein an oleate. The sodium soaps are hard, and those of potassium are soft. In the discussion of intestinal digestion it will be seen that the process of saponification takes place in the small intestine, and that the soap there formed aids in the important functions of that portion of the alimentary canal.

Emulsification.—Besides being saponifiable, fats are also emulsifiable—capable of forming an emulsion. If oil and water be poured into a test-tube, they will at once separate, the oil floating on the water. If the mouth of the tube be closed by the thumb and the tube firmly shaken, the oil and water will form a milky mixture, but will separate again when the agitation ceases; if a small amount of an alkali be added and the tube be again shaken, the separation will not take place as before, but the milky appearance will continue for some considerable time. If a drop of the mixture be placed under the microscope, it will be found that the oil-globules have been broken up into an exceedingly fine state of subdivision, some of the particles being too small to measure even with a very high magnifying power. This more or less permanent subdivision and suspension of the oil-globules constitutes an emulsion. The change is not a chemical one, but is purely physical. A similar process takes place in the small intestine during intestinal digestion, and is a necessary preliminary to the absorption of fat.

Lactic Acid is found in the alimentary canal, especially when large quantities of carbohydrates have been ingested. It occurs also in muscles, and has been said to exist in the nerve-cells of the brain. It has already been mentioned as the product of lactic fermentation.

Sarcolactic Acid occurs in blood and in muscles; to the latter it gives their acid reaction.

Cholesterin.—Chemically, this substance is an alcohol, the only one found free in the human body. It occurs in the bile, in the blood, in white nervous matter, and in the crystalline lens. It is a constituent also of the yolk of egg, of wheat, Indian corn, peas, and beans. It has some characteristics of the fats, such as insolubility in water and solubility in ether and chloroform, but it is not saponifiable, and is in other most important respects unlike them. It is classified here more for purposes of convenience than for any affinity with other members of the class.

D. Proteids.

These ingredients compose the principal parts of the muscles, the glands, and the nervous tissues, and of the solids of the blood they are the most important. Their percentage composition is as follows:

Carbon	50. –55.	Hydrogen . .	6.9– 7.3
Nitrogen . . .	15. –18.	Oxygen . . .	20. –23.5
Sulphur			0.3– 2.

When proteids are burned, there is found in the ash a certain quantity of salts—from the ignition of egg-albumin, for instance, chlorides of sodium and potassium result, and salts of calcium, magnesium, and iron in small quantities. It is still undecided whether these salts are integral parts of proteids or impurities.

Reactions of Proteids.—The presence or absence of proteids is determined by certain reactions, three of which are given:

Xanthoproteic Reaction.—When proteids are heated with strong nitric acid, they turn yellow, the color becoming deep orange on the addition of ammonia, caustic soda, or potash.

Millon's Reaction.—Proteids when heated with Millon's reagent give a white precipitate which becomes brick-red on cooling. This reagent is prepared by dissolving mercury in nitric acid and adding water. The precipitate which forms is allowed to settle, and the fluid is the reagent. Very small amounts of proteids give the red color without the precipitate.

Piotrowski's Reaction.—When a proteid is mixed with an excess of concentrated solution of sodium hydrate and one or two drops of a dilute solution of cupric sulphate, a violet color is produced which becomes deeper on boiling.

Classification.—The proteids are classified as follows:

1. Native albumins . . . . . { Egg-albumin. Serum-albumin.
2. Derived albumins . . . . { Acid-albumin. Syntonin. Alkali-albumin. Casein.
3. Globulins . . . . { Crystallin. Vitellin. Paraglobulin. Serum-globulin. Fibrinogen. Myosin. Globin.
4. Albumoses.
5. Peptones.
6. Albuminoids.
7. Enzymes.
8. Intermediate products.
9. Waste products.
10. Coloring matters.

1. Native Albumins.

Native albumins are found in the solids and fluids of the body. They are soluble in water, and are coagulated by heat at from 65° to 73° C., coagulation taking place more readily if dilute acetic acid be present. They are not precipitated by alkaline carbonates, by chloride of sodium, the solution of neutral salts in general, or by dilute acids.

Egg-Albumin.—As its name implies, egg-albumin is obtained from the white of egg. If much of it be taken in the food or if it be injected into the blood, part of it appears in the urine. When shaken with ether it is precipitated. Nitric acid, heat, and the prolonged action of alcohol coagulate egg-albumin, and mercuric chloride, nitrate of silver, and lead acetate precipitate it, forming insoluble compounds.

Serum-Albumin.—Serum-albumin occurs in the blood, in lymph, in chyle, in milk, and in some pathological fluids. When albumin is found in the urine it is generally serum-albumin. Serum-albumin differs from egg-albumin in not readily being coagulated by alcohol or precipitated by ether, and in not appearing in the urine when injected into the blood.

2. Derived Albumins.

The members of this group are sometimes spoken of as "albuminates." They are insoluble in distilled water and in dilute neutral saline solutions, but are soluble in acids and alkalies. Their solutions are not coagulated by boiling.

Acid-Albumin.—When a solution of either of the native albumins is treated with a dilute acid—hydrochloric acid, for instance—it is converted into acid-albumin. In this conversion it undergoes important changes. Its solution is not coagulated by heat, and when it is neutralized the proteid is precipitated. The conversion from the native to the acid-albumin is gradual, and is hastened by heat, care being taken that the temperature is not sufficiently high to coagulate it. Globulins are likewise converted into acid-albumins by the same means, but more readily, while coagulated proteids or fibrin require the acid to be concentrated. Each proteid produces its own special acid-albumin, although the difference between them is very slight.

Syntonin.—Syntonin is the special acid-albumin which results from the action of acids on myosin—the globulin which occurs in muscles. It is of special interest as being the acid-albumin formed in the stomach during the digestion of muscular tissue. It is soluble in lime-water, and this solution is partially coagulated by boiling; it is insoluble in acid sodium phosphate (NaH_2PO_4), while other acid-albumins are soluble. It differs from alkali-albumin in that when acid sodium phosphate is present and an alkali is added it does not pass into solution until the whole of the acid phosphate salt has been converted into the neutral phosphate (Na_2HPO_4), while alkali-albumin is soluble before this change takes place.

Alkali-Albumin.—If a native albumin be treated with a dilute alkali in the manner described in the treatment with a dilute acid, it will be converted into alkali-albumin, as in the former instance when an acid was used it was changed into acid-albumin. The alkali-albumin, like the acid-albumin, is not coagulated by heat; when neutralized the proteid is precipitated, and the precipitate, which is insoluble in water and in neutral solution of sodium chloride, is dissolved by dilute acids or alkalies.

Some writers have regarded acid- and alkali-albumin as differing from each other only in that in the one case the proteid is united with an acid, and in the other case with a base; but more recent investigations seem to show that, though closely related, they are in reality distinct, and that what was said of the product of the action of acids on proteids is probably true of that of alkalies—namely, that each proteid yields its own product, although as yet they cannot well be distinguished. Acid-albumin can be converted into alkali-albumin by strong alkalies, but alkali-albumin cannot be changed into acid-albumin by the action of acids. In 1838, Mulder described a substance which he called "protein." This designation is now abandoned. It has been suggested that what he called "protein" might have been alkali-albumin.

Casein exists in human milk in from 0.18 to 1.90 per cent., the mean being 0.63 per cent., and in that of the cow in from 1.17 to 7.40 per cent., 3.01 per cent. being the mean. This derived albumin occurs only in milk. It has been suggested that this physiological ingredient should be called "caseinogen," and that the term "casein" should be restricted to the curd formed when milk coagulates under the influence of rennin, the ferment in rennet. Inasmuch as we speak of "fibrinogen" and "fibrin," the former before and the latter after coagulation, the suggestion is well worthy of consideration as tending to simplification. Casein is precipitated by acids and by rennet at 40° C., and it contains 0.847 per cent. of phosphorus. When pure it is a fine snow-white powder insoluble in water, but is soluble in alkalies, carbonates and phosphates of the alkalies, lime- and baryta-water.

As has already been stated, casein clots under the influence of the enzyme rennin, but alkali-albumin, which has been regarded by some as identical with casein, does not. Milk from which casein has been removed by precipitation still contains a small amount of a coagulable proteid—*lactalbumin*—very similar to serum-albumin, but not identical. Upon the surface of milk exposed for some time to a temperature above 50° C. a pellicle forms, which is stated by some chemists to be casein, by others lactalbumin. This formation takes place more rapidly if a stream of air be blown over the surface of the milk.

What has been said of casein applies especially to that obtained from cow's milk. The differences between cow's milk and human milk, so far as regards casein, are as follows: 1. Human milk, when it clots at all with rennin, does so less firmly than cow's milk; 2. Acids very imperfectly precipitate the casein from human milk: to do this completely magnesium sulphate must be used to the point of saturation; 3. The casein of human milk is less soluble in water than that of cow's milk.

3. Globulins.

Globulins are insoluble in distilled water, but are soluble in dilute saline solutions, as, for instance, 1 per cent. sodium chloride, in very dilute acids and alkalies. If the saline solutions be saturated, the globulins will be precipitated. If the acid or the alkali be not dilute, but strong, the globulins will be converted into acid-albumin or into alkali-albumin.

Crystallin (globulin) is the globulin of the crystalline lens.

Vitellin is the proteid of the yolk of eggs. An identical globulin has been obtained from vegetable protoplasm. In the egg, vitellin is associated with lecithin, and indeed up to the present time vitellin has never been obtained free from lecithin. It has been said to occur in the chyle and in the amniotic fluid.

Paraglobulin (serum-globulin; fibrino-plastin; serum-casein) exists in blood-plasma to the amount of from 2 to 4 per cent., and also in lymph, in chyle, and in serous fluids like the fluid in hydrocele. In urine there has been found a globulin which is apparently identical with paraglobulin.

Fibrinogen.—The plasma of blood contains fibrinogen, as do also chyle and serous fluids. Like paraglobulin, it is contained in the fluid of hydrocele. It is of great physiological interest, as the clotting of blood consists in the conversion of fibrinogen into fibrin. For purposes of study fibrin is usually obtained by whipping blood with twigs or with wires. The material that clings to these is fibrin, together with some of the white and red corpuscles of the blood, which are entangled in the meshes of the fibrin. When washed in water the red coloring-matter is washed out and the fibrin is colorless. Fibrin is insoluble in water and in dilute saline solutions. In dilute acids—as, for instance, hydrochloric acid—it swells up and becomes transparent. If it be left in the acid for a long time or if the temperature be raised to 40° C., it is changed into acid-albumin.

Myosin.—When a muscle passes into the condition known as *rigor mortis* or "cadaveric rigidity," this change is due to a coagulation or clotting of the material of which the muscle consists, the clot being myosin. It has been suggested that this substance should, before coagulation, be called "myosinogen," and after coagulation "myosin," just as "fibrinogen" and "fibrin" are spoken of. It will be remembered that an acid acting on myosin converts it into syntonin.

Globin.—When exposed to the air for a sufficient time hæmoglobin, the red coloring-matter of the blood, decomposes, and globin is one of the products. Globin is very slightly soluble in dilute acids, alkalies, and solutions of sodium chloride, but is converted into acid- and alkali-albumin by strong acids and alkalies respectively.

4. Albumoses.

If a proteid be acted upon by pepsin in the presence of 0.2 per cent. of hydrochloric acid, a portion of it is changed into an acid-albumin. Some writers regard this as syntonin, but the tendency at the present time is to apply the name of "syntonin" only to that particular acid-albumin formed by the action of acid on myosin. It has also been spoken of as "parapeptone," but the two are not identical, as is evident from the fact that parapeptone is incapable of being converted into peptone by the action of pepsin. Subsequently, if the action of the pepsin be continued, this acid-albumin disappears and parapeptone and albumoses are produced. Still later in the process these albumoses are changed into peptones.

If instead of pepsin and hydrochloric acid the proteid be treated with trypsin, one of the enzymes of pancreatic juice, and a 0.25 per cent. solution of sodium carbonate, alkali-albumin is formed, and later albumoses, which are changed into peptones, some of which still later are converted into leucin and tyrosin. The albumoses, then, are intermediate products in the conversion of proteids into peptones. The theory of Kühne is that in the digestion of a proteid two albumoses are formed, anti-albumose and hemi-albumose.

Anti-albumose is practically not distinguished from acid-albumin or syntonin; the further action of the digestive ferment converts it into antipeptone.

Hemi-albumose is identical with what has been called "propeptone." It occurs occasionally in the urine, and is found also in the marrow of bones and in cerebrospinal fluid. Under the further influence of the ferment it passes into hemipeptone. Hemi-albumose is regarded by some writers as being composed of four forms of albumose: 1, protalbumose; 2, deutero-albumose; 3, hetero-albumose; 4, dysalbumose; but this is not yet determined. This subject is further discussed in treating of *Digestion*.

Albumoses have of late assumed a position of great importance, for the reason that they have been found to possess peculiar properties which were never before suspected. The poison of the cobra, regarded as the most virulent of animal poisons, is an albumose. When certain albumoses are injected into the blood its coagulability may be destroyed and death may result. This action was formerly attributed to peptones, but it is now believed to be due to the albumoses in the peptones. Immunity from certain diseases has been brought about by the protective influence of certain albumoses which have been produced by the action of the germs of those diseases, so that in this group of substances there is a variety of members, some beneficial and some poisonous. Albumoses also occur in plants, as wheat and the papaw.

5. Peptones.

In no part of physiological chemistry has more valuable work been done than in the study of this group of physiological ingredients, one important result being to show that what have been described as peptones are in reality mixtures of albumoses and peptones.

True peptones are very soluble in water, and are not precipitated by boiling nitric acid, by acetic acid, or by potassium ferrocyanide. They are, however, precipitated from neutral or feebly-acid solutions by mercuric chloride, tannic acid, bile-acids, and phospho-tungstic acid. They give Millon's and the Biuret reaction, are very diffusible, and are lævo-rotatory. In stating that peptones are very diffusible it must also be stated that this is true when they are compared with other proteids, but when the comparison is made with crystalline substances, such as sodium chloride, peptones are not very diffusible.

As has already been seen, antipeptone is the peptone which results from the action of the digestive ferments —pepsin or trypsin—on anti-albumose, and hemipeptone is that which results from their action on hemi-albumose. The latter yields leucin and tyrosin with the further action of trypsin; the former does not, though the action of the ferment be prolonged.

E. Albuminoids.

The albuminoids resemble the proteids in their composition; some of them contain no sulphur. They are neither crystallizable nor diffusible.

Mucin.—Mucus, the product of mucous glands, owes its peculiar ropy consistency to the ingredient *mucin.*

Mucin contains carbon, hydrogen, nitrogen, and oxygen, but no sulphur. It is derived from the proteids, and exhibits Millon's and the Xanthoproteic reactions. When treated with mineral acids an acid-albumin is formed, and at the same time there is produced a carbohydrate which may yield, when treated with acid, a reducing sugar. On account of these two products which result from the action of an acid on mucin, it has been regarded by some, although probably incorrectly, as a mixture of a proteid and a carbohydrate.

It has been assumed that the mucin of different fluids is the same substance, but that it is slightly modified in each instance. This has not been proved; indeed, the weight of evidence rather favors the view that there are several mucins, differing in certain particulars. Mucin is an ingredient of bile, but is not found in that fluid while it is still in the liver. It is added to the bile while in the gall-bladder, and is secreted by the lining membrane thereof. Mucin dissolves in water and is precipitated by acetic acid and by alcohol.

Gelatin.—When connective tissues are boiled in water for a considerable time, especially in a Papin digester, they yield a substance which is called "gelatin." It has been assumed that there is in bone a substance which has been named "ossein," and that in the ordinary connective tissues there is another substance called "collagen;" moreover, that the gelatin is not an original constituent of the tissues, but is the product of these two substances after the boiling. This assumption has much to sustain it, for if tendons be treated with trypsin, everything will be dissolved but the collagen, and if bones be treated with cold dilute acid, the salts will be dissolved and the ossein will remain. These two substances—collagen and ossein—are insoluble in water, in saline solutions, in cold dilute acids, and in alkalies. If, however, they be boiled in water for a long time, they are changed into gelatin, which when it cools forms a jelly or "gelatinizes." When this gelatin is dry it forms a transparent brittle substance which is familiar as glue or as the gelatin used in food.

Gelatin is insoluble in cold water, but swells up in it, and, when the water is warmed, dissolves. It is precipitated by tannic acid and mercuric chloride, but not by acids, by alum, nor by the salts of silver, iron, copper, or lead. Its percentage composition is carbon, 50.76; hydrogen, 7.15; oxygen, 23.21; nitrogen, 18.32; sulphur, 0.5. The sulphur is believed to be due to impurities, and is not regarded as a constituent of pure gelatin. By comparing this analysis with that of the proteids the difference will be seen.

If collagen be boiled in water for a longer period than is sufficient to convert it into gelatin, the latter will be converted into gelatin-peptones. This same change takes place if gelatin be treated with pepsin in presence of an acid or with trypsin, and the same conversion takes place in the stomach. Gelatin-peptones are more soluble than gelatin, and are diffusible. It will be remembered that in noting the action of the enzymes, pepsin and trypsin, upon proteids, albumoses were formed as intermediate products before the final formation of peptones. Likewise, when gelatin is changed into gelatin-peptones there are intermediate products, to which the name of "gelatoses" has been given. Gelatin is digested and absorbed in man and is a valuable food-stuff, but does not supply the tissues with nitrogen, as its nitrogen cannot be built up into that of a proteid.

Chondrin.—As gelatin is looked upon as a product of the prolonged boiling in water of collagen and ossein, so chondrin is regarded as resulting from a similar treatment of "chondrigen," the matrix of hyaline cartilage. Chondrigen is insoluble in water, but when boiled in a Papin digester it is dissolved gradually and is transformed into chondrin, which gelatinizes on cooling. The percentage composition of chondrin is carbon, 50.9; hydrogen, 7.1; nitrogen, 14.9; oxygen, 29; sulphur, 0.4. It is precipitated by acetic acid, which does not redissolve the precipitate. Mineral acids in small amounts produce a precipitate which dissolves in excess of the acids. Chondrin is also precipitated by alum and by the salts of silver, iron, and lead. There is some evidence showing that chondrin is a mixture of mucin and gelatin, but this combination is not conclusively determined.

Elastin.—This substance is an ingredient of elastic tissue, as, for instance, the ligamentum nuchæ. Its percentage composition is carbon, 55.6; hydrogen, 7.7; nitrogen, 17.7; oxygen, 21.1; it does not contain sulphur. Elastin is soluble only when boiled in strong alkalies at 100° C. If boiled with sulphuric acid at 100° C., it is not only dissolved, but is also decomposed, yielding from 30 to 40 per cent. of leucin and 0.25 per cent. of tyrosin. Elastin is digested under the influence of pepsin in an acid, and trypsin in an alkaline medium, but it is doubtful whether elastin passes into the stage of peptone, but rather does not go beyond the intermediate stage of what may be termed "elastoses."

Keratin.—This substance is found in all horny tissues, such as hair, nails, and epidermis. Its percentage composition is carbon, 52.5; hydrogen, 7; nitrogen, 17;

oxygen, 25; sulphur, 5. Keratin is dissolved by alkalies, and the sulphur forms sulphides of the metals. It is unaffected by the action of pepsin or trypsin.

F. Enzymes.

There are two classes of enzymes or ferments: (1) organized ferments, of which yeast is an example, and (2) unorganized or soluble ferments, of which pepsin is an example. It has been proposed to limit the term "ferment" to the *organized* class, and to denominate the changes which its members cause in substances upon which they act as "fermentation," while to the soluble or *unorganized* class to apply the name of "enzyme," and to give to the process for which its members are responsible the term "zymolysis." There will here be discussed only the unorganized ferments or enzymes.

Some of the enzymes on analysis have been found to be very similar in their composition to the proteids, although containing less carbon. This similarity is shown in the percentage composition of trypsin. The unorganized enzymes are soluble in water and in glycerin, and are precipitated by an excess of absolute alcohol, but are not diffusible. Minute quantities of unorganized enzymes under proper conditions will bring about zymolytic changes in considerable quantities of the substances upon which they act, apparently without diminishing. The conditions under which they act vary for each enzyme, but as a rule high temperatures destroy and low temperatures inhibit, while for each there is a temperature at which its action is the most pronounced; this is called the "optimum" temperature. Thus for pepsin the optimum temperature is from 35° to 40° C., while below 1° C. its action ceases, as it does also at

70° C., while boiling permanently destroys it. It has been determined, however, that when perfectly dry the enzymes may be heated to 160° C. without destroying their power.

An interesting fact also connected with the enzymes is, that when they have produced a considerable amount of their product their action is diminished, and that if this new product accumulates still more, the zymolytic action of the enzymes may be brought to an end, although their power to act would still be present if these products were removed. In some instances the enzyme is not the direct product of the cells, but the cells form what is termed a "zymogen," which is afterward converted into the enzyme. Each zymogen is named from the enzyme which it produces: thus the zymogen of trypsin is "trypsinogen," that of pepsin is "pepsinogen," etc. It is an interesting and valuable fact that chloroform inhibits the action of the organized ferments, but does not interfere with that of the unorganized. As it is very important to have a clear idea of the meaning of certain terms which occur repeatedly in the discussion of the enzymes and their action, these terms will here be defined—namely:

Amylolytic Enzyme.—The conversion of starch into sugar is an *amylolytic* change, and an enzyme which has the power of producing this change is an amylolytic enzyme.

Diastatic or Diastasic Enzyme.—There exists in barley an enzyme, diastase, which has the power of changing starch into sugar; the change itself, and also the enzyme, are spoken of as *diastatic* or *diastasic*. It will be seen, therefore, that amylolytic, diastatic, and diastasic are synonymous.

Proteolytic Enzyme.—The conversion of a proteid into a peptone is a *proteolytic* change, and any enzyme which causes it is a proteolytic enzyme.

Hydrolytic Enzyme.—It is now generally accepted that in the conversion of starch into sugar and of proteids into peptones the change consists in the assumption of a molecule of water; thus,

$$\underset{\text{Starch.}}{(C_6H_{10}O_5)_n} + \underset{\text{Water.}}{H_2O} = \underset{\text{Sugar.}}{C_6H_{12}O_6}$$

This change is called "hydrolysis," and the action is said to be *hydrolytic*. Both amylolytic and proteolytic changes are hydrolytic. Indeed, there are reasons for believing that the enzymes produce their action in every instance by causing the substances upon which they act to unite with water.

Ptyalin.—This enzyme is found in saliva, and is one of its important constituents. It is an interesting fact that from many of the tissues and fluids of the body a similar enzyme may be obtained. This is especially marked in the pig. When ptyalin is obtained from saliva it is a white powder which dissolves in water and converts starch into maltose. This action markedly takes place in solutions that are neutral. So far as known, ptyalin is formed directly by the cells, and there is no intermediate stage of a zymogen. If such a substance should be discovered, it would, by analogy, be called "ptyalinogen." Ptyalin is an amylolytic enzyme, but acts only on cooked starch.

Amylopsin.—This substance is also an amylolytic enzyme, and acts on both cooked and raw starch. Its action is more rapid than that of ptyalin, and further it changes the maltose into dextrose, in which form sugar is absorbed during the digestive process.

Pepsin.—This substance is the enzyme of the gastric juice, and is proteolytic in its action. There exists for pepsin a true zymogen, pepsinogen, which is formed by the cells of the gastric glands, and under the influence of the hydrochloric acid of the gastric juice the pepsinogen becomes pepsin. Pepsin exerts its proteolytic action only in the presence of an acid, of which, for experimental purposes, hydrochloric acid, 0.2 per cent., is the best.

Trypsin.—This substance is the proteolytic enzyme of pancreatic juice. Considerable study has been made of trypsin, its composition being given as follows: carbon, 47.22 to 48.09; hydrogen, 7.15 to 7.44; nitrogen, 12.59 to 13.41; sulphur, 1.73 to 1.86. Trypsin acts most promptly in the presence of an alkali, but it will act also in neutral solutions or even when 0.012 per cent. of hydrochloric acid is present; but its action ceases when free hydrochloric acid is present to the amount of 0.1 per cent.

In connection with this enzyme it is interesting to note that the contents of the small intestine, into which the pancreatic juice is discharged, are not invariable in their reaction. Sometimes they are alkaline, at other times neutral, and they may even be acid. When this acidity exists in the upper part of the small intestine, it is due to the hydrochloric acid produced by the stomach, but when it is found elsewhere it is attributable to lactic or butyric acid formed as a result of fermentation of the carbohydrates of the food. It is claimed that a small amount of lactic acid, less than 0.05 per cent., is an aid to the proteolytic action of trypsin, but that more than this percentage puts a stop to the process. Trypsin has its zymogen, which is called "trypsinogen."

Pialyn (Steapsin).—This enzyme is sometimes spoken of as the "fat-splitting ferment," because its action is to decompose the neutral fats, the result being a fatty acid and glycerin. The optimum temperature for the action of pialyn is 40° C., and the most favorable reaction is a slightly alkaline one.

Rennin.—In cheese-making the casein of milk is coagulated by rennet, which is an infusion in brine of the fourth stomach of the calf. This coagulating property of rennet is due to an enzyme to which has been given the names of "rennet ferment," "milk-curdling ferment," and "rennin." Rennin may be extracted from the mucous membrane of the stomach of most animals, including man. The zymogen of rennin is denominated "renninogen."

Fibrin-ferment.—The clotting of blood is due to the change of its fibrinogen into fibrin under the influence of an enzyme, fibrin-ferment. The theory that this clotting is produced by the breaking down of the white corpuscles seems to be the most reasonable one at the present time. In the consideration of the coagulation of the blood this subject will again be referred to.

Muscle-enzyme.—The clotting of the plasma of muscle is attributed to this enzyme, which is regarded as distinct from fibrin-ferment. It is sometimes spoken of as "myosin-ferment."

G. Intermediate Products.

There exists in the body a class of substances which, after they are formed by the tissues, perform some office in the economy of the body, but what this office is, exactly, is not understood. These substances are not permanent, but undergo changes into other forms, and are therefore known as "intermediate products" or "by-products."

Sodium Glycocholate ($C_{26}H_{43}NO_6Na$) is one of the ingredients of the bile of man, of the ox, and of other animals, only traces of it being found in the carnivora, some authorities claiming it to be absent. This salt consists of glycocholic acid united with sodium. Glycocholic acid is composed of glycin and cholalic acid, and is sometimes found in the urine in jaundice.

Sodium Taurocholate ($C_{26}H_{45}NSO_7Na$) and sodium glycocholate are known as the "bile-salts." Sodium taurocholate, which is composed of taurocholic acid and sodium, exists in both human and ox bile. In the bile of carnivora it exists without the glycocholate. Taurocholic acid is composed of taurin and cholalic acid. Cholalic acid or cholic acid, which is produced by the decomposition of the bile-acids, is formed in the small intestine, and still more abundantly in the large intestine. Taurocholic acid precipitates ordinary proteids from their solutions, but has no such action on peptones. When the contents of the stomach, therefore, enter the small intestine, the proteids are thrown down and the enzymes can act upon them more readily, while the peptones are absorbed. This acid is said also to possess antiseptic properties to a marked degree.

Pettenkofer's Test for Bile-acids.—This test consists in the production of a cherry-red color, which changes to a purple, when a few drops of a 20 per cent. solution of cane-sugar are added to a solution of bile-acids or the biliary salts and followed by concentrated sulphuric acid. Other substances, such as morphine and salicylic acid, will give the same color reactions, so that to exclude them it is necessary to evaporate to dryness the fluid to be examined, to extract with absolute alcohol, and to precipitate by the addition of ether in excess. To this precipitate, when dissolved in water, the test may be applied as already indicated.

Lecithin ($C_{44}H_{90}NPO_9$).—This ingredient is sometimes known as "phosphorized fat." It is a constituent of the red and white blood-corpuscles, of the bile, brain, nerves, semen, and pus. It occurs also in yeast and in other vegetable cells, in the yolk of egg, and in milk.

Cerebrin ($C_{17}N_{33}NO_3$).—This substance is found in the brain, in nerves, and in pus-corpuscles.

Protagon ($C_{160}H_{308}N_5PO_{35}$).—This substance is also found in the brain. It is still undecided whether protagon is an independent substance or is a mixture of lecithin and cerebrin, although evidence is accumulating which indicates that it is not a mixture.

H. WASTE PRODUCTS.

This class includes substances which are the result of the disintegrative changes that occur in the tissues of the body and in the food. After being formed they are eliminated, being of no use.

Kreatin ($C_4H_9N_3O_2$).—This substance is one of the characteristic ingredients of the muscles, and in the metabolism of these tissues ultimately becomes converted into urea. Kreatin occurs also in nervous tissues. It is not a constituent of urine, although it is sometimes so regarded. When found in this fluid it has doubtless been produced from kreatinin by the methods used to obtain it from the urine. Kreatin readily becomes converted into kreatinin by giving up a molecule of water.

Kreatinin ($C_4H_7N_3O$).—A comparison of the formulæ

of kreatin and kreatinin shows that the latter is a dehydrated form of the former. Kreatinin readily unites with water, forming kreatin; it exists in the urine in proportions which vary according to the amount of proteids eaten—from 0.5 to 4.9 grammes per diem.

Urea ($(NH_2)_2CO$) is the principal waste product in the urine of mammals, although it occurs in small amounts in that of birds, especially when they are fed on meat. In the urine of man it is present to the amount of 2.5 to 3.2 per cent., 30 grammes on an average being daily excreted. In blood it occurs in the proportion of 0.025 per cent., and it may also be obtained from lymph, perspiration, and from the liver. Urea is soluble in water and alcohol, but insoluble in anhydrous ether. Under the influence of bacteria, urea undergoes alkaline fermentation, in which two molecules of water are taken up and carbonate of ammonia is formed. This change is expressed by the formula

$$\underset{\text{Urea.}}{(NH_2)_2CO} + \underset{\text{Water.}}{2H_2O} = \underset{\text{Carbonate of ammonia.}}{(NH_4)_2CO_2}$$

The source of urea is from the kreatin of muscular tissue, and the liver is, in all probability, the organ in which take place the transformations that result in its production, so that when this organ is diseased there is likely to be a diminished amount of urea excreted.

Uric Acid ($C_5H_4N_4O_3$) is found in small quantities in human urine, only from 0.2 to 1 gramme being daily excreted. This acid is, however, abundant in the urine of birds and of reptiles. It is found constantly in the spleen, and it has been found also in the lungs, the heart, the pancreas, the brain, and the liver. The calculi which form in the urinary organs frequently consist of uric acid or of salts formed from it. The so-called "concretions" which form in the joints of persons suffering from gout are composed of uric acid. The principal salts into the formation of which uric acid enters are sodium, potassium, and ammonium urates. In the production of urea uric acid is regarded as one of the steps.

$$\underset{\text{Uric acid.}}{C_5H_4N_4O_3} + \underset{\text{Water.}}{H_2O} + \underset{\text{Oxygen.}}{O} = \underset{\text{Alloxan.}}{C_4H_2N_2O_4} + \underset{\text{Urea.}}{(NH_2)_2CO}$$

Hippuric Acid ($C_9H_9NO_3$).—This ingredient of human urine is excreted to the amount of but from 0.1 to 1.0 gramme per diem. It is much more abundant in horses and in other herbivora.

Leucin ($C_6H_{10}(NH_2)O.OH$) occurs in the pancreas, spleen, thymus, thyroid, salivary glands, and liver. It is sometimes found in urine, especially in certain diseases of the liver, such as acute yellow atrophy. Leucin occurs also in the bulbs, tubers, and seeds of some plants. It is found in the small intestine during the digestion of proteids.

Tyrosin ($C_9H_{11}NO_3$).—This is an ingredient of the pancreas and pancreatic juice and of the spleen. Tyrosin is intimately associated with leucin, being found with it during the pancreatic digestion of proteids; also in urine during diseases of the liver, and in plants.

Indol (C_8H_7N) occurs in the fæces, and is one of the ingredients which gives them their peculiar odor. Indol is a product of the decomposition of proteids which occurs in the intestines.

Skatol (C_9H_9N) occurs in the fæces with indol, and it contributes to produce the fæcal odor.

I. Coloring-matters.

Hæmoglobin (Reduced Hæmoglobin) ($C_{600}H_{960}N_{154}FeS_3O_{179}$).—Hæmoglobin with oxyhæmoglobin gives the characteristic color to the blood. In the blood of an asphyxiated animal the coloring-matter is almost entirely hæmoglobin; in venous blood it is both hæmoglobin and oxyhæmoglobin, while in arterial blood the oxyhæmoglobin is in excess. It is probable that there are various hæmoglobins, as this ingredient obtained from the blood of different animals varies in important particulars. The percentage composition of that of the dog is as follows: carbon, 53.85; hydrogen, 7.32; nitrogen, 16.17; sulphur, 0.390; iron, 0.430; oxygen, 21.84. The great physiological interest which attaches to this substance is due to its affinity for, and the readiness with which it gives up, oxygen.

Oxyhæmoglobin is a compound of one molecule of oxygen and one molecule of hæmoglobin. The power of hæmoglobin to take up oxygen depends upon the iron it contains. When oxyhæmoglobin is treated with acids or with strong alkalies it is decomposed, the products being a proteid, globin, and hæmatin. This change takes place in extravasated blood and also during digestion. Hæmatin may be found in the fæces, especially after a meat diet. If to dried blood a crystal of common salt be added, and on this be dropped glacial acetic acid, and heat be then applied, there form crystals which are called "hæmin crystals." Chemically speaking, they are chloride of hæmatin.

Carbon-monoxide Hæmoglobin.—A union of one molecule of hæmoglobin and one of carbon monoxide produces the coloring-matter carbon-monoxide hæmoglobin.

If a current of carbon monoxide be passed through a solution of oxyhæmoglobin, the gas will displace the oxygen and carbon-monoxide hæmoglobin will be formed. An important difference is to be noted in the behavior of this gas as compared with oxygen: while oxygen is easily replaced, carbon monoxide is not. Carbon monoxide is the gas formed when combustion is incomplete, such as is produced by the charcoal furnace used in France for suicidal purposes; the charcoal fumes when inhaled in sufficient quantity produce fatal results. The combinations of hæmoglobin with oxygen, carbon monoxide, and other gases are definite compounds, each of which crystallizes in its own characteristic form and has its own spectrum.

Bilirubin ($C_{16}H_{18}N_2O_3$).—The bile of man and of carnivora owes its golden-red color to bilirubin. This coloring-matter is insoluble in water, but is very soluble in solutions that are alkaline. Bilirubin is identical with what was formerly called "hæmatoidin," a coloring-matter found in old blood-clots, in corpora lutea, and sometimes in urine.

Biliverdin ($C_{16}H_{18}N_2O_4$), which is the coloring-matter of the bile of herbivora, is characterized by its bright-green color. Its formula shows that it is oxidized bilirubin, and when the golden-red bile of carnivora is exposed to the air it becomes green, its bilirubin having been changed into biliverdin. Any oxidizing agent produces the same effect, and on this fact are based tests for the presence of the bile-pigment. Gmelin's test is as follows: Nitric acid, which contains nitrous acid, is poured into a test-tube, and upon it is poured the fluid suspected of containing the coloring-matter, care being taken not to mix the two, but to permit the fluid to float on the acid. If the bile-pigments be present, colored rings appear where the two fluids join, the ring nearest the acid being yellow, and those above being red, violet, blue, and green. This test is sufficiently delicate to detect the presence of 1 part of bilirubin in 70,000 parts of the solvent.

Hydrobilirubin ($C_{32}H_{40}N_4O_7$) is another coloring-matter in the bile, and exists also in fæces, in which it has been described as "stercobilin." The identity of hydrobilirubin and urobilin, a coloring-matter of the urine, may now be regarded as established. It gives to the urine a red or reddish-yellow color, and is especially abundant in highly-colored urine, as in fevers. One authority at least believes that the urobilin of normal urine and that of pathological urine have certain essential points of difference.

All these bile-pigments are regarded as being derived from hæmoglobin, and the liver-cells are probably the structures endowed with the power of their formation.

Urochrome.—This coloring-matter of the urine is regarded by some as distinct from, and by others as identical with, urobilin.

Melanins.—There is a group of substances to which the name melanins might well be given, as its members differ somewhat from one another. In general this group comprises the black or dark pigments, as in the choroid, the skin, etc.

Fuscin is the melanin of the cell-substance and processes of the retinal epithelium.

Urinary melanin is the name given to the coloring-matter of the dark-brown or black urine of persons suffering with melanotic tumors; that is, tumors which are dark-colored from containing a melanin.

Lutein is the yellow pigment of the corpus luteum. *Serum-lutein* is the pigment which gives the yellowish color to the serum of blood. This fluid may sometimes owe part of its color to bile-pigments.

FOOD.

THE human body is constantly wasting. In a single day this waste is estimated to be at least eight pounds. If this loss were not compensated for, death would result from starvation, the length of time necessary to produce this fatal result depending much on circumstances. In one instance, in which one hundred and fifty persons in 1816 were wrecked on the "Medusa," after being thirteen days without food either solid or liquid all were dead but fifteen. It is, however, to be said that in this case there was not only absence of food, but as an additional factor in hastening the result there was also exposure to the elements. It may be said, in general, that death will supervene when the body has lost four-tenths of its weight. To supply the waste of the body and to maintain it in its physiological condition food is taken.

There is a process of oxidation taking place in the body in which the oxygen taken in by the lung oxidizes some of the fats, carbohydrates, and proteids, and as a result there are formed carbon dioxide, water, and urea; that is, complex substances are broken up into simpler forms and energy is produced. Besides this, the body is constantly the seat of certain activities, as movements of the muscles, the production of vital heat, and nervous activity, and for this food is also required. *Food, then, may be defined as material taken into the body to repair the waste of tissues and to produce energy.* Foods are made up of food-stuffs and other substances associated with them, which latter, being indigestible, are of no value either for purposes of nutrition or for the generation of energy.

Food-stuffs are divided into four classes, and they have already been discussed in treating of the physiological ingredients. The classes of food-stuffs are:

1. Inorganic, including water and salts.
2. Carbohydrates.
3. Fats or oils.
4. Proteids.

1. INORGANIC FOOD-STUFFS.—*Water* is, as has been pointed out, one of the most important ingredients of the body, and is therefore one of the most essential of the food-stuffs. It is the solvent of many of the constituents of the food and the salts, and by its softening action on the dry parts aids in the processes by which they are masticated and swallowed. It is important to remember that water should be free from such impurities as render it harmful. Thus, if it be too "hard"—that is, contains too much *lime*—there is liability to the production of gastric or intestinal derangements; if it contain the *germs* of disease, sickness may follow its use. It is by drinking water infected with the germs of cholera or of typhoid fever that these diseases are often produced. To avoid this danger, when there is any doubt as to the purity of the water it should be boiled. In one family known to the writer no water that has not been boiled has been drunk for many months.

The impression that boiled water is unpalatable is erroneous. But boiling the water will be of no avail in avoiding the danger of infection if impure ice be used in connection with it. Nothing is more clearly settled than that freezing does not destroy all disease-producing germs. The typhoid-fever epidemic which occurred in 1885 at Plymouth, Pa., where, of a population of 8000, 1153 persons were stricken with the disease, 114 of them dying, is a striking instance of the vitality of the typhoid germs. The drinking-water of Plymouth became contaminated from the fæces of a patient having typhoid fever, although these fæces had been frozen for a long time during the winter months. Laboratory experiments have demonstrated that the germs of this disease may be frozen for more than one hundred days and still retain their vitality.

The writer investigated an epidemic of dysentery in which the disease was traced to ice used in drinking-water. The ice had been cut from a pond in which during the summer hogs wallowed, and in which they deposited their excreta. When melted this ice had a most offensive odor. Other instances might be given showing the danger from the use of impure ice, but the one cited will suffice. Fortunately, there is now furnished for use in many of our cities artificial ice, which, if properly prepared, is free from all contamination. In this process of manufacturing ice the water is not only boiled, but is distilled, and when ready for freezing is absolutely pure. With boiled water and artificial ice all danger of infection through these channels may surely be prevented.

Salts.—The list of salts taken in with the food has already been given, the most important being sodium chloride, calcium phosphate, and the alkaline carbonates and phosphates. The offices which these salts perform in the economy of the body vary. By some of them the solubility of certain ingredients is made possible, as is the globulin in the blood by virtue of the presence of sodium chloride. Salts are stimulants also to the glands, causing the latter to secrete more actively; thus the digestive fluids are more abundantly poured out when the food is properly salted, and the kidneys more completely perform their functions under the stimulation of the salts.

2. CARBOHYDRATES.—These food-stuffs, in the form of starch and sugar, are especially abundant in vegetable foods and in milk, and less so in animal foods.

3. FATS OR OILS.—These food-stuffs are found in milk, in butter, in cheese, in the fatty tissues of meat, and also in some vegetables, such as nuts. The following table shows the amount in some of the ordinary foods:

Meat	5 to 10 per cent.
Milk	3 to 4 " "
Eggs	12 " "
Cheese	8 to 30 " "
Butter	85 to 90 " "

4. PROTEIDS.—This class contains some of the most valuable of the food-stuffs. The importance of this class is readily understood when it is recalled that the principal ingredients of the blood and the muscles are supplied by the proteids of the food. This is the only class whose members contain nitrogen, and it has therefore been sometimes spoken of as the "nitrogenous" class. The albuminoids contain nitrogen also, but this class has little nutritive value, except gelatin, which is valuable, but, as has already been stated, its nitrogen is not available for the tissues. The proteids are represented in eggs by albumin, in milk by casein, in

meat by myosin, in peas and in beans by legumin, and in the cereals by gluten. The amount of proteids varies in different foods; thus there is in

Meat	15 to 23	per cent.
Milk	3 to 4	" "
Peas and beans	23 to 27	" "
Grains (flour)	8 to 11	" "
Bread	6 to 9	" "
Potatoes	1 to 4	" "

The following diagram (Fig. 4) shows the amount of the principal food-stuffs in some of the more generally used foods:

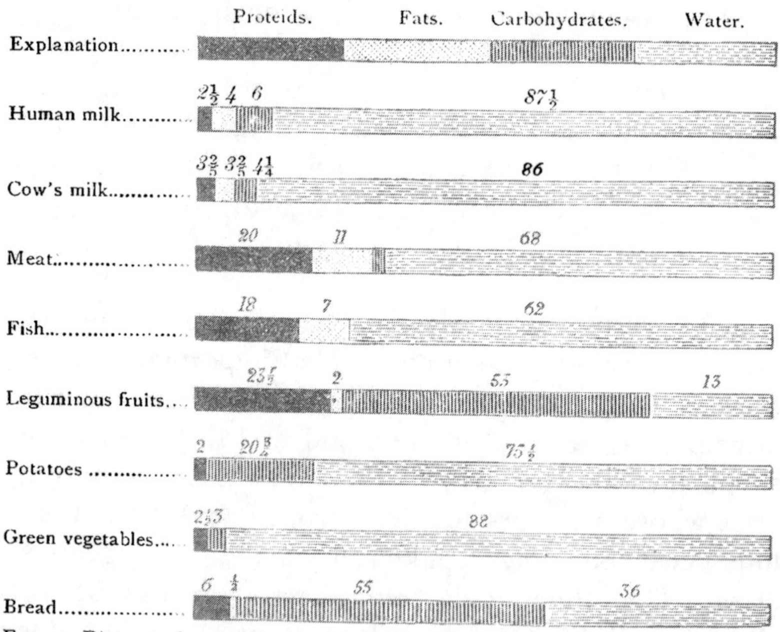

FIG. 4.—Diagram showing the proportion of the principal food-stuffs in a few typical comestibles. The numbers indicate percentages. Salts and indigestible materials omitted. (After Yeo.)

From the above consideration of the food-stuffs it is seen that they are in most respects the same as the tissues of the body; yet it would be erroneous to infer that the fats and the proteids of the food go directly into the tissues as such, and take the place of the fats and proteids which are wasted. There are many intermediate steps, some of which are known and will be discussed, and others of which we are entirely ignorant. Experience has abundantly demonstrated that in order to maintain the body at its physiological standard, representatives from all these four classes of food-stuffs must be supplied. If man be deprived of water, death speedily results; it comes as surely, though not so quickly, if fats or carbohydrates or proteids be cut off from the food-supply. Indeed, a man may be starved to death by withholding the salts.

Whenever, therefore, it is found that life can be maintained physiologically for a long period of time on any diet, it is certain that this diet contains representatives of all the classes enumerated. Thus, milk, which is the sole food of young children—among some of the Eskimos to the sixth year of life—is found on analysis to contain such representatives, the inorganic class being represented by water and salts, the carbohydrates by milk-sugar, the fats by butter, and the proteids by casein and some albumin. It is not, however, sufficient that each class should be represented, but the proportions of the ingredients must be proper. It is possible that any given food may have the requisite constituents, but may have too much of one and too little of another. It has been determined that the daily waste of the body is 4500 grains of carbon and 300 grains of nitrogen, or 15 to 1, so that in the food the nitrogen should be to the carbon as 1 is to 15.

In the table given above it is seen that in the proteids

there are three times as much carbon as nitrogen, so that should proteids only be supplied to the body there would have to be given an enormous amount of nitrogenous food in order to supply enough of the carbonaceous. The effect of this excess of nitrogenous food would be to injure the digestive and eliminating organs. Imagine, for instance, the effect upon the digestive apparatus if man's exclusive diet were potatoes. It will be seen by the table that in potatoes there are 2 per cent. of proteids and 20.75 per cent. of carbohydrates. Therefore, to obtain enough proteids from potatoes to sustain life it would be necessary to eat daily at least ten pounds, or thirty good-sized potatoes. In some parts of the world this has been put into practice, the effect being to distend the stomach and to derange digestion to a harmful degree.

If the diet were exclusively of meat, then in order to supply the body with the necessary amount of carbonaceous material a very large quantity of meat would be required, and to meet this requirement there would be taken in an excess of nitrogenous constituents, thus placing a serious burden on the eliminating organs to get rid of them. Experience demonstrates that a mixture of foods is the true physiological method of supplying the wants of the human body: from meat is obtained the proteids necessary for nutrition; from the potato is derived the starch; and from butter is secured the fat. Experience shows also that a higher standard of efficiency is maintained by a variety of food, a change being made from one kind of meat to another and from one vegetable to another, always, however, giving the body the food-stuffs in the proper quantities to supply its demands.

There are individuals who believe that meat-eating is not only unnecessary to, but that it tends also to degrade, man; they consequently confine themselves to vegetable diet: this exclusive dietary practice is called "vegetarianism." It is true that vegetables contain all the physiological ingredients necessary for nutrition, but, as above noted in the case of potatoes, the proportion is not such as will subserve the best interests of the body, and physiologists have decried the system as being irrational. The following extract from a letter of Dr. Alanus, a vegetarian, published in the *Medical and Surgical Reporter*, gives his experience in this matter:

"Having lived for a long time as a vegetarian without feeling any better or worse than formerly with mixed food, I made one day the disagreeable discovery that my arteries began to show signs of atheromatous degeneration. Particularly in the temporal and radial arteries this morbid process was unmistakable. Being still under forty, I could not interpret this symptom as a manifestation of old age, and being, furthermore, not addicted to drink, I was utterly unable to explain the matter. I turned it over and over in my mind without finding a solution of the enigma. I, however, found the explanation quite accidentally in a work of that excellent physician, Dr. E. Monin of Paris. The following is the verbal translation of the passage in question: 'In order to continue the criticism of vegetarianism we must not ignore the work of the late lamented Gubler on the influence of a vegetable diet on the chalky degeneration of the arteries. Vegetable food, richer in mineral salts than that of animal origin, introduces more mineral salts into the blood. Raymond has observed numerous cases of atheroma in a monastery of vegetarian friars, amongst others that of the prior, a man scarcely thirty-two years old, whose arteries were already considerably indurated. The naval surgeon, Treille, has seen numerous cases of atheromatous degeneration in Bombay and Calcutta, where many people live exclusively on rice. A vegetable diet, therefore, ruins the blood-vessels and makes one prematurely old, if it is true that a man is as old as his arteries. It must produce at the same time tartar, the senile arch of the cornea, and phosphaturia.' Having, unfortunately, seen these newest results of medical investigation confirmed by my own case, I have, as a matter of course, returned to a mixed diet. I can no longer consider purely vegetable food as the normal diet of man, but only as a curative method which is of the greatest service in various morbid states. Some patients may follow this diet for weeks and months, but it is not adapted for everybody's continued use. It is the same as with the starvation cure, which cures some patients, but is not fit to be used continually by the healthy. I have become richer by one experience, which has shown me that a single brutal fact can knock down the most beautiful theoretical structure."

Another factor to determine the nutritive value of any food is its digestibility. The chemical analysis of cheese would place it high among the foods, but experience shows that its constitution is such as not readily to permit the action of the digestive fluids, and its availability as a food is therefore low.

In regard to meats, it may be said that veal is not of such nutritive value as beef. Indeed, to many persons it seems almost poisonous. It is certainly much less digestible than beef or mutton, though more digestible when roasted.

In conclusion, then, the following table is given as showing a simple daily diet for an adult:

Butter or fat	100	grammes.
Meat	453	"
Bread	540	"
Water	1530	"

With this diet life could doubtless be maintained for a long time, but for reasons already given it should be varied.

II. NUTRITIVE FUNCTIONS.

1. Digestion.

Having considered the composition of the body and food, there may now be taken up the study of the nutritive functions.

As has already been noted, the body is constantly producing *energy* and undergoing *waste*, both of which require the taking of food. But food is absolutely of no use to the body until it reaches the blood and by this fluid is conveyed to the tissues. So long as the food remains within the alimentary canal it is as much outside the body, so far as nutrition is concerned, as if it had never been taken inside. To be of any service the food must enter the blood, and it does this by being absorbed.

In some forms of animal life the food is of such a nature that it readily and without further change undergoes absorption; that is, passes through the walls of the absorbing vessels. In other forms of animal life this is not the case: in the latter form of animals, unless certain changes take place, the food passes out of the alimentary canal as waste material, without having contributed to the nutrition of the body in the slightest degree. Unless, therefore, some provision were made to obviate this, such animals would die of starvation. The provision which has been made consists in the presence of certain organs whose duty is to change the form of the food-substances from that in which they will not, into that in which they will, be absorbed. Substances that are not in a condition to be absorbed—that is, will not pass through animal membranes—are said to be "non-diffusible;" those that are in a condition to pass through are said to be "diffusible." The above change, then, consists mainly in the alteration from a non-diffusible to a diffusible state. The only exception to this rule is that of the fats, which are otherwise prepared. It is this change (its preparation for absorption) which constitutes food-digestion, and the organs concerned in bringing about these necessary changes in the food are the digestive organs.

Manifestly, these organs will be simple or be complex according to the amount of change which it is necessary to bring about in the food in order that absorption may take place. Thus, if the food on which an animal relies for its sustentation be already in a diffusible form, no change will be needed, and the animal will therefore have no digestive organs. If the requisite change be a slight one, the number of the digestive organs will be few and their structure will be simple. But if the food be varied in its composition, and largely made up of non-diffusible food-stuffs, then the digestive apparatus—that is, the group of organs concerned in digestion—will be complex. Such is the character of the food of man, and, consequently, such is the character of his digestive apparatus (Fig. 5).

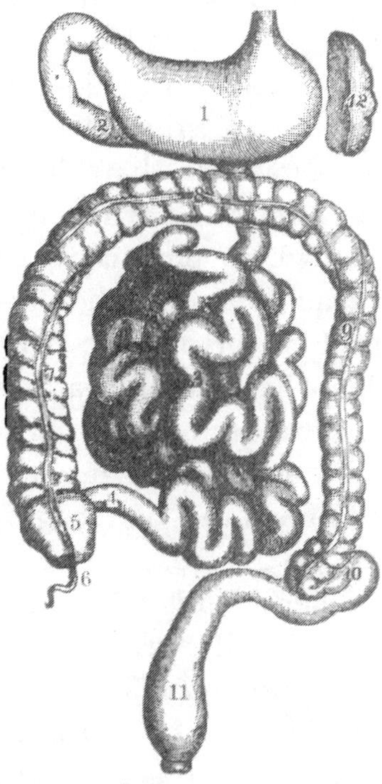

FIG. 5.—1. Stomach; 2-4. Small intestine: 5. Cæcum; 6. Vermiform appendix; 7, 8, 9. Colon; 10. Sigmoid flexure; 11. Rectum; 12. Spleen.

The human digestive apparatus consists of the alimentary canal and the other digestive organs, which, although outside, still communicate with this canal by ducts through which their secretion is poured. The alimentary canal consists of the mouth, the œsophagus, the stomach, and the small intestine. The digestive organs which are outside, but discharge their secretion into, this canal are the salivary glands, the liver, and the pancreas.

The digestive process is subdivided into three parts: (A) That which takes place in the mouth—mouth digestion; (B) that which takes place in the stomach—stomach or gastric digestion; and (C) that which takes place in the small intestine—intestinal digestion. Formerly, when digestion was spoken of it was always *stomach* digestion which was referred to, because it was supposed that the entire process took place in that organ, and when digestion was impaired the remedies which physicians employed were directed to the stomach alone. There is, unfortunately, too much of this kind of practice even now, but the study of physiology has taught that indigestion may be due quite as much to the improper performance of mouth and intestinal digestion as to that which takes place in the stomach, and unless this be recognized many cases will unsuccessfully be treated.

When food is taken into the mouth it has, presumably, been as fully prepared as possible by the removal of those portions which are of no nutritive value. No one eats the husks of corn, the shells of nuts, the gristle of meat, or similar substances, because experience has shown that they are of little or of no nutritive value and that their digestion is practically impossible. Such extraneous matters, therefore, are removed, and the food is further prepared, provided this preparation be necessary, by the process of cooking. In the form, then, in which the food is taken in it is as fully prepared as it can be outside the body. Whatever remains to be done in order that the food may be prepared for absorption must be effected after it enters the alimentary canal.

Some of the ingredients of human food are already in a diffusible form—that is, in a condition to be absorbed by the blood-vessels of the alimentary canal—and therefore they need to undergo no change. Such ingredients are water, salts, and dextrose, and were they the only constituents of the food, no digestive organs would be needed; but, as already seen, this is not the fact. The greater part of the food is in a non-diffusible form, and must be converted into a diffusible form before it can be absorbed. The first step in this conversion is that which takes place in the mouth.

A. Mouth Digestion.

When food enters the mouth it consists of a mixture of various food-stuffs. In order that the changes which these food-stuffs undergo may be traced thoroughly, let it be supposed that representatives of all classes of food-stuffs are present—namely, (1) *inorganic*, salts and water; (2) *carbohydrates*, starch and sugar; (3) *fats*, or oils; and (4) *proteids*.

The water and salts are absorbed directly by the blood, for the most part from the stomach, although there is doubtless some absorption in the mouth. If the food remained in the mouth a longer time than it usually does, more of these ingredients would there be absorbed, but the duration of time is so short that the amount absorbed cannot be very great. All the food of a fluid nature, no matter what classes of food-stuffs it comprises, passes immediately from the mouth into the pharynx, and thence through the œsophagus into the stomach. Such food undergoes no chemical changes whatever during this time; thus, milk, chocolate, and beverages of various kinds are unchanged in this part of digestion. If, however, fluids be taken into the mouth when it contains solid food, the latter will be softened by them, and the two will be mixed, and will come under the influence of the agents concerned in carrying on mouth digestion. These agents are the teeth and the salivary glands.

Mastication.—The chewing of the food, or mastication, is performed by the teeth, of which there are two sets. The first set of teeth, which are known as "temporary," "deciduous," or "milk-teeth," and which exist during early childhood, are twenty in number, and the second or permanent set, which begin to take the place of the first set at about the sixth year of life, remain to a greater or lesser extent until old age. The latter set is composed of thirty-two teeth—four incisors, two canines, four bicuspids, and six molars—in each jaw. The incisors, or cutting teeth, are adapted to bite the food; the molar teeth, or grinders, are adapted to grind the food, while the canines and bicuspids in man aid the incisors and molars. In the carnivora, the canines—or "tushes" as they are called—are very long and pointed, and are admirably adapted to pierce the body of their prey, even to the vitals, thus killing and subsequently tearing the animal preparatory to feeding upon it. The herbivora need no such aggressive weapons, and in them the molars are so constructed as to grind the food, their teeth resembling the grindstones of the miller. The teeth of man have characters which resemble those of both carnivora and herbivora, and from this fact it may be inferred that it was designed that man should have a mixed diet.

The function of the teeth in man is to thoroughly subdivide and comminute the food; and this function is an essential part of the process of digestion. As will be seen later, during digestion certain fluids are poured into the alimentary canal to contribute their part toward the process. These fluids cannot act properly on large, compact masses of food. While their action is not entirely that of solution, still, in order to fulfil perfectly their office they must come in direct contact with every portion of the food. This contact is the more essential because the given time in which to act is not unlimited, and if the process be not completed within the allotted time, digestion will be performed incompletely. When the chemist desires to dissolve a substance quickly and completely, he first thoroughly pulverizes it in a mortar. Likewise, in digestion one of the most important steps is this process of comminution or mastication. If mastication be insufficiently performed, the succeeding steps in the process of digestion are seriously interfered with, and indigestion or dyspepsia results.

Insufficient mastication is one of the commonest causes of indigestion, and many dyspeptics are drugged with remedies prescribed to overcome some fancied trouble in the stomach when they should be sent to a dentist. Defective mastication may be due to various causes. The teeth may be so decayed as to expose sensitive surfaces, and when food which is at all hard is taken into the mouth, the discomfort, or sometimes the pain, caused their possessor in chewing it makes the performance of the act incomplete, and the food is swallowed half masticated; or the eater may be in too great a hurry and not give enough time to this important act. Whatever the cause, the result is the same; therefore too much attention cannot be given to this process, which is so simple as often to be overlooked.

Insalivation.—Coincident with mastication is the act of insalivation or the incorporation of saliva with the food. Saliva is the secretion of the salivary glands (Fig. 6), which comprise the parotid, submaxillary, and sublingual; and their products, together with that of the mucous glands of the mouth, form the saliva. The salivary glands are known as "compound racemose;" they are made of lobes, and these, again, of lobules which end in alveoli. These glands are of two kinds: one is called "mucous," because its cells secrete a fluid of which *mucin* is a constituent, and the other is called "serous," because the product of its cells is more watery in its nature, or is called "albuminous," because it contains *serum-albumin*. The sublingual gland is of the mucous kind, the parotid gland is of the albuminous, while the submaxillary gland is of a mixed character, its secretion being both mucous and serous, the alveoli of the serous kind being more numerous. The mucous glands of the mouth—"buccal," as they are

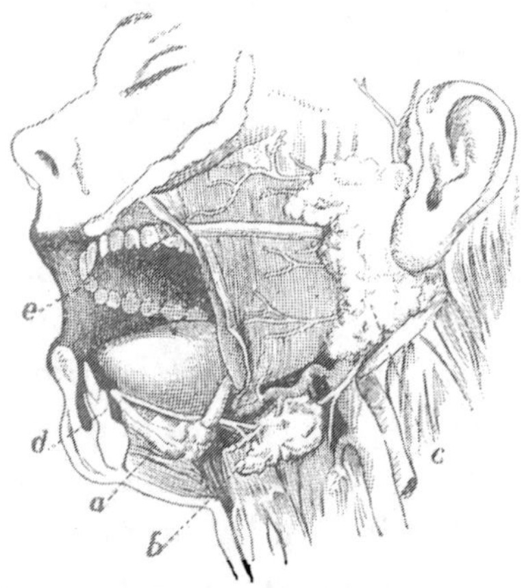

FIG. 6.—Dissection of the Side of the Face, showing the salivary glands (after Yeo): *a*, sublingual gland; *b*, submaxillary gland, with its duct opening on the floor of the mouth beneath the tongue at *d*; *c*, parotid gland and its duct, which opens on the inner side of the cheek.

called—secrete mucus only, their office being to moisten the mouth when mastication is not going on. Mucus from the buccal glands mixes also with the products of the salivary glands.

Saliva is an alkaline fluid with a specific gravity of 1004, and is secreted to the amount of 1½ litres daily. It is occasionally acid a few hours after a meal, and may be slightly acid between midnight and morning. The greatest acidity is observed two or three hours after breakfast and four or five hours after dinner. Saliva is composed of 99.5 per cent. of water and 0.05 per cent. of solids. Of the solids, one-half is inorganic, the salts being principally sodium chloride, calcium carbonate, and calcium phosphate. It is these latter two salts which accumulate on the teeth, forming the "tartar." They likewise occasionally form "salivary calculi" in the interior of the salivary glands or their ducts, and require removal by the surgeon. Another salt—which, however, is not invariably present in the saliva—is potassium sulphocyanide, which has, so far as known, no physiological importance. The remaining constituents of the saliva are mucin, serum-albumin, serum-globulin, ptyalin, and some carbon dioxide in solution. Examined under the microscope, there are seen epithelial scales from the mucous membrane of the mouth, and leucocytes, probably from the tonsils and elsewhere, described usually as "salivary corpuscles." Bacteria and portions of food are commonly found in saliva, but they are not constituent parts, but rather impurities.

Office of Saliva.—The office of saliva is twofold: (1) chemical; and (2) mechanical.

The Chemical Action of Human Saliva is due to the enzyme ptyalin, which has already been described. This enzyme is found in the parotid gland of new-born children, but not in the submaxillary gland, and it is not found as an ingredient of the saliva of animals other than man. It will be recalled that ptyalin has the power of changing hydrated starch into dextrin and maltose. If the action of the ptyalin be long continued, some of the maltose becomes dextrose; but as the time required to accomplish this change is longer than the ptyalin continues to act during ordinary digestion, this change probably takes place only occasionally. Ptyalin has no action on raw starch. It will be seen, therefore, that the contribution which the chemical action of saliva makes to the process of digestion is not very great, and yet it is not wholly to be ignored.

Mechanical Office of Saliva.—The principal office of saliva is undoubtedly mechanical. While the teeth are thoroughly comminuting the food, they are at the same time working saliva into the interstices which they make between the particles of the food. This process not only facilitates the chemical action of the ptyalin, but it tends also to keep the particles separated, so that when the food reaches the stomach the gastric juice may the more readily permeate it and produce its characteristic action. Saliva aids also in softening the food, thus enabling the process of deglutition, or swallowing, more easily to be performed. The secretion of the mucous glands of the mouth is of special importance in this act, the consistency of the mucus secreted being "ropy" and possessing great lubricating properties. Saliva is intimately connected with the sense of taste. Only soluble substances are sapid; that is, excite the sense of taste. Insoluble substances have no taste. It is for this reason, among others, that calomel is such an excellent cathartic for children;

being insoluble, it is tasteless, and they readily swallow it. Soluble substances not already in a state of solution are dissolved by the saliva, and in this condition excite the sense of taste. When in a febrile or other state, in which the secretion of saliva is greatly diminished, deglutition is difficult and the sense of taste is markedly deteriorated.

A portion of the food having been thoroughly masticated and insalivated, it is collected by the tongue and cheeks into a small mass known as the "alimentary bolus," which now undergoes the process of deglutition.

Deglutition, or the act of swallowing, consists in the passage of the food from the mouth, through the pharynx and œsophagus (Fig. 7) to the stomach. Deglutition is divided into three stages or steps. In the first stage the alimentary bolus is carried by the tongue back into the pharynx; as the bolus passes over the soft palate it receives a coating of the very viscid secretion of the mucous glands, which are here situated. This first step is purely voluntary, entirely under the control of the will, and may be performed or not as desired. After the bolus, however, reaches the pharynx, it passes from the control of the will. If one were informed at this stage of the act that the bolus contained the most virulent poison, it could not be rejected, but he would be compelled to swallow it. In this, the second stage, the bolus passes through the pharynx, under the

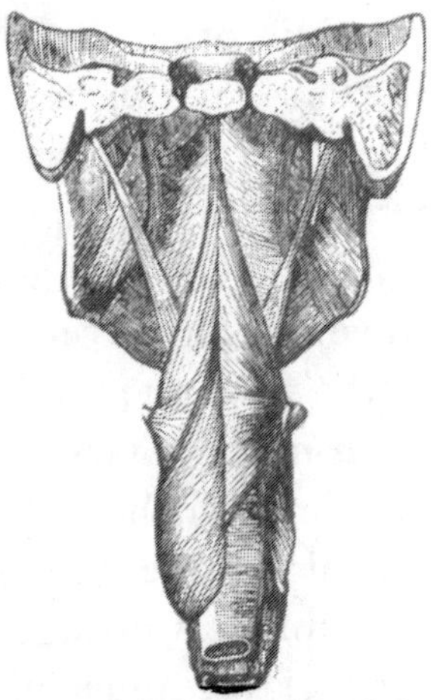

FIG. 7.—Muscular Coat of the Pharynx and Œsophagus.

influence of the constrictor muscles, into the œsophagus. The tongue is drawn backward, the isthmus of the fauces is contracted, and the soft palate, the larynx, and the pharynx are elevated, so that the entrance of food into either the posterior nares or the larynx is prevented; the constrictor muscles then contracting, the food is carried through the pharynx into the œsophagus.

It was formerly thought that the function of the epiglottis was to prevent the entrance of food into the larynx, and its relations would seem to justify such a view, but observation shows that this view is not true. In the first place, this organ is present only in mammals, and is absent in other vertebrates, although the process of deglutition is performed as well in the former as in the latter. Then, too, a dog whose epiglottis has been excised experiences no difficulty in swallowing either solids or liquids. The elevation of the larynx and the backward drawing of the tongue are alone sufficient to protect the glottis from the entrance of food.

From the pharynx the food passes into the œsophagus, and through the latter into the stomach; this constitutes the third stage, which is also involuntary in its character, and which is brought about by the successive contractions of the muscular coat of the œsophagus. In the act of rumination, which is characteristic of the ruminants, and in vomiting, there is a reversal of this action, so that the contents of the stomach are carried to the pharynx.

In deglutition the food does not pass through the œsophagus by virtue of the force of gravity. This is shown by the fact that deglutition may be performed as successfully when an individual is standing on his head as when he is on his feet, and many animals, such as the horse and dog, always perform the act in opposition to gravity. This act is brought about by a series of muscular contractions which begin in the mouth and end at the stomach. During deglutition the ptyalin continues its action on the starch; other than this action no chemical change takes place in the food while it is passing through the œsophagus. The mucous membrane of this canal furnishes a mucus which has no digestive action, but is simply a lubricant.

B. Stomach Digestion.

The food, having reached the stomach, now undergoes stomach or gastric digestion. The stomach in the human adult is about 35 centimetres in length and 12 in width, and when distended it may contain 3 litres.

Coats of the Stomach.—The stomach is composed of four coats: serous, muscular, submucous, and mucous. The serous coat is a reflection of the peritoneum. The submucous coat, which contains the nerves and blood-vessels, is of special interest as giving to the mucous coat great mobility and as permitting it to form folds, called "rugæ," when the cavity is empty. This structure is in striking contrast with the anatomical structure of the uterus, in which organ, the submucous coat being absent and the mucous lying directly upon the muscular coat, there is a total want of mobility in the membrane. Aside from this statement neither the serous nor the submucous coat has any special physiological interest. The muscular coat is composed of three layers: longitudinal, circular, and oblique. The *longitudinal* layer is made up of fibres continuous with similar fibres of the œsophagus, and is most external—that is, immediately beneath the peritoneum. These fibres radiate from the œsophageal or cardiac orifice, and are especially abundant in the region of the greater and lesser curvatures. They extend to the intestine, where they form a layer of the muscular coat of that organ. The *circular* layer is situated internal to the longitudinal, and, as the name implies, its fibres encircle the stomach—that is, are in general at right angles to the longitudinal axis of the stomach. At the pyloric orifice of the stomach, where the duodenum begins, these circular fibres are aggregated in such number as to receive the name of "pyloric muscle." Their projection into the interior of the organ at this location with its covering of mucous membrane constitutes the pyloric valve. The oblique layer is found especially at the cardiac extremity of the stomach.

The mucous coat, or mucous membrane, is soft and velvety. Near the cardiac orifice the membrane is about 1½ millimetres in thickness, and near the pylorus 2 millimetres, while in general between these two points its thickness is about 1 millimetre. Its surface is composed of columnar epithelium, which secretes the mucus found in the stomach in the intervals of digestion, this mucus being a constituent of the gastric juice.

In the mucous membrane, and forming a part of it, are two sets of glands, the "pyloric" glands, so called from their abundance in the pyloric portion of the stomach, and the "cardiac" glands (Fig. 8), which are so called because of their occurrence in the cardiac region. The ducts of both sets are lined by columnar epithelium continuous with that covering the mucous membrane. In the tubes of the pyloric glands are granular cells called "chief cells." The same kind of cells is found in the tubes of the cardiac glands, and beneath these cells —that is, between them and the basement membrane—are, besides, larger cells, which are ovoid in shape and which

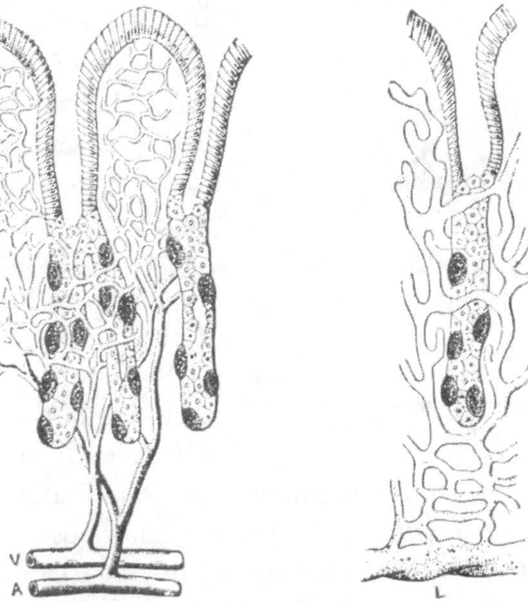

FIG. 8.—Cardiac Glands.

Diagram showing the Relation of the Ultimate Twigs of the Blood-vessels, *V* and *A*, and of the absorbent radicals, *L*, to the glands of the stomach, and the different kinds of epithelium—namely, above, cylindrical cells; small pale cells in the lumen, outside which are the dark ovoid cells.

are known as "parietal cells." These cells cause the basement membrane against which they lie to bulge out. The chief cells are regarded as producing the pepsinogen which is converted into the pepsin of the gastric juice, and the parietal cells as producing the hydrochloric acid. The vascularity of the stomach is very great. In the intervals of digestion the mucous membrane is of a pale pinkish color, while during active digestion its color is a bright red. This change in color is due to the greatly increased amount of blood present in the blood-vessels of the organ at this time.

Prior to 1822 the process of stomach digestion was little understood. During that year Alexis St. Martin, a Canadian boatman, was so injured by the accidental discharge of a gun that when the wound healed there remained in his side a permanent opening (nearly 2½ centimetres in diameter), which communicated with the cavity of the stomach (Fig. 9). Dr. Beaumont, the surgeon in charge of the case, and subsequently others, carried on a series of experiments and observations extending through years, and the present knowledge of stomach digestion is largely based upon this remarkable case.

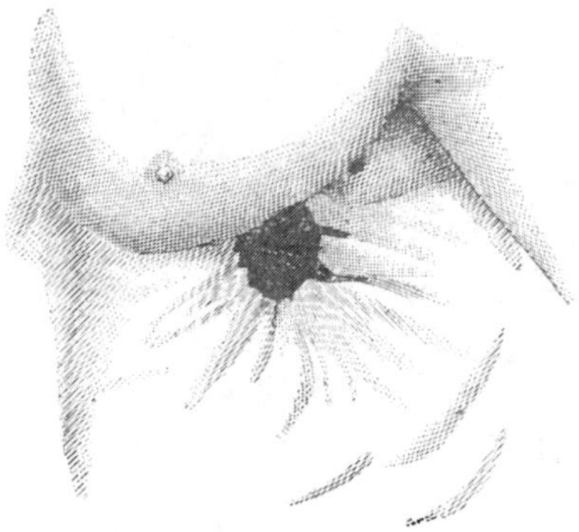

FIG. 9.—Left Breast and Side (erect position), showing perforation of the walls of the stomach of Alexis St. Martin.

During the intervals of digestion the mucous membrane of the stomach is pale in color, and is covered with a transparent and viscid mucus which is neutral or alkaline in reaction. This mucus is the product of the epithelium of the mucous membrane. After food has entered the stomach drops of gastric juice appear at the mouths of the glands.

Quantity of Gastric Juice.—The amount of gastric juice daily secreted is difficult of determination, and it is not surprising that authorities should differ so much on this point. Dr. Beaumont estimated it to be 180 grammes in the case of St. Martin, while others place it as high as 7 litres, or one-tenth of the weight of the body. The gastric juice is never in large quantity in the stomach at any one time. It is secreted gradually by the glands, is poured out into the cavity of the stomach, where it permeates the food, is passed on into the small intestine, where it is absorbed by the blood-vessels, and is then returned to the circulation, from which its constituents were derived. It has the following properties: it is clear, slightly yellowish in color, and strongly acid. Its specific gravity is from 1001 to 1010.

Composition of Human Gastric Juice mixed with Saliva.—As can readily be understood, it is impossible to obtain gastric juice unmixed with particles of food or saliva or other foreign substances, hence an accurate analysis cannot be given. The analysis of Schmidt of gastric juice from a women having a gastric fistula is as follows:

	Percentages.
Water	99.4400
Organic substances (pepsin, peptones, and rennin)	.3195
Free hydrochloric acid	.0200
Calcium chloride	.0061
Sodium "	.1464
Potassium "	.0550
Calcium, Magnesium, Ferrum } phosphates.	.0125
Loss	.0005
	100.0000

The constituents of the gastric juice of any special physiological interest are hydrochloric acid, pepsin, and rennin. It was at one time a matter of dispute whether the acidity of this fluid was due to hydrochloric or to lactic acid, but there is now a unanimity of opinion that it is the former. If lactic acid be present, it is probably due to lactic fermentation which has taken place in the carbohydrates of the food when these are in excess. This fermentation may go on to the formation of acetic and butyric acids, these changes being doubtless due to the presence of micro-organisms.

Hydrochloric Acid.—The amount of free hydrochloric acid in human gastric juice varies from 0.05 to 0.3 per cent. Several of the best authorities give the average as between 0.2 and 0.3 per cent.

Pepsin.—The "chief" cells of both the cardiac and the pyloric glands, during the intervals of digestion, produce the zymogen *pepsinogen*, which has no digestive action upon proteids. The parietal cells produce hydrochloric acid, the action of which upon the pepsinogen converts the latter into pepsin. This acid is formed from the chlorides which are brought to the glands by the blood. The action of pepsin upon proteids in presence of hydrochloric acid has already been studied. To recapitulate: The proteid is first converted into acid-albumin, or syntonin (some authorities, it will be remembered, limit the term "syntonin" to that particular acid-albumin which is produced from myosin), which passes into albumose, and this into peptone or peptone with some albumose.

Rennin.—There is in human gastric juice another enzyme, *rennin*, which is produced from renninogen, a zymogen which, like pepsinogen, is the product of the "chief" cells of the gastric glands. It is interesting to note in this connection that some observers have found that this enzyme was absent from the gastric juice in carcinoma of the stomach, atrophy of its mucous membrane, and in some cases of gastric catarrh. It will be remembered that rennin coagulates the casein of milk. In the gastric digestion of this important food the coagulation of the casein is a preliminary step. Mothers are sometimes frightened when their children, seemingly in perfect health, vomit curdled milk, but this curdling of milk is a normal process, and the only abnormality consists in its regurgitation, which is usually due to over-feeding.

As matter of secondary interest there is some evidence that in gastric juice there is a lactic-acid ferment which changes the lactose of milk into lactic acid; another ferment which converts cane-sugar into glucose; and still another, a fat-splitting one, which breaks up fats into glycerin and fatty acids, but the amount of these materials changed in the stomach is not very great. Gastric juice does not change starch.

The albuminoids are, some of them, as has been seen, converted into peptones, but they have little nutritive value. The one which is more than any other looked upon as contributing to nutrition is gelatin. But gelatin is not available directly for the growth and repair of tissues. It has an "albumin-sparing" action. Much less flesh is required by an animal if fat be taken with the flesh, this being spoken of as the "albumin-sparing" action of fat. The same is true of gelatin. Gelatin forms urea, and when present in the food in large amount the kidneys are excited to increased action.

Chyme.—The mixture of food and gastric juice is called "chyme." Chyme is not a mixture having a constant composition: it varies according to the articles of food ingested.

There are, in addition to the presence of pepsin and hydrochloric acid, two other requisites for normal digestion. The temperature must be favorable, and this is found in the stomach where the thermometer indicates 38° C;

the other requisite is the muscular movements of the stomach.

Muscular Movements of Stomach.—In the empty condition of the stomach the direction of the greater curvature is downward and that of the lesser curvature upward; but as food enters and begins to fill this organ, it rises upward in such a manner that when filled the greater curvature is forward and the lesser curvature backward. From the time that food enters the cavity of the stomach until it has all passed out the muscular coat of the stomach is in action. The walls are in contact except where separated by food, and are constantly rubbing against each other, or against that which separates them, with a rotatory motion. The masses of food are by this means broken up and the gastric juice is incorporated with them. In the stomach of the cow it is not unusual to find balls of considerable size, made up of hair which the animal has licked from her hide and swallowed. These balls are perfectly spherical, and are undoubtedly formed by this rotatory or churning motion of the muscular coats of the stomach. There is, besides this, a movement which carries the food toward the pyloric orifice, and which is known as "vermicular" or "peristaltic." If any portion of the food as it reaches this part of the stomach be sufficiently liquid, the pyloric muscle relaxes and permits it to pass through into the duodenum; otherwise it is carried back, and is again brought under the influence of the rotatory movements of the stomach. While during the greater part of stomach digestion the pyloric muscle keeps the pylorus closed, only relaxing to permit the prepared material to pass, at the close of the act it remains so relaxed that solid particles can pass into the duodenum without difficulty.

Self-digestion of Stomach.—One of the interesting and still unexplained physiological enigmas is: Why does not the stomach, which is proteid in its nature, undergo self-digestion during life? It is known that when death takes place during the period of active stomach digestion erosion of the mucous membrane, and even perforation of the wall of the stomach, may occur. As this takes place at the most dependent portion, where the gastric juice naturally gravitates, the explanation is simple. But if this self-digestion can occur after death, why not during life? No satisfactory answer to this question has yet been given, although many theories have been advanced.

Results of Stomach Digestion.—The following, then, are the results of stomach digestion: The proteids are converted into peptones; in the case of milk the proteid casein is first coagulated, and then changed into peptone. Starch is not changed by the gastric juice, though the action of the ptyalin, which commenced in the mouth and was continued in the œsophagus, does not cease in the stomach until the food becomes so acid as to prevent the further action of the enzyme. Some of the carbohydrates may, as has been seen, undergo the lactic fermentation.

If fat be present in the food in the free state, as in oil, it is made more fluid by the heat of the stomach; if it be in the form of adipose tissue, in which the fat is enclosed in sacs, forming the adipose vesicles, these sacs, being proteid in their nature, are acted upon by the gastric juice as are other proteids, and the fat is set free, when it is acted upon in the same manner as the free fat just referred to. Some of the fat may be split up into glycerin and fatty acids, but the greater part passes on into the duodenum.

The stomach contains gases which in the dog have been found to be nitrogen, oxygen, and carbon dioxide. The hydrochloric acid that is normally present in gastric juice prevents the formation of gases from fermentative changes in the food. The stomach-gases are attributable to the air incorporated with the food in the mouth, and to the saliva, in which, as we have seen, carbon dioxide exists in solution. It is also probable that there is some escape of gases from the intestine into the stomach.

Duration of Stomach Digestion.—The duration of stomach digestion is variable, and depends upon several circumstances, among which is the composition of the stomach-contents. Some kinds of food remain in the stomach longer than others. Stomach digestion may in general be said to be from one and a half to five and a half hours, according to the nature of the food. The following table contains a list of some of the substances with which Dr. Beaumont experimented, and the length of time they remained in the stomach:

Kind of Food.	Time.
Pig's feet and tripe	1 hour.
Salmon	1 "
Milk	2 hours.
Potatoes, roasted	2 "
Roast turkey	2½ "
Soft-boiled eggs	2½ "
Beefsteak, broiled	2½ "
Hard-boiled eggs	3 "
Potatoes, boiled	3½ "
Pork, boiled	4½ "
" roast	5¼ "

The above table, and others of like nature, are to be very cautiously made use of in determining the digestibility of the different foods. The observations here recorded simply indicate the length of time the respective articles remained in the stomach, and nothing more. Substances are *digested* when they are in condition to be absorbed, and not until then. Whenever any portion of the food is rendered sufficiently liquid, it is liable to pass out from the stomach, although there are other factors than this liquid character of the food. If two different articles of food were in the stomach at the same time, one might pass out from that organ into the small intestine in one hour, while the other might remain in the stomach two hours. From this fact alone one would not be justified in assuming that the one substance was twice as digestible as the other, for the former might not at the time it left the stomach have been prepared for absorption, but might require several hours for such a change after it reached the small intestine; while the latter, although it remained in the stomach an hour after the former had left it, might at the time it left the stomach have been in a condition to pass at once into the blood.

The practical use of tables showing the length of time that different substances remain in the stomach seems to be to determine of what the food should consist when this organ is unable to perform its function in a normal manner and it is considered wise to lighten its labors as much as possible. For this purpose such food should be selected as will remain in the stomach but a short time, even though it pass out in an undigested state, for, as will hereafter be seen, the peptonizing function is as well carried on in the small intestine as in the stomach, and in a disabled condition of the latter organ the former will supplement it. In the dog so thoroughly may digestion be performed by the intestines alone, without the aid of the stomach, that this latter organ has been almost completely removed, yet the animal has been kept alive in excellent health and strength. The proper foods under these circumstances are those that are liquid when ingested or are readily liquefied in the stomach.

As above stated, the length of time that food remains in the stomach is not determined by its consistency alone. One of the important factors is the amount of hydrochloric acid present; thus when this acid is relatively great it seems to act as an irritant, and the pyloric muscle relaxes more readily than when the amount is less.

Some light has been thrown on this question of the duration of stomach digestion by the application of methods of obtaining and examining the contents of the stomach for diagnostic purposes. To ascertain how far the digestive process is interfered with, "trial" meals are given. The stomach is evacuated by means of a soft-rubber stomach-pipe after a proper time, and inspection shows how far the process of digestion has advanced. Ewald's "trial" meal consists of one water-roll weighing 35 grammes and a cup of tea or 300 or 400 cc. of water. After this food has been two and a half hours in the stomach that organ will be found empty; in one case the food had disappeared after one hour. Riegel's "trial" meal consists of a cup of broth, 400 grammes; beef, 60 grammes; and bread, 50 grammes. After seven hours the stomach will be found empty.

Artificial Gastric Juice.—In addition to the observations of Beaumont and others upon cases of gastric fistula, many experiments have been made with an artificial gastric juice made by extracting the pepsin from the mucous membrane of the stomach of the pig with glycerin, and adding to this glycerin-extract 0.2 per cent. of hydrochloric acid. The results of these experiments are, however, not to be regarded as identical with those that take place in the stomach of a living human being. The factors in the problem are many, and some of them are still undetermined, as, for instance, the action of the gastric juice on the different proteids.

Effects of Alcohol on Digestion.—Much has been written on the effects of alcoholic and other beverages upon digestion, and the testimony is very conflicting. Thus one authority states that the action of pepsin is retarded temporarily by the presence of alcohol, but after the latter is absorbed, which occurs very rapidly, there is an increased flow of very active gastric juice; another says that alcohol retards, and even prevents, digestion; while a third maintains that it aids digestion from the beginning of its entrance into the stomach. The fact probably is that in each of these opinions there is some truth, and that the effects of alcohol vary according to the conditions present. The first principle which may be laid down is that alcohol, under ordinary circumstances, is not needed to aid digestion, but it is to be regarded as an agent which, under the direction of the physician, may be employed to assist him in the treatment of diseased conditions. About 95 per cent. of the alcohol taken into the body is oxidized, carbon-dioxide and water resulting. To this extent it serves to produce heat, and whenever, therefore, the supply of food is insufficient, alcohol is of value in preventing so far as possible the using up of the tissues of the body. The above statement is true if an amount not exceeding two ounces be taken daily, but when an abundance of food can be obtained the use of alcohol offers no advantages. Alcohol in small doses excites the nervous system, and if this stimulation be kept up harm must result, for after the stimulation there is a depressing reaction. The action of alcohol on the vascular system is to excite the latter and to increase the circulation of the blood; thus in a given time both nerves and muscles are supplied with more blood. It is this action which produces the sense of warmth when alcohol has been taken, but this warmth is purely subjective, the thermometer showing that alcohol, even in moderate amount, actually lowers the temperature. The blood-vessels of the skin dilate under the influence of alcohol, and there is a loss of heat by radiation from the blood. The pulse is smaller and is increased in rate, while its strength is diminished, showing action upon the heart. One who has made a special study of the action of alcohol upon the nervous system says that it seems to induce progressive paralysis, the judgment being affected first, although the imagination and emotions may be more than usually active; the motor centres and speech are next affected, then the cerebellum, then the spinal cord; and finally, if the quantity taken be large, death may result.

An instructive lesson may be obtained by observing the effect of alcohol upon animal tissues immersed in it. It is known that such tissues are dried up and shrivelled; in the same way, although to a very much less degree, the proteids of the cells of the mucous membrane are affected in the form of coagulation when alcohol is taken into the empty stomach in concentration, as in whiskey or in brandy. When diluted the action of alcohol is less pronounced. When the stomach contains food the liability of injury is less, as then the alcohol is diluted by the liquids, and, if there be proteids in the food, some of these are coagulated, the mucous membrane thus being doubly protected. The frequent imbibing of spirituous liquors on an empty stomach, as practised by so many, is the most injurious form of alcohol-taking. Not only are the nervous and vascular systems affected, but a catarrhal condition of the digestive organs is also produced. If the alcohol contain impurities, such as fusel oil, its action is still more harmful.

Before leaving the process of stomach digestion it may be well to call attention to the fact that the hydrochloric acid of the gastric juice has a germicide action on some of the pathogenic bacteria. This action, on the one hand, is not true of all pathogenic bacteria, for those which produce tuberculosis and anthrax are not destroyed by gastric juice; on the other hand, the cholera spirillum, the germ of Asiatic cholera, is destroyed in normal gastric juice. Experiments have demonstrated this fact, and also that if a solution of soda be injected into the stomach, the vitality of this micro-organism is not destroyed. It is therefore of the utmost importance, during the prevalence of cholera, to keep the digestive organs in normal condition. Anything which tends to produce a catarrhal condition of the stomach, as alcohol in excess, will be likely to increase the alkaline mucus, and thus make the conditions favorable should the spirilla find their way into the stomach in solid or in liquid food. It is probably by interfering with normal digestion, inhibiting the production of hydrochloric acid, that fear conduces toward the spread of this disease. Dr. Beaumont in the case of St. Martin observed that when his temper was irritated the secretion of gastric juice was greatly interfered with or even suspended. Unusual fatigue and a condition of fever would produce the same results. It is a matter of common experience that fear, worry, anger, the receipt of unexpected news, either joyous or sorrowful, will oftentimes seriously interrupt gastric digestion. Therefore at all times the endeavor should be to keep the mind, during the period of digestion at least, free from these disturbing agencies.

The acidity of gastric juice, even in comparative health, is not always the same: it may be in excess or it may be deficient. In the latter condition, the antifermentative action of the acid being diminished, there occurs fermentation of the carbohydrates, and lactic, acetic, and butyric acids appear, together with hydrogen and other gases. These acids and gases give rise to heartburn, waterbrash, and other conditions indicative of disordered digestion.

C. Intestinal Digestion.

The small intestine, in which intestinal digestion takes place, is about 22 feet long, extending from the stomach to the ileo-cæcal valve, where it passes into the large intestine.

Coats of the Intestine.—Like the stomach, the small intestine is composed of four coats: 1, serous; 2, muscular; 3, submucous; 4, mucous. It is divided into three portions: (*a*), duodenum; (*b*), jejunum; (*c*), ileum. As in the stomach, the two coats which have physiological interest are the *muscular* and the *mucous*. The muscular coat is made up of two layers: an external or longitudinal and an inner or circular.

Valvulæ Conniventes.—The mucous coat of the intestine is covered by a single layer of columnar epithelium. It is arranged in folds to which the name "valvulæ conniventes" has been given (Fig. 10). These folds, which begin about 2 centimetres below the pylorus, are present throughout the length of the small intestine, excepting in the lower part of the ileum. They are more abundant in the upper half of the intestine, where they have been counted to the number of six hundred, than in the lower half, where only two hundred and fifty have been found. These folds are arranged around the interior of the intestine at right angles to its long axis. They do not completely encircle it like a ring, but vary in length, some extending two-thirds and others only one-third the distance around. The widest of them is not more than half an inch in width, projecting into the calibre of the intestine to this extent. Each fold is mucous membrane, and between these reduplications of mucous membrane is connective tissue, which so binds the folds together that even in the condition of distention the valvulæ conniventes are not obliterated, as is the case with the rugæ of the stomach. By means of these foldings the extent of the mucous membrane is greatly increased over what it would be did it simply line the intestine.

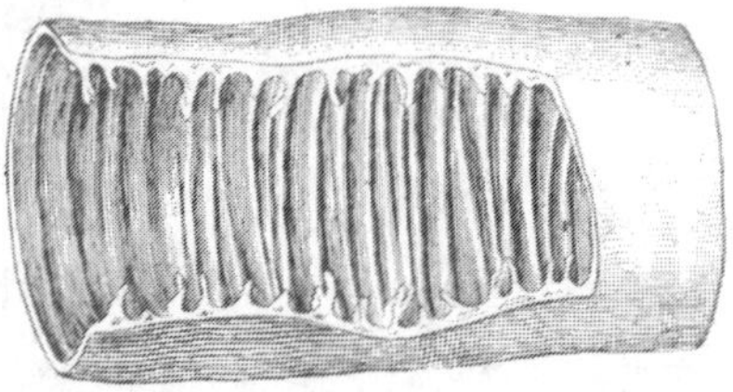

FIG. 10.—Portion of the Wall of the Small Intestine, laid open to show the valvulæ conniventes (Brinton).

Villi.—Projecting from the mucous membrane including the valvulæ conniventes are the "villi" (Fig. 11), which are so numerous as to give to it a velvety appearance. These villi are prominences, some triangular, some conical, and some filiform in shape, and in length are about 1 mm., and in width at their base about one-fourth their length. They are most numerous in the duodenum and the jejunum, although present throughout the whole extent of the small intestine. It has been estimated that there are no less than five millions of these villi in an intestine. They are intimately connected with the process of absorption, and their further description will therefore be deferred until that subject is discussed.

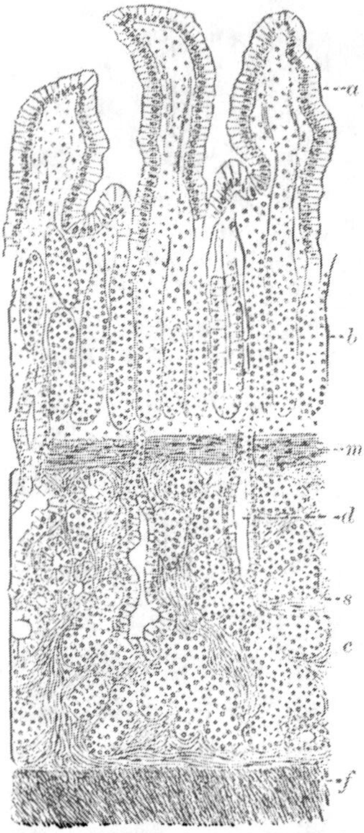

FIG. 11.—Vertical Section of Duodenum, showing villi (*a*); crypts of Lieberkühn (*b*), and Brunner's glands (*c*) in the submucosa (*s*), with ducts (*d*); muscularis mucosæ (*m*), and circular muscular coat (*f*), (Schofield).

Brunner's Glands.—In the submucous coat of the upper part of the duodenum, and, to a less extent, in that of the lower part and in the beginning of the jejunum, are certain glands known as the "glands of Brunner," or the duodenal glands. These are racemose glands, similar to those in the œsophagus and also to the lobules of a salivary gland. They discharge through ducts which open upon the surface of the mucous membrane of the intestine. Their secretion is mucus having a slightly alkaline reaction, but it has never been successfully obtained so pure as to admit of its being analyzed. These glands are so few in number, comparatively, that their product cannot be very abundant nor very important in its action upon the food, although a ferment has been described as one of its constituents which has the power of converting maltose into glucose. The secretion of these glands, together with that of the follicles of Lieberkühn, constitutes the intestinal juice. These glands are inflamed and ulcerate whenever the body is burned to any great extent.

Follicles of Lieberkühn.—The follicles or crypts of Lieberkühn, which are found throughout the entire length of the small intestine, are tubular glands in the mucous membrane, and not beneath it, as is the case with the glands of Brunner. Their lining is a layer of columnar epithelium. Besides these tubular glands there are solitary glands scattered throughout the mucous membrane of the intestine, and agminated glands, commonly known as "Peyer's patches," which number about twenty-five, and which are most numerous in the ileum. These glands have no excretory ducts, but they produce a secretion which probably oozes through the walls of the glands and contributes something to the intestinal juice. In typhoid fever Peyer's patches become inflamed and often undergo ulceration.

Intestinal Juice.—The intestinal juice, "succus entericus," is the product of all the glands, but the follicles of Lieberkühn, being vastly more numerous, contribute by far the greater part of this fluid. It is an alkaline secretion having a specific gravity of 1010, and containing about 95 per cent. of water, salts, and at least one ferment, invertin. As to the presence of other ferments there is doubt.

Action of Intestinal Juice.—The action of intestinal juice upon the food has not been thoroughly determined.

The property which it possesses in the most marked degree is that of changing cane-sugar into invert-sugar, which, as will be remembered, is a mixture of lævulose and dextrose. This inversion is due to the ferment invertin. The intestinal juice also converts starch,

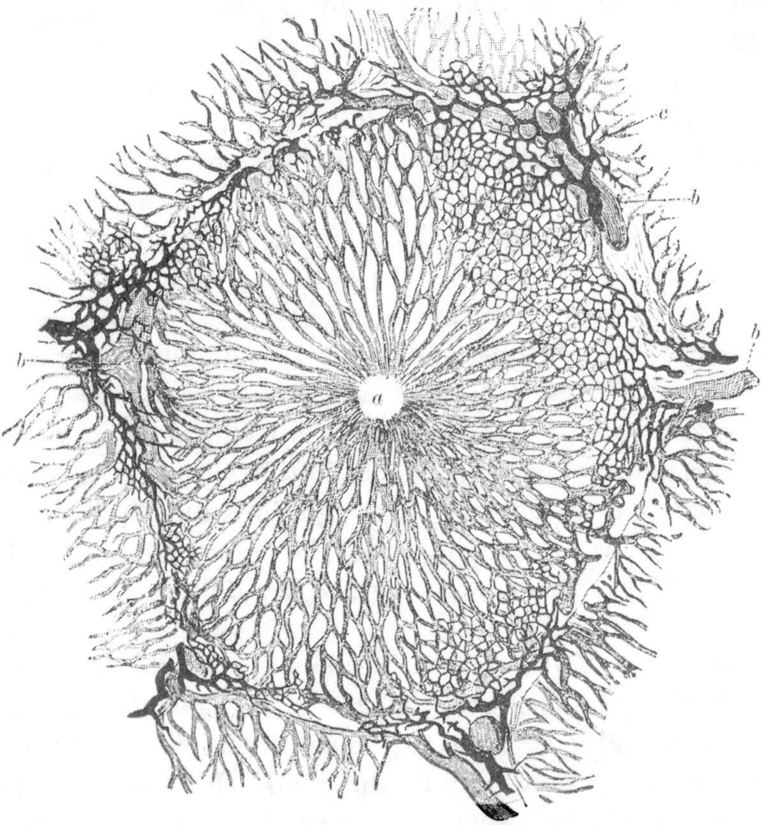

FIG. 12.—Section of Lobule of a Rabbit's Liver, in which the blood and bile-capillaries have been injected (after Cadiat): *a*, intralobular vein; *b*, interlobular veins; *c*, biliary canals beginning in fine capillaries.

both raw and cooked, into sugar. Maltose is changed into glucose, and the viscid secretion of Peyer's patches brings about the latter change very quickly. The neutral fats are not decomposed by intestinal juice, but this fluid, by virtue of its alkalinity, does emulsify them. Its action on proteids is not determined, some experimenters reporting that it possesses proteolytic powers, others denying it.

From the above considerations the intestinal juice may be regarded as possessing some digestive action upon the food-stuffs, the most marked of which action is its power of inversion. It is not an abundant secretion, and perhaps its most important office is to lubricate the mucous membrane of the small intestine.

The Bile.—The bile is one of the products of the cells

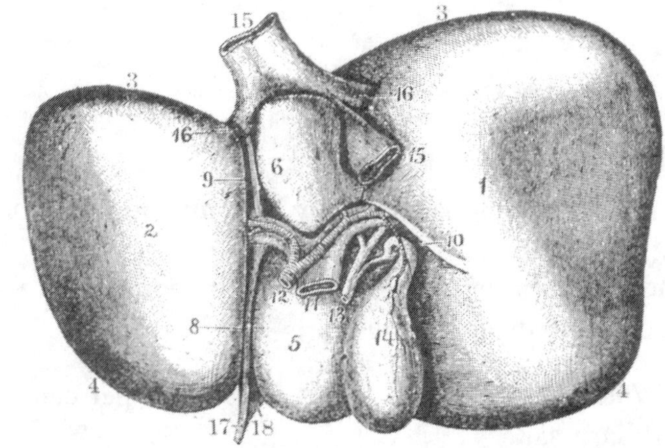

Fig. 13.—The Liver: 1, right lobe; 2, left lobe; 3, posterior border; 4, anterior border; 5, lobus quadratus; 6, lobus Spigelii; 7, lobus caudatus; 8, 9, longitudinal fissure; 10, transverse fissure; 11, portal vein; 12, hepatic artery; 13, ductus communis choledochus; 14, gall-badder fissure; 15, inferior vena cava; 16, hepatic vein; 17, round ligament; 18, suspensory or broad ligament.

of the liver, and as it is secreted it passes into the gall-bladder through the hepatic and cystic ducts, where it is stored until needed at the time of intestinal digestion. Bile when discharged from the gall-bladder is a viscid fluid, having in man a golden-brown color, a specific gravity of

1018, and an alkaline reaction. Its viscidity is due to mucus, which is not present when the bile leaves the liver, but which is added to it while it is stored in the

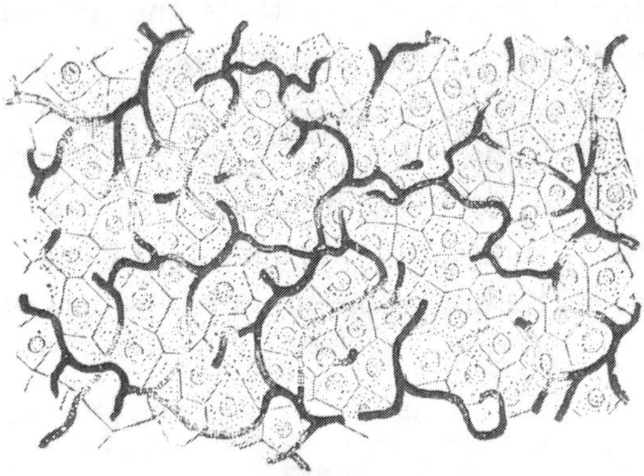

FIG. 14.—Section of the Liver of the Newt, showing the bile-ducts injected, forming a network of fine capillaries around the liver-cells, the outlines and nuclei of which can be seen.

gall-bladder, being secreted by the mucous membrane lining that organ.

The quantity of human bile daily secreted is about 1500 cc., and its composition is—

Water	86. per cent.
Biliary salts	9. "
Cholesterin	0.3 "
Mucus and coloring matters	3. "
Salts and other ingredients	1.7 "
	100.

The ingredients of the bile have already been discussed in the section treating of Physiological Chemistry, and the offices of this fluid will be considered later.

Pancreatic Juice.—The pancreatic juice is the product of the pancreas, and is discharged into the duodenum at about its middle, through the pancreatic duct—or ducts more properly, as there are usually two. One of these, the main duct, discharges by an opening common to it and the common bile-duct. During the intervals of digestion no pancreatic juice flows into the intestine, but during stomach digestion the flow begins, even before any food has passed from the stomach into the duodenum. It is a viscid fluid, alkaline in reaction, having a high specific gravity. The quantity secreted daily is variously estimated, some placing it at 150 cc., others at a much higher figure. The composition of pancreatic juice (dog) is as follows:

Water	90 per cent.
Organic matter (including albumin and ferments)	9 "
Salts (sodium carbonate, sodium chloride, potassium chloride, calcium phosphate)	1 "
	100

Pancreatic Ferments.—Special interest attaches to the pancreatic ferments, of which there are three—amylopsin, steapsin, and trypsin.

Amylopsin is a diastatic or amylolytic ferment, and is sometimes spoken of as "pancreatic diastase." It is not produced in the human subject until one month after birth. It converts both raw and cooked starch into maltose and some dextrose.

Steapsin is a lipolytic or fat-splitting ferment. The fatty acids unite with the carbonate of soda of the pancreatic juice, forming soaps, so that there is an actual process of saponification taking place in the intestines.

Trypsin is a proteolytic ferment having the power to change the proteids, which have not already been peptonized by the gastric juice, into peptone, and also of changing in the same way the acid-albumins and albumoses, the partial products of stomach digestion. Trypsinogen is first formed by the pancreas, and this is later changed into trypsin. The action of trypsin is in some respects like that of pepsin, but in other respects differs from it. Thus pepsin requires the presence of an acid reaction, while trypsin acts when the reaction is alkaline or neutral, the most energetic action being when the alkali, carbonate of soda, is present to the amount of from 0.3 to 0.4 per cent. Mineral acids prevent the action of the ferment, but lactic and other organic acids do not as seriously interfere with it. It has been noted that salicylic acid in large quantities will inhibit its action. In the process of pepsin-digestion an acid-albumin is first formed; in trypsin-digestion the first product is an alkali-albumin. By the further action of the enzyme hemi- and anti-albumose are formed, and still later hemi- and anti-peptones. To distinguish the product of the action of trypsin from that of pepsin some writers speak of the former as "tryptone." The hemi-peptones may, by the continued action of the trypsin, be decomposed into leucin and tyrosin. This power is not possessed by pepsin. It may, perhaps, be questioned whether this formation of leucin and tyrosin ordinarily takes place during pancreatic digestion, as it requires some time for its accomplishment, and the peptones may have been absorbed before this change can take place; but it undoubtedly does occur when the proteids have been taken in in excess of the demands of the body. There is doubtless a rennet-ferment in the pancreatic juice, but it probably is rarely called upon to exert its specific action, as the casein of milk is thoroughly coagulated before entering the intestine by the ferment of the gastric juice.

After the above consideration of the intestinal fluids we are in a position to understand the process of intestinal digestion as a whole. As the chyme leaves the stomach its reaction is markedly acid, and unless this acidity is overcome the ferments of the intestine, having no power in acid media, can exert no action upon the food. It is essential, therefore, that this acidity should be neutralized. The presence of the chyme in the small intestine, causes through nervous agency, the gall-bladder to empty itself of the contained bile, which is discharged through the common bile-duct into the duodenum. The action of the bile on the chyme is such as to cause the peptones and acid-albumins to be precipitated, and with them the pepsin, so that all further action of this ferment is prevented. At the time the discharge of bile takes place into the intestine the secretions of the glands, which have just been studied, are also poured out, and begin to exercise the characteristic properties already mentioned—the conversion of starch into sugar, of proteids into peptones, and the saponification of a part of the fat. In addition to this action there is an emulsification of so much of the fat as is not saponified. This does not seem to be due to any special enzyme, but is attributable to the alkalinity of the fluids and the presence of proteids and soap. If the interior of the small intestine were examined at this stage of digestion, its mucous membrane would be seen covered by a layer of material much resembling cream.

The bile, then, so far as its influence in digestion is concerned, has for its special purposes the termination of the digestion taking place in the stomach and the preparation of the food for intestinal digestion. It also stimulates the muscular coat of the small intestine to more efficient action, thus materially aiding in propelling the food along this canal, and in bringing it thereby into contact with the secretions concerned in digestion. This muscular action is of importance also in the process of absorption. Bile aids also in emulsifying the fats, although the principal factor in that process is doubtless the pancreatic juice. The absorption of the fats after being emulsified is materially aided by the bile. Some claim has been made for its antiseptic properties, but the presence of bacteria in it would seem to controvert this. It is, however, a noteworthy fact that when a biliary fistula is made, and the bile, instead of pursuing its normal route into the intestine, is withdrawn directly from the gall-bladder, the fæces become very offensive. The bile probably prevents the excessive formation of those ingredients which give the characteristic odor to the fæces, and these are produced to a greater degree when the discharge of bile into the small intestine is interfered with. The bile is also, in part, an excrementitious fluid, as is shown by the blood-poisoning which occurs when the bile is not normally formed by the liver, or when, after having been formed, it is reabsorbed.

After the bile has performed its part in the intestine it undergoes disintegration. The mucin, cholesterin, and part of the coloring matter in the form of hydrobilirubin pass off into the fæces. A part of the coloring matter is excreted in the urine as urobilin. The biliary salts are reabsorbed and enter the blood.

All the food-stuffs requiring it, excepting the fats, having been made diffusible by the various digestive processes, the process by which they are rendered available for nutrition may now be studied; that is, the process of absorption, for, as has been stated, until they reach the blood they are of no use to the economy of the body.

The Large Intestine.—Before taking up the subject of absorption the functions of the large intestine will be considered.

The innutritious portions of the food are carried along by the action of the muscular coat of the small intestine into the large intestine, together with those bile-constituents which are not reabsorbed. Here they are added to by the secretion of the mucous-membrane glands, some of which closely resemble the follicles of Lieberkühn. This secretion is an alkaline fluid, but its digestive power, if it possess any, is unimportant. Although this fluid is alkaline, still the contents of the large intestine are acid, owing to the fermentative process.

While the large intestine has no digestive power, it has considerable power of absorption. This absorptive power is constantly being exercised by the withdrawal of the liquid portion of the intestinal contents as they pass along, making them more and more consistent until they are discharged at the anus. This power possessed by the large intestine is made use of in certain diseases of the stomach, in which diseases that organ is unable to perform its function, when by means of nutrient enemata, skilfully administered, life may be maintained for a long time. In a case of circumscribed peritonitis from perforated gastric ulcer a female patient was nourished on the following rectal enema for ninety-four days, during which time she lost but 2700 grammes in weight:

Lean beef . . . . 300 grammes.
Pancreas . . . . 150 "

These were well rubbed up in a mortar and strained, and then there were added:

Water . . . . q. s.
Carbonate of soda . . . . . 5 grammes.
Fresh ox-gall . . . . 25 "

This sufficed for four enemata a day when diluted with a sufficient amount of tepid water.

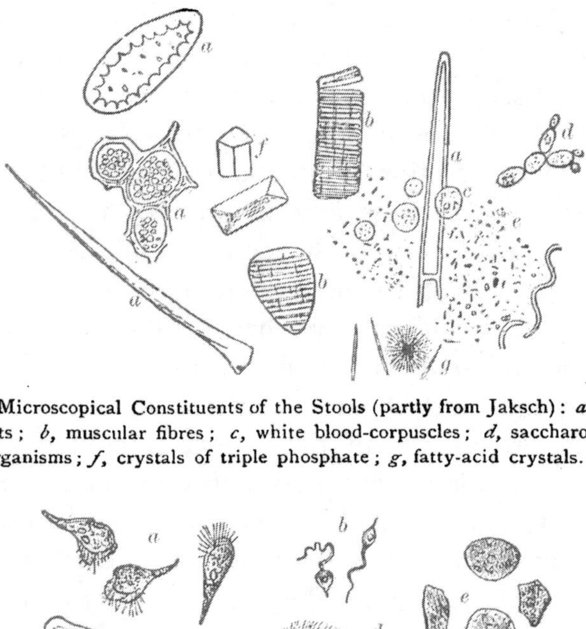

FIG. 15.—Microscopical Constituents of the Stools (partly from Jaksch): *a*, vegetable fragments; *b*, muscular fibres; *c*, white blood-corpuscles; *d*, saccharomyces; *e*, micro-organisms; *f*, crystals of triple phosphate; *g*, fatty-acid crystals.

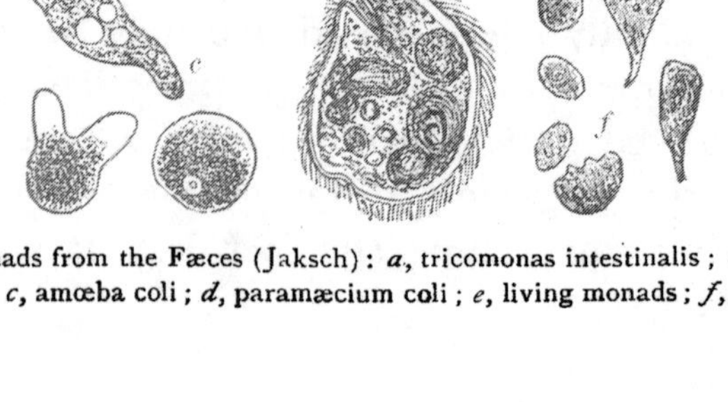

FIG. 16.—Monads from the Fæces (Jaksch): *a*, tricomonas intestinalis; *b*, cercomonas intestinalis; *c*, amœba coli; *d*, paramæcium coli; *e*, living monads; *f*, dead monads.

The contents of the large intestine are called the "fæces" (Figs. 15, 16), and are made up of useless portions of the food, of certain ingredients of the bile, mucus, stercorin, skatol, indol, and other excretory products, and some salts. Nitrogen, carbon dioxide, and carburetted hydrogen are almost always found, and sometimes hydrogen and hydrogen monosulphide. These gases doubtless are the result of decomposition of the food. The amount of fecal matter daily evacuated by an adult is about 160 grammes, 74 per cent. of which is water.

2. Absorption.

Absorption takes place in the mouth, in the stomach, and in the small intestine. The epithelium lining the mouth is not well adapted for absorption, yet that this does occur is proved by the fact that cyanide of potassium taken into, and remaining in, the mouth will cause death. As has been noted, the amount of absorption of food taking place in the mouth is very small, while that taking place in the stomach is much greater. Salts, dextrose, and some peptones here find their way into the blood through the walls of the veins, and it is a well-known fact that some poisons are absorbed from the stomach. It has been claimed that when milk is taken in large amount some of its fatty portions are absorbed by the vessels of the stomach. But to the small intestine must be referred the accomplishment of the greatest part in absorption; for here there is not only a very large area of absorbing surface, it having been estimated to be 10 square metres, but here also are those structures which are especially adapted to perform this function—namely, the *villi.*

Structure of the Villi.—The general characteristics of the villi and their enormous number have been already referred to. Each villus (Fig. 17) is composed of a single layer of columnar epithelium, lying upon a basement membrane, beneath which is a plexus of capillary blood-vessels. Interior to this are non-striated muscular fibres which cover a lacteal. Between the basement membrane and the contained structures, and intertwined with them, is a network of connective tissue in which are cells, including leucocytes, and which is called "lymphoid tissue." The lacteal, which is in the centre of the villus, is a lymphatic vessel; that in some villi is single, and in some double, and begins by a blind extremity. The connection between the lacteal and the columnar epithelium is made by the network spoken of above.

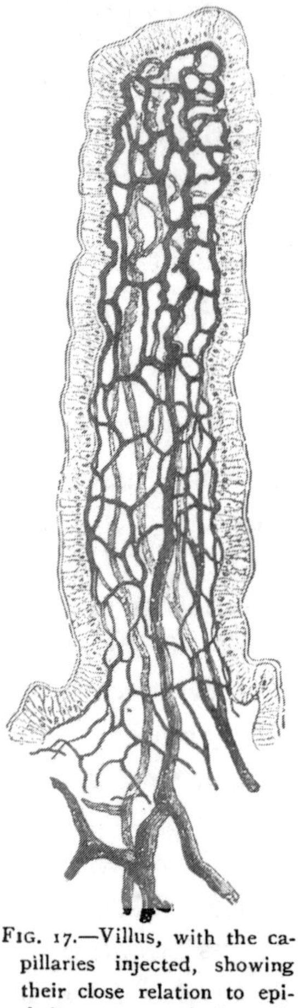

FIG. 17.—Villus, with the capillaries injected, showing their close relation to epithelium, some of the cells of which are distended with mucus (Cadiat).

The lacteals are so called because during the period of absorption of the digested food they contain a material resembling milk in appearance, this material being the *chyle*. The lacteals in reality are lymphatic vessels, and in the intervals of digestion they contain lymph as do other lymphatics. When containing chyle, the lacteals, as they course through the mesentery, appear like minute white threads, by reason of the milky fluid showing through their transparent walls. At other times, when carrying

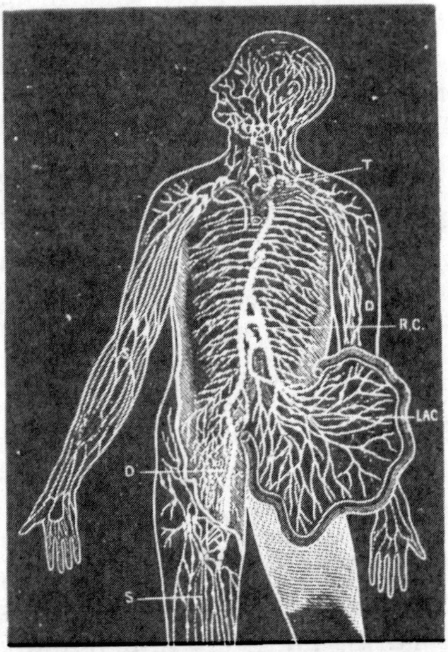

Fig. 18.—Diagram showing the Course of the Main Trunks of the Absorbent System: the lymphatics of lower extremities (D) meet the lacteals of intestines (LAC) at the receptaculum chyli (RC), where the thoracic duct begins. The superficial vessels are shown in the diagram on the right arm and leg (S), and the deeper ones on the left arm (D). The glands are here and there shown in groups. The small right duct opens into the veins on the right side. The thoracic duct opens into the union of the great veins of the left side of the neck (T).

lymph alone, they cannot be distinguished from the surrounding tissue.

Lymph.—Lymph is the fluid which remains after the tissues have taken from the blood the materials needed for their nutrition. This fluid has still nutritive properties which are too valuable to be lost; hence provision is made for its return to the circulation. The vessels by which it returns are the lymphatics. The following table gives the composition of human lymph:

Water	93.99
Fibrin	.06
Albuminous (caseous) matter (with earthy phosphates and traces of iron)	4.27
Fatty matter	.38
Hydro-alcoholic extract (containing sugar, and leaving after incineration sodium chloride, with sodium phosphate and carbonate)	1.30
	100.00

Lymph contains the same ingredients as the blood from which it is derived, except that the red corpuscles are absent. The proportion, however, in which the ingredients exist is not the same.

Chyle.—If the composition of the chyle be examined it will be found that chyle contains more albuminous matter, more fibrin, and very much more fatty matter than the lymph. The following table shows the composition of chyle from a donkey:

Water	90.24
Albuminous matter	3.51
Fibrinous matter	.37
Fatty matter	3.60
Salts	.71
Extractive matter	1.57
	100.00

The efficient agents in absorption are the blood-vessels and the lacteals. All the blood from the stomach and the small intestine passes into the portal circulation of the liver. By this channel most of the peptones find their way into the circulation, as do also the salts and sugar, as well as some fat. By the lacteals the greater part of the emulsified fat is absorbed, as are also some of the peptones and some of the sugar. By the lacteals a portion of the water taken in as drink is absorbed, although the greater part of the latter is taken up by the blood-vessels. In general it may be said that all the products of digestion are absorbed by each of the sets of absorbents, but the lacteals absorb most of the fat, and the blood-vessels most of the sugar and peptones.

Absorption of Fat.—Much interest attaches to the method by which the fatty portion of the food reaches the lacteals. It has been seen that the fat is emulsified in the small intestine; that is, broken up into an exceedingly fine state of subdivision—so fine, indeed, that the size of the globules is from 1 to 2 m.mm. Although the statement that these globules pass into and through the epithelium of the villi has been contradicted, the weight of evidence at the present time seems to be in favor of this explanation. It is not to be supposed that the fat or other substances absorbed by the villi passes into them by a sort of filtering process; there is undoubtedly a selective power exercised by the epithelial covering. From the epithelium through the lymphoid tissue to the lacteal is a continuous path which is followed by the fat. The presence of the bile undoubtedly aids in the process, as experiment shows that membranes moistened with bile permit substances the more readily to pass through them. Some fat, probably a very small portion, is also absorbed as soap.

The changes which the products of digestion undergo after being absorbed are exceedingly obscure, very little being known of them. The sugar which is the product of the changes that have taken place in the carbohydrates is dehydrated by the liver-cells, and is deposited in them as glycogen. This glycogen is gradually re-converted by the liver-cells into sugar and is taken up by the blood. It is carried by the blood to the muscles, where it is utilized in their activities, being broken up ultimately into carbon dioxide and water, in which form it is eliminated from the body. This production of sugar by the liver is its glycogenic function. The peptones are converted into albumin while passing through the mucous membrane, probably in the epithelium, and in that condition are taken up by the blood. The fat and other materials taken up by the lacteals find their way into the thoracic duct, and thence into the venous system.

It is deemed important to direct attention to the fact that at the present time more regard is paid by authorities to the selective power of the epithelium of the villi as absorbing agents than to the older idea of osmosis.

Blood.—The office of blood is twofold: 1. It carries to the tissues of the body the materials which they need for their nourishment, and, in the case of glands, for their secretion; and 2. It takes from the tissues the materials which result from their destructive metabolism —waste materials—which it carries to those structures whose office it is to eliminate them, as, for instance, urea to the kidneys. The blood may be likened to a river which bears to the inhabitants along its banks their daily food, and into which at the same time their waste is discharged and carried to the sea.

Physical Properties of Blood.—Blood is in general red in color and alkaline in reaction, and has a specific gravity of 1055. The specific gravity of the corpuscles is 1105, that of the plasma 1027.

Color of Blood.—Although generally blood is said to be red, still this color is subject to considerable variation. Thus, venous blood is variously described as bluish-red, reddish-black, deep purple, dark purplish-red, dark blue, and dark purple, while arterial blood is a bright scarlet. The color of blood depends on hæmoglobin or its derivatives. In the blood of an animal that has been suffocated, where the purplish or blackish color is most pronounced, the coloring matter is almost entirely hæmoglobin, while in arterial blood the oxyhæmoglobin predominates, and in ordinary venous blood there is a mixture of hæmoglobin and oxyhæmoglobin.

Reaction of Blood.—The alkalinity of blood is a property essential to life. It depends upon the presence of disodic phosphate and sodium bicarbonate. It is said that the blood becomes acid immediately before death in cases of cholera.

Odor of Blood.—Blood has an odor which is said to be characteristic of the species of animal from which it is taken. This odor is usually very slight, but it may be brought out by the addition of sulphuric acid.

Taste of Blood.—The sodium chloride which blood contains gives to it a salty taste.

Quantity of Blood.—The amount of blood in the body of a human adult is about one-thirteenth of his weight; some authorities state one-eighth, and others one-fourteenth. In a new-born child it is about one-nineteenth. During the latter half of the period of pregnancy it is increased, and it is also increased during digestion.

Distribution of Blood.—The distribution of the blood in the body is as follows:

In the heart, lungs, and great blood-vessels, one-fourth.

In the skeletal muscles, one-fourth.

In the liver, one-fourth.

In the rest of the body, one-fourth.

Temperature of Blood.—The temperature of blood varies greatly in the different parts of the circulatory apparatus. The mean temperature may be stated as 39° C.; that of the superior vena cava, 36.78° C.; the right side of the heart, 38.8° C.; the left side of the heart, 38.6° C.; the aorta, 38.7° C.; the portal vein, 39.9° C.; the hepatic vein, 41.3° C. The temperature of the blood in the hepatic vein is the highest in the body, and it varies from 39.5° C. at the beginning of digestion to 41.3° C. at the time when the process is the most active. The blood in the right side of the heart is made warmer by its proximity to the liver, while in its circulation through the lungs it loses heat, and is therefore cooler in the left side of the heart. In the portions of the body exposed to the air, as in the skin, the temperature of the blood is doubtless as low as 36.5° C.

Microscopical Structure of the Blood.—When examined by the microscope the blood is seen to be composed of a fluid portion, *plasma* or liquor sanguinis, in which are suspended bodies called "corpuscles." The plasma is a straw-colored fluid, the color being due to lutein, whose chemical composition will be hereafter discussed.

Blood-corpuscles are of three varieties: (1) Red corpuscles; (2) white corpuscles; and (3) plaques.

Red corpuscles in human blood are circular, biconcave, non-nucleated disks, having an average diameter of 7.7 m.mm., some of them being as small as 4.5 m.mm., while others are 9 m.mm. In chronic anæmic conditions some have been found as large as 14 m.mm., and others as small as 2.2 m.mm.

Number of Blood-corpuscles.—The number of red corpuscles in a millimetre of the blood of a male adult has been reckoned at 5,000,000; in that of a female, 4,500,000. In anæmia this number has been reduced

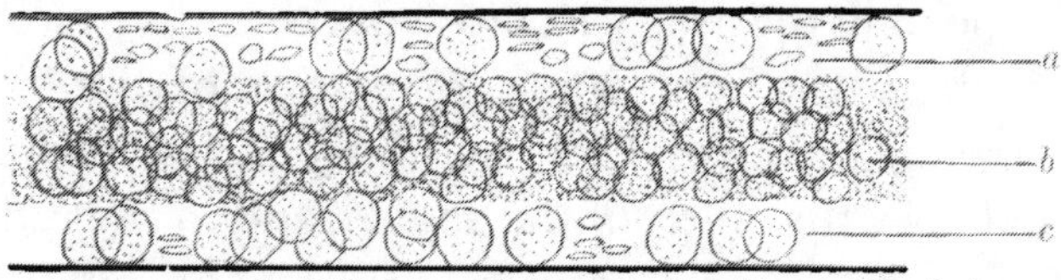

FIG. 19.—Blood-corpuscles (Eberth and Schimmelbusch): *a*, blood-plaques or third corpuscles; *b*, red corpuscles; *c*, white corpuscles.

to 1,000,000. In all the blood of the body in health their number is consequently enormous.

Color of Red Corpuscles.—A single corpuscle is of a yellowish or amber color, and the red color of the blood only appears when the corpuscles are in thick layers or in masses. They are exceedingly flexible, as may readily be seen by watching them in the circulation of the web of a frog's foot. At times they will be so stretched out as to pass through a vessel whose diameter is smaller than is theirs when in a circular shape, or sometimes they may be seen bent over the projection made by the junction of two vessels, one portion being within each, until, one current being the stronger, they are carried into it, resuming their circular shape as soon as that is possible.

Structure of Red Corpuscles.—The red corpuscles are composed of a substance called the "stroma" and of the coloring matter. Some of the constituents of the stroma have been determined. These constituents are lecithin, cholesterin, and cell-globulin. Potassium, sodium, phosphoric acid, and chlorine have also been obtained. The coloring matter has already been spoken of. During a portion of fœtal life the human red blood-corpuscle has a nucleus, but this disappears at about the fourth month, and it is wanting in the adult.

Development of Red Blood-corpuscles.—The corpuscles are developed in the area vasculosa of the embryo from the cells which result from the segmentation of the vitellus. These divide, and thus form new corpuscles. They are formed also in the liver, in the spleen, and in the red marrow of bones, being found in the red marrow after birth. This red marrow occurs in the bones of the skull and in the trunk. In the bones of the extremities the marrow is yellow and is largely fatty. If any red marrow be found in the bones, it is in their heads. It is said that after severe hemorrhages, when the production of red corpuscles is very active, this yellow marrow becomes red and produces red corpuscles. Some have claimed that they are also formed from white corpuscles, but this claim is doubtful.

Destruction of Red Blood-corpuscles.—The duration of a red blood-corpuscle is undetermined, but it is doubtless limited. Some authorities place its life at from three to four weeks. Old corpuscles constantly undergo disintegration and new ones appear. The fact that fewer corpuscles are found in the blood of the hepatic than in that of the portal vein, and the additional fact that biliary pigment is formed from the coloring matter of the blood, indicate that in the liver a part, at least, of these destructive changes takes place. These same changes take place also in the spleen. If, as there is reason to believe, the pigment of the bile and the urine be formed from that of the blood, the number of the corpuscles daily destroyed must be very great.

Function of Red Blood-corpuscles.—The red corpuscles

are the carriers of oxygen to the tissues, without which oxygen they could exist but for a short time. The blood can absorb at least ten times as much of this gas as can the same amount of water, and this absorption is due principally to the affinity which the hæmoglobin has for it. While oxygen is mainly in the corpuscles, carbon dioxide is in the plasma.

White blood-corpuscles are sometimes spoken of as "colorless corpuscles," and sometimes as "leucocytes." The last term is, perhaps, the best, as under it are included cells which are found in lymph, chyle, pus, connective tissue, and elsewhere, and which cannot be distinguished from those found in the blood. The *size* of white corpuscles is variable, from 4 to 13 m.mm., averaging perhaps 10 m.mm. The *shape* of these corpuscles is said to be spherical, but by virtue of their power of amœboid movement their form is constantly changing. They consist of masses of protoplasm containing a nucleus, and sometimes more than one. Their *number* is commonly said to be, compared with the red corpuscles, as 1 to 350 or 1 to 750, but these figures are of but little value, so greatly does the proportion vary under different conditions and in different portions of the circulatory apparatus. Thus, after eating this proportion is much increased, as is also the case after the loss of blood, during suppurative processes, and after the use of bitter tonics; while in a state of hunger or deficient nourishment it is diminished. In the splenic vein the proportion has been found to be as 1 to 60; in the splenic artery, 1 to 2260; hepatic vein, 1 to 170; and portal vein, 1 to 740. As a rule, white corpuscles are more numerous in the veins than in the arteries. The great difficulty encountered in attempting to ascertain the number of white corpuscles is due to the fact that in the shedding of blood large numbers disappear. One authority estimates that only one-tenth of the number that existed in the blood when it was circulating remains after it has left the blood-vessel.

Composition of White Blood-corpuscles.—White corpuscles contain myosin, serum-globulin, glycogen, lecithin, cholesterin, nuclein, salts of sodium, potassium, calcium, and magnesium. Besides these ingredients they contain a zymogen which produces fibrin-ferment.

Function of White Blood-corpuscles.—But little is known of the function of the white corpuscles of the blood, except that concerned in the process of coagu-

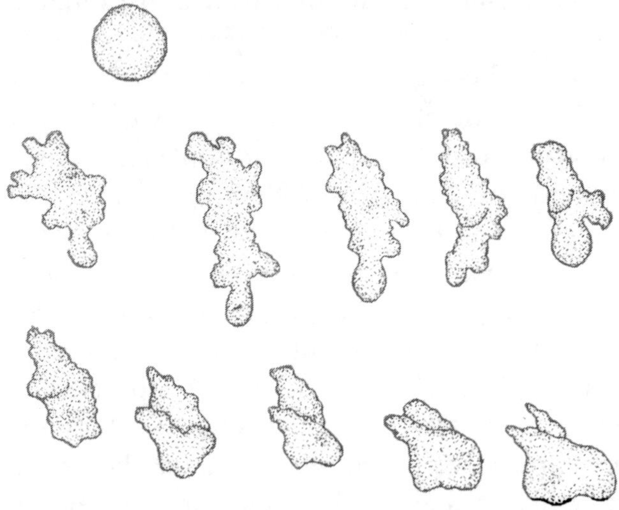

FIG. 20.—Changes in the Leucocyte of a Frog during ten minutes (*Am. Text-book of Surgery*).

lation. As already stated, it is doubtful if they have anything to do with the formation of the red corpuscles.

Blood-plaques are known also as "blood-plates" and

"hæmatoblasts." The latter name has been given them because they are regarded by some authorities as an early stage in the development of the red corpuscles. Blood-plaques are round or oval in shape and are colorless. Their size is very variable, averaging perhaps 3 m.mm. Their number, compared with the red corpuscles, is as 1 to 25 or 180,000 to 250,000 per cubic millimetre of blood.

The *function* of blood-plaques is undetermined.

Blood-plasma and liquor sanguinis are synonymous terms, but serum, which is often used as interchangeable with them, is a different fluid, having a different composition, which will be described in discussing the coagulation of blood.

Composition of Plasma.—Blood-plasma contains the following constituents: water, fibrinogen, paraglobulin, serum-albumin, fat, soaps, cholesterin, lecithin, glucose, urea, uric acid, creatin, lutein, sodium chloride, sodium carbonate, calcium phosphate, and some others which need not be specified. Blood-plasma also contains the following gases: carbon dioxide, nitrogen, and oxygen.

Coagulation of Blood.—When blood is withdrawn from the circulation it undergoes coagulation, consisting in the production of a clot from which is subsequently expressed a fluid called the "serum." The length of time required for coagulation varies in different animals. In human blood the change manifests itself in about two or three minutes. When the blood is withdrawn from the vessel it is fluid, but at the end of two or three minutes its fluidity is so much diminished that it will not flow; this consistency increases until at the end of eight or ten minutes the entire quantity of blood becomes a mass resembling currant jelly in color and consistency. This jelly-like mass becomes more and more consistent, squeezing out upon its surface a few drops of a straw-colored fluid—the serum. As the shrinking of this gelatinous mass—the clot—continues, it separates from the sides of the vessel in which the blood was received, and the serum is squeezed out on all sides, until at length there is a more or less solid clot floating in a considerable quantity of serum. When examined the clot is found to be made up of fibrin and corpuscles, the red corpuscles giving to it the red color. The serum has the same composition as the plasma, minus the fibrinogen.

Although the corpuscles are denser than the plasma, still the difference is so slight and the process of coagulation so rapid that before they can settle they are entangled in the meshes of the fibrin as it forms, and thus become a part of the clot. If anything occur to delay coagulation, the corpuscles settle, and the clot is then less red and more yellowish. This delay may be brought about by the addition of a solution of magnesium sulphate; it occurs also in inflammatory processes, and hence in the olden time, when venesection was commonly practised, this *crusta phlogistica*, or "buffy coat," was always looked for by the physician, and when it formed was considered as evidence that the bleeding was justifiable. That the physicians of that period were not always right in this judgment is now known, for a buffy coat will form in blood which is hydræmic, a condition in which bleeding is contraindicated. In horses' blood, which normally coagulates very slowly, this "buffy coat" always forms. It is simply the fibrin without the corpuscles, or at least without enough of them to give the red color which the clot usually possesses.

Influences which Retard Coagulation.—Coagulation is retarded by cold, by solutions of sodium or magnesium sulphate, by a diminished amount of oxygen, by an increased amount of carbon dioxide, by acids or alkalies, by egg-albumin, by oil, by a solution of albumose, and by an infusion of the leech, which doubtless contains an albumose. Venous blood coagulates more slowly than arterial, because of the lessened amount of oxygen and the increased amount of carbon dioxide. It is said that blood from the capillaries does not coagulate at all.

It is the prevalent opinion that menstrual blood does not clot; this, strictly speaking, is not true. If the blood as it comes from the uterine vessels were collected, it would doubtless coagulate as does other blood, but when it is mixed with the acid vaginal mucus its coagulation is then impeded. Then, too, during the menstrual period some of the blood undergoes clotting within the uterine cavity or in the vagina: that which escapes and which is regarded as menstrual blood is for the most part only serum, which of course does not coagulate.

Influences that Hasten Coagulation.—Coagulation is promoted by warmth and by contact with roughened surfaces.

Causes of Coagulation.—Perhaps no physiological question has excited more controversy than that which deals with the cause of blood-coagulation. Normally, blood remains fluid within the blood-vessels, but within three minutes after withdrawal it begins to undergo coagulation. What is the explanation?

It has been suggested that blood-coagulation is due to exposure to the air. It is true that contact with the air hastens coagulation, but that this is unnecessary to the process is shown by the fact that coagulation will take place under mercury, when all air is excluded. Nor can it be due to the cooling the blood undergoes when it is exposed to the air, for, as already noted, cold retards coagulation, while heat aids it. It has also been suggested that the fluid condition of the blood in the circulation is due to its motion, and that it clots when it comes to a state of rest. But experiment shows that motion, such as the beating of blood with agitation, hastens coagulation.

Experiments demonstrate that the fluidity of the blood is maintained only when the blood is in contact with the normal lining membrane of the blood-vessels: when this relation is interrupted, either by disease, or by death or injury of the membrane, or by withdrawal of the blood from the vessel, this fluidity ceases and the blood coagulates.

The clot that forms in the coagulation is fibrin, in the meshes of which the corpuscles become entangled. This fibrin is the coagulated fibrinogen of the blood, and the factor which causes it to coagulate is fibrin-ferment. The preponderance of evidence at the present time points to the white corpuscles as the source of this ferment, although this has not been definitely proved to be its origin.

The presence of lime-salts in the blood is very important in the process of coagulation, although it cannot perhaps be said that they are absolutely essential, as is the case with casein, which is not coagulated by rennin unless these salts be present.

The property of coagulation possessed by blood is of great service in arresting hemorrhage. There are individuals in whom bleeding, which to most people would be only slight, amounts to a dangerous hæmorrhage, often requiring surgical skill for its arrest, and in some instances being so uncontrollable, even by the most skilful treatment, that death results. Such persons are called "bleeders," and on them surgeons hesitate to perform any operation, however trivial, the extraction of a tooth even being often followed by an alarming loss of blood. This condition is spoken of as "hæmophilia" or "hæmorrhagic diathesis." It is probable that in such cases the fibrinogen is very deficient.

Blood, then, before coagulation consists of plasma and corpuscles; after coagulation, of serum and clot, the serum having the same composition as the plasma, save that it has lost the fibrinogen, which, having assumed a new form, fibrin, exists in the clot together with the corpuscles.

Gases in the Blood.—The blood contains nitrogen, oxygen, and carbon dioxide. The first of these gases exists in the proportion of from 1 to 2 per cent., and is practically the same in both arterial and venous blood. Nitrogen has no special physiological interest. The amount of carbon dioxide and of oxygen varies greatly in different portions of the circulatory apparatus and under different circumstances. The variations, indeed, are so great that it is possible to give only general averages. The amount in human arterial blood has been given as 21.6 volumes per cent.; that is, in every 100 volumes of arterial blood there are 21.6 volumes of oxygen. In venous blood the percentage is but 6.8. Another estimate gives the oxygen in arterial blood as 20 per cent., and in venous blood as from 8 to 12 per cent. The blood in these estimates is presumed to be at 0° C. and the pressure to be 760 mm. of mercury.

The following figures illustrate the difference in the amount of this gas in the different vessels and in the same vessel under different circumstances: Oxygen in carotid artery, 21 per cent.; in renal artery, 19; in renal vein (kidney active), 17; in renal vein (kidney at rest), 6. In the blood of asphyxiated animals oxygen may entirely be absent.

The difference between the amount of oxygen in the renal vein when the kidney is active and when it is at rest (and what is true of the kidney is true of other glands) needs some explanation. When the kidney is at rest only enough blood goes to it to nourish it and to supply the small amount of oxygen which it needs in a resting state; the blood that returns from it is venous blood, in which the amount of oxygen is but 6 per cent. When, however, the gland is actively at work, the amount of blood which goes to the kidney is greatly in excess of the amount needed for nutritive purposes, the surplus being for the specific purposes of the gland; and, although more oxygen is taken from it than when the gland is quiescent, still the proportion thus taken, compared with the amount of blood which traverses the gland, is so small that when it leaves the gland it contains nearly as great a percentage of oxygen as before. Thus, the oxygen in the renal artery under these circumstances is 19 per cent., and in the renal vein 17 per cent.

It has already been stated that this oxygen is combined with the hæmoglobin in the red corpuscles, the amount in the plasma being 0.26 per cent.—no more than would be found in an equal amount of distilled water.

Carbon dioxide exists in human arterial blood to the amount of about 40 per cent., and in venous blood about

48 per cent. This may be greatly increased in asphyxia, when it has been found to be 69.21 per cent. One-third of the carbon dioxide is in the corpuscles, a small part of this being in the leucocytes, the remaining two-thirds being in the plasma, some simply absorbed (perhaps one-tenth), and some combined to form sodium carbonate and bicarbonate.

3. Respiration.

One of the most important processes carried on in the body is that by which the tissues receive oxygen. In animals whose structure is exceeding simple, and so constituted that all portions of their bodies are bathed by the oxygen-carrying medium, the oxygen is directly absorbed, but in those in which there are tissues remotely situated as regards this medium, some provision must be made for conveying the oxygen from the medium to the tissues. This condition exists in man, many of whose tissues are so deeply situated that without such provision the maintenance of life would be impossible. In man this medium is the blood. But additional provision must be made for the renewal of the oxygen abstracted by the tissues. That part of the process by which the tissues take oxygen from the blood is internal respiration, and that part by which the renewal is accomplished is external respiration. Ordinarily, when respiration is spoken of without qualification it is external respiration that is referred to.

Respiratory Apparatus.—The group of organs concerned in external respiration is collectively spoken of as the "respiratory apparatus," which consists of the nose, larynx, trachea, bronchial tubes, lungs, and thorax.

The nose is the beginning of the air-passages, for,

although it is regarded by many as the organ of smell only, it has another function as well. The mouth belongs to the alimentary canal, and should only be opened to take in food or to speak, never to take in air. The proper channel for the admission of air is the nose, and the use of the mouth for this purpose is not physiological. Indeed, man is said to be the only animal that breathes through the mouth. If the nursing child should attempt to use its mouth for the admission of air to the lungs, sucking could not be performed without great difficulty, and after a few moments the child would be compelled to let go the breast in order not to suffocate.

Mouth-breathing.—There is no more pernicious habit, so far as health is concerned, than breathing through the mouth. If this be due simply to habit and nothing else, it may be overcome, but if, as is often the case, it be due to some diseased condition of the nose, or to the presence in the nasal cavities of tumors, or to the existence of enlarged tonsils, its relief can only be accomplished by surgical means. The function of the nose in respiration is to warm the air and to filter out from it dust and other extraneous matter which would otherwise enter the air-passages and cause irritation. When air is taken in by the mouth these advantages are lost.

Mouth-breathing causes dryness of the mouth and the pharynx, which dryness is very noticeable on awaking from sleep. The mucous membrane becomes congested and inflammation is likely to follow. A chronic inflammatory condition of the larynx may also result from this cause, and the evidence is very conclusive that the hearing becomes affected in these cases. The deformity known as *pigeon-breast* is not an uncommon sequel. Indeed, the consequences of mouth-breathing are numerous, widespread, and serious, and the subject has never received the attention which its importance demands.

The anatomical structures in the larynx having special physiological interest in connection with the process of respiration are the arytenoid cartilages, the vocal cords, and the posterior crico-arytenoid muscles. The

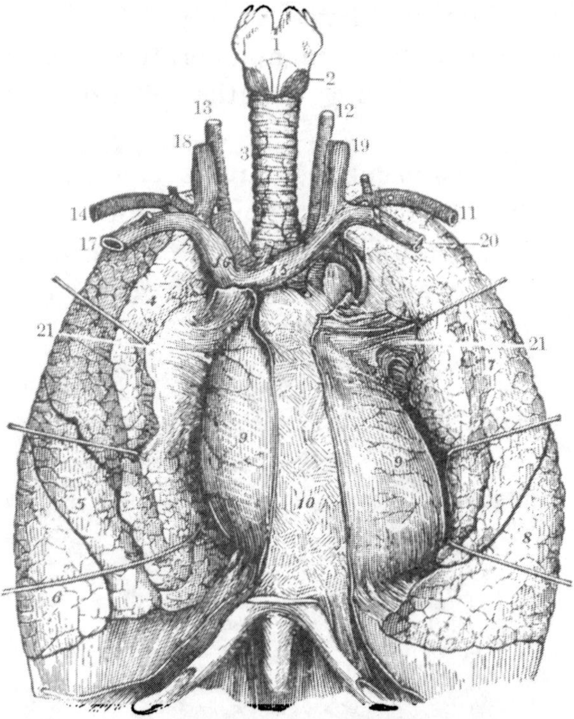

FIG. 21.—1, larynx; 2, crico-thyroid muscles; 3, trachea; 4–6, right lung; 7, 8, left lung; 9, pericardium; 10, mediastinum; 11 and 14, subclavian arteries; 12, 13, carotid arteries; 15, 16, innominate veins; 17, 20, subclavian veins; 18, 19, internal jugular veins; 21, root of lung. The lungs naturally cover the pericardium, but in the figure are represented as held back by hooks.

space between the vocal cords is the *rima glottidis*, or glottis.

The trachea, or windpipe, is a tube about 11.5 cm. inches in length, and it extends from the larynx to the bronchi, into which it divides (Fig. 21). It is made up of rings of cartilage which are incomplete behind, their ends being joined by fibrous membrane; here the trachea is in contact with the œsophagus. The cartilages are joined to one another by similar membrane. The trachea is lined with mucous membrane, the epithelium of which is of the columnar ciliated variety.

The bronchi are two in number, the right bronchus going to the right lung, and the left bronchus to the left lung.

The lungs, two in number, are covered by the visceral layer of the pleura. Each bronchus as it enters the lungs divides, the branches which result from this division again divide, and so on, until the last subdivision is

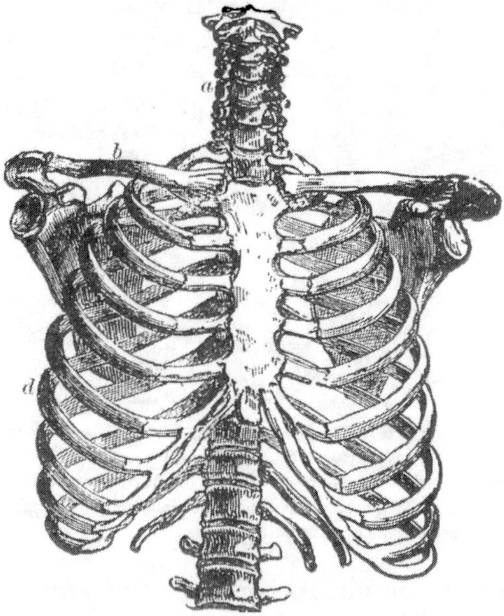

FIG. 22.—*a*, vertebral column; *b*, clavicle; *d*, ribs; *e*, sternum.

reached, the ultimate or lobular bronchial tube, which passes into a lobule which is made up of air-cells. The walls of the air-cells are composed of elastic tissue, and in them are the capillary blood-vessels.

The thorax, the cavity in which the lungs are situated, is composed of the vertebral column, the ribs, the sternum, the diaphragm, and the muscles (intercostals) between the ribs and those which cover them (Fig. 22). The vertebral column is rigid, and takes no part in any of the movements connected with respiration, but with a portion of it the heads of the ribs articulate. The ribs are connected posteriorly with the vertebral column, as stated, and anteriorly with the sternum by means of the costal cartilages. The general direction of the ribs is such that their vertebral extremities are higher than the sternal. The diaphragm (Fig. 23) is the lower boundary

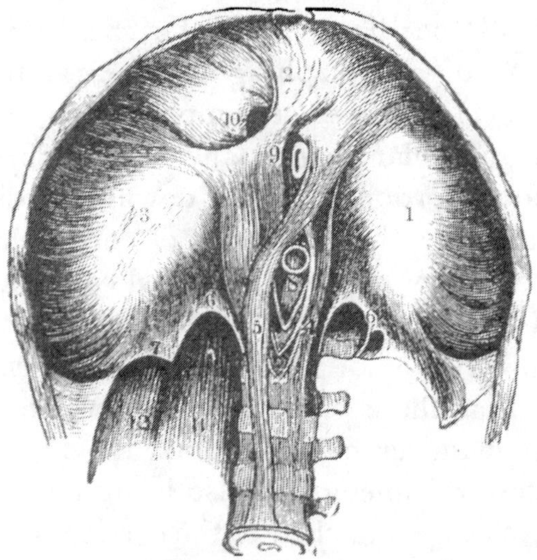

Fig. 23.—Interior View of the Diaphragm: 1–3, the three lobes of the central tendon surrounded by the fleshy fasciculi derived from the inferior margin of the thorax; 4, 5, the crura; 6, 7, the arcuate ligaments; 8, aortic orifice; 9, œsophageal orifice; 10, quadrate foramen; 11, psoas muscle; 12, quadrate lumbar muscle.

of the thoracic cavity, separating it from that of the abdomen. The central portion is tendinous in structure, while the peripheral portion is muscular. It is attached to the interior of the thorax, and forms an arch with its convexity directed upward, the summit of the arch being at the level of the fifth rib. The intercostal muscles, as their name implies, are between the ribs. The fibres of the external intercostal muscles are directed downward and forward, while the direction of those of the internal is upward and forward.

Respiratory Movements.—The respiratory movements are of two kinds—inspiratory and expiratory.

Inspiratory Movements.—By virtue of the inspiratory movements the air passes into the lungs. During their performance the thorax expands under the influence of the diaphragm and the external intercostal muscles. In inspiration all the diameters of the chest are increased. The descent of the diaphragm increases the vertical diameter (Pl. 1). This is accomplished by the contraction of the muscular portion, and as the fibres shorten the tendinous portion is drawn downward, diminishing very considerably the convexity of the arch. In this descent the organs of the abdominal cavity are pressed down and are also compressed. This displacement causes a protrusion of the abdominal walls. At the same time that these changes are going on, increasing the vertical diameter of the thorax, the transverse and antero-posterior diameters are also being increased. The scaleni muscles are attached to the cervical vertebræ and the first and second ribs. By their contraction these ribs are firmly fixed, and then, the external intercostals contracting, the ribs are raised, rotating at their articulation with the vertebræ. The shape and direction of the ribs are such that when they are raised their convexities are carried outward, and thus the transverse diameter of the thorax is increased. But this movement also carries the sternum forward, thereby increasing the antero-posterior diameter. Under some circumstances, as when there is some obstruction to the entrance of air, additional muscles, called "extraordinary muscles of inspiration," are brought into action. In this way most of the muscles about the thorax may be called upon. This is known as "forced inspiration." It should be noted that inspiration is an active process; that is, one that requires for its performance the action of muscles.

Expiratory Movements are for the most part passive in their nature; that is, are not due to muscular contraction. During the descent of the diaphragm, referred to in describing the inspiratory movements, the elastic abdominal organs and their attachments and the abdominal walls are put upon the stretch. At the end of the inspiratory act the diaphragm ceases to contract, and by virtue of the elasticity of these structures the contents of the abdomen return to the position they occupied at the beginning of the diaphragm's descent, and in so doing this structure is carried back to its original position. The elevation of the ribs by the contraction of the external intercostals during inspiration twists the elastic costal cartilages which join the ribs to the sternum: as soon as these muscles cease to contract these cartilages untwist, and in so doing aid in the return of the ribs. In describing the structure of the lungs it was stated that the walls of the lobules were rich in elastic tissue: in inspiration these lobules are greatly distended, their walls being put on the stretch. When the inspiratory forces cease to act, then this tissue, by virtue of its elasticity, returns to its former condition, and in so doing expels the air, constituting expiration. Contractility may be said to be the inspiratory force; elasticity, the expiratory force.

As in inspiration, so in expiration, there are occasions when obstruction to the outgoing air exists, and forced expiration becomes necessary. The muscles concerned in this act are the internal intercostals, and others known as "extraordinary muscles of expiration," whose arrangement is such that in their contraction the capacity of the thorax is diminished. The abdominal walls, by exerting pressure on the abdominal viscera, and thus on the diaphragm, still further diminish the thoracic cavity and force out the contained air.

Movements of Glottis.—There are in connection with the process of respiration certain movements of the glottis which are important. On examination of the interior of the larynx it will be seen that during inspiration the vocal cords separate, and during expiration approach each other. During deep breathing (Fig. 25) the separation of the cords is greater than in quiet breathing (Fig. 24).

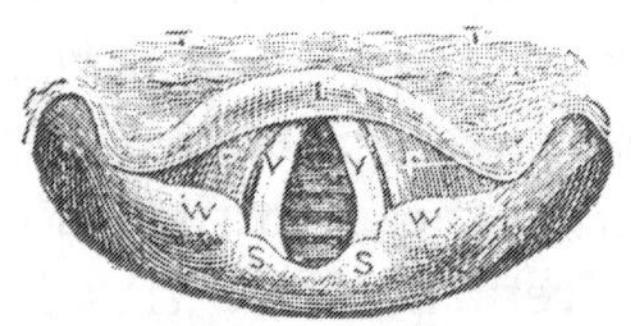

FIG. 24.—The Larynx in Gentle Breathing (Lennox-Browne): L, epiglottis; V, vocal cords; S, cartilages of Santorini, which surmount the arytenoid cartilages; P, P, ventricular bands.

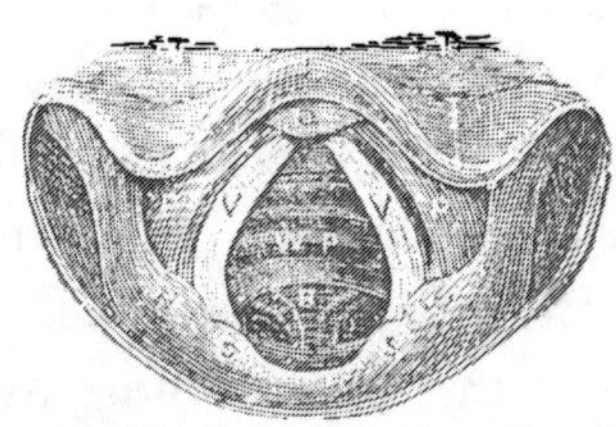

FIG. 25 —The Larynx in Deep Breathing (Lennox-Browne): W,P, tracheal rings; B, openings of bronchi; P, P, ventricular bands.

The area of the trachea is nearly three times that of the space between the cords at the beginning of inspiration. The separation of these cords is effected by the contraction of the posterior crico-arytenoid muscles, which by their attachment to the arytenoid cartilages rotate these outward, and thus separate the posterior ends of the cords which are attached to them, increasing the area nearly twofold. When these muscles cease their contraction, as they do at the end of the inspiratory act, then the elasticity of the cartilages brings the muscles back to the position they occupied at the beginning of inspiration. These movements of the glottis occur synchronously with the respiratory movements of the thorax.

Capacity of the Lungs.—At the beginning of an ordinary inspiration the lungs contain 3280 cc. of air, which so distends the lungs that the visceral layer of the pleura is in contact with the parietal layer. As the thorax enlarges the air in the lungs distends them still more, so that they are still kept in contact with the thoracic walls. This contact between the visceral and parietal layers of the pleura is constant, irrespective of the amount of distention of the lungs. The expansion of the air in the lungs makes it of less density than the external air with which it is in communication through the air-passages, and immediately there is a flow of external air into these passages to establish an equilibrium: this inflow constitutes *inspiration.* The amount of air which thus flows in is ordinarily 500 cc. During expiration this amount is forced out by the mechanism already described. To the air which flows in and out during ordinary respiration the name of "tidal air" is given, from the resemblance which the process bears to the ebb and flow of the tide. At the end of an ordinary expiration there remain in the lungs, as already stated, upward of 3000 cc. of air. By a forced expiration 1640 cc. of air may be expelled; this is the reserve or supplemental air. When this expulsion has been accomplished there still remains 1640 cc. of "residual" air, which cannot be expelled, no matter how great the effort. Since this residual and supplemental air ordinarily remains in the lungs during respiration, it is spoken of as the "stationary air." After breathing in the tidal air there may, however, be taken in, by forced inspiration, about 1600 cc. of air; this is the "complemental air."

Vital Capacity.—The volume of air over which an individual can exert control is known as his "vital capacity." It is the sum of the complemental, tidal, and supplemental air, and excludes the residual.

Frequency of Respiration.—In the new-born child the number of respirations per minute is 44; at five years of age, 26; at twenty years, 20; and at thirty years, 16. These figures represent an average during a quiescent condition. Should the respirations be counted during sleep, they would be one or two less per minute; during great activity they would be increased considerably, in the adult running up to 30 or more.

Cause of Respiration.—The discussion of the cause of respiratory movements will be deferred until the function of the respiratory centre of the medulla oblongata is considered.

Types of Respiration.—It has been the practice among physiological writers to speak of the "costal," or female, type of respiration, and the "abdominal," or male, type. The following condensed statement from one of the best text-books on this subject represents the views of these writers: "In children, as well as in the adult male, under ordinary conditions, the diaphragm performs most of the work, and the movements of the abdomen are the only ones especially noticeable. . . . In the female the movements of the chest, particularly of its upper half, are habitually more prominent than those of the abdomen, and this difference in the mechanism of respiration is characteristic of the sexes." The costal type of respiration here spoken of as characteristic of the female was supposed to be a wise provision of nature, in order that when pregnancy should occur the respiratory movements would not be interfered with, as they would be had the female possessed the abdominal type of respiration seen in the male.

Very careful and complete studies of women in and out of civilization, the lower portions of whose chests have never been compressed with corsets or with other devices calculated to prevent expansion of those parts, have demonstrated that the supposed respiratory difference in male and female does not exist naturally, and that when it is found it is due to the corset and not to any peculiarity of sex. Indeed, if the male chest be encased in the corset the abdominal type becomes changed at once into the costal. It is also of interest to note that in one case at least where the observation was made abdominal respiration was well marked in a pregnant woman within one week of her confinement.

Chemistry of Respiration.—The air contains 20.96 parts by volume of oxygen, 79.02 parts of nitrogen, and 0.03 parts of carbon dioxide. Watery vapor is also present, the amount varying under different circumstances, being greater the higher the temperature of the air. The term *absolute humidity* has reference to the total amount of watery vapor which a volume of air contains, irrespective of the question of temperature; the term *relative humidity* is used to express the proportion of watery vapor present in the air at certain temperatures as compared with air fully saturated, saturation being expressed by 100. Absolute humidity is expressed in grammes per cubic metre or in grains per cubic foot, while relative humidity is expressed in percentages. Thus if the temperature of the air be 4°, and it is saturated with watery vapor, its relative humidity would be said to be 100; if, now, its temperature were raised to 27°, its relative humidity would be only 24, because the higher the temperature the more vapor can a given volume of air contain, and the air at 27° would hold a much greater amount than when its temperature was 4°.

The amount of moisture present in air is an important factor in the preservation of health. If it be too dry, the air-passages are irritated, while if too moist there is produced a feeling of oppression. A relative humidity of 70 is, as a rule, very agreeable. Traces of ammonia are also found in the atmospheric air. Besides these constituents, which are universal, there are many others that may or may not be present as the result of processes of manufacture.

Expired Air.—When the atmospheric air has been breathed its composition is markedly changed in the following particulars: 1. It has gained carbon dioxide, the amount being increased from 0.03 parts per cent. to 4.38. 2. It has lost oxygen, the 20.96 volumes per cent. being reduced to 16.03, or about 5 per cent. It should be noted that the loss of oxygen is greater than can be accounted for by the amount of that gas returned in the carbon dioxide, the difference representing the amount used up in processes of oxidation constantly going on in the body. 3. It has gained watery vapor, the expired air being saturated. The actual amount of vapor which it receives while in the lungs will of course vary. If the air when inspired be cool and dry, it will take more moisture from the body than if it be moist and warm. The daily loss to the body through this channel is 255 grammes. 4. The expired air is, as a rule, warmer than the inspired, under ordinary circumstances being 36° C. Thus, if the temperature of the air be 21° C., it will gain 15° C. while in the lungs. The temperature of the expired air is very nearly 36°, whatever that of the atmospheric air may be. 5. The expired air contains certain volatile organic matters which are at once recognized by the sense of smell, although the chemist has not yet made us acquainted with their exact composition. These organic constituents are of great importance, and will be discussed later.

Ventilation.—It is manifest that if at each inspiration oxygen be abstracted from the air, in the course of time the amount of this gas will be so reduced as to make its want seriously felt. It is necessary, therefore, in order to keep the amount of oxygen up to the standard, that some provision should be made to supply it. Besides the removal of the oxygen, the air is still further rendered unsuited for respiratory purposes by the carbon dioxide, and especially by the organic matter thrown off by the expired air; the oxygen being still further diminished by stoves and lights, and the air being vitiated by the products of combustion. To supply oxygen and to remove these impurities is the object of ventilation.

A common test to determine whether the air of an apartment contains sufficient oxygen for respiratory purposes is to see if a candle will burn in it. This test is used to determine whether the air in vaults or in excavations is fit for respiration. A candle will not burn if the air contain only 17 per cent. of oxygen. A man could breathe, however, if this amount were present, but if it were reduced to 10 per cent., asphyxia would be produced. So far, then, as the question of oxygen is concerned, a man could breathe where a candle would not burn, but it does not necessarily follow that it is always safe for a man to venture where a candle *will* burn, for sometimes, although there may be oxygen sufficient to sustain life, poisonous gases may also be present in an amount sufficient to produce a fatal result. It would be a surer test to place a dog in the suspected place and leave him there for twenty minutes. If he survive, it will be safe for a man to enter.

It is a general impression that the carbon dioxide which accumulates in a room where a large number of persons is congregated is the ingredient of the air which makes its use in respiration so injurious; but this is not the fact. An atmosphere containing as much as 2 per cent. of carbon dioxide, as in factories where so-called "soda-water" is made, may be breathed without injury or even inconvenience, while one in which this gas exceeds 0.07 per cent., provided it have its origin in the lungs, is regarded by sanitarians as containing the maximum amount that should be permitted. In other words, it is not the carbon dioxide that causes the injurious results, but it is the organic matter thrown off from the body in the expired air: the carbon dioxide which accompanies the organic matter is only the index. In testing the purity of the air it is easy to ascertain the amount of carbon dioxide present, and very difficult to measure the amount of organic matter; hence it is the former which is looked for in lecture-rooms, factories, or churches, and when it is found to exceed 0.07 per cent. it is known that there is a hurtful amount of organic matter present. As much as eighteen times the normal amount of carbon dioxide has been found in school-rooms.

To maintain the air sufficiently pure for respiratory purposes, 90 cubic metres of fresh air should be supplied per hour to each individual. It would seem to be an easy thing to accomplish this, but as a matter of fact it is one of the most difficult problems. To supply this amount of air without producing such draughts as to endanger health requires that to each individual should be allotted a certain amount of air-space, practically not less than 30 cubic metres per person in health, while for the sick, as in hospitals, double this amount is none too great. It seems hardly necessary to say that due attention must be paid to the source from which the introduced air is drawn. If it be taken from filthy cellars or from dirty streets, it may be as impure as that which it is designed to replace.

Changes in the Blood due to Respiration.—The blood when it reaches the lungs from the heart is venous, and when it leaves the lungs to return to the heart it is arterial. The conversion of the venous blood into arterial, then, takes place while the blood is traversing the pulmonary capillaries. As previously noted, the inspired air loses oxygen during its stay in the pulmonary air-cells, and arterial blood contains more oxygen than venous blood; the loss, then, which the air sustains is a gain to the blood. The expired air, while it contains less oxygen than the inspired air, contains more carbon dioxide and watery vapor, and a comparison of the blood going to the lungs and returning from them shows that during its passage it loses these very ingredients.

Internal Respiration is the process by which the tissues receive oxygen from the blood, and is very obscure.

There are no means of ascertaining just how much oxygen is taken up by any given tissue ; it is only known that it is essential this gas should be supplied and in sufficient quantity, and that when this does not occur the tissues suffer. When the tissues are at rest the amount needed is less than when they are active, but under the latter condition more oxygen is eliminated in carbon dioxide than is supplied during the same time, showing that when at rest the tissues store up oxygen, undoubtedly as a part of their structure, and that the destructive changes in the tissues taking place to a greater extent when they are active than when quiescent result in the production of an increased amount of carbon dioxide. This is true of all activity, both that of glands and of muscles as well as of other structures.

Respiration is a process of oxidation, the principal product of which is carbon dioxide. The oxygen is not converted directly into carbon dioxide, but becomes an integral part of the tissues, and in their destructive metabolism carbon dioxide is one of the products.

4. Vital Heat.

The temperature of a lifeless object is approximately that of the air which surrounds it; the temperature of a living object is independent of the temperature of the air, although it may be modified by it. This difference is due to the fact that living things produce heat within themselves: this is called "vital heat." Many, perhaps most, authorities speak of it as "animal heat," but, though it is most striking in members of the animal kingdom, yet inasmuch as its production is not confined to animals, but also occurs in plants, the writer prefers the term *vital heat* as indicating that the phenomenon is peculiar to the living condition, irrespective of the question whether it occurs in an animal or in a vegetable.

Warm-blooded Animals.—The term "warm-blooded" was applied to certain animals because their temperature was so high as to make them warm to the touch, while others were spoken of as "cold-blooded" because they were cold to the touch. Thus, man with a temperature of 37° C., the dog, 39°, the cat, 39°, the swallow, 44° or even higher, are among the warm-blooded, while reptiles and fishes, whose temperature is from 1.70° to 4.5° C. above that of the medium in which they exist, are cold-blooded. The terms warm-blooded and cold-blooded are, however, now not so frequently used as formerly, but in their stead are used the terms *homoiothermal* and *poikilothermal.*

Homoiothermal animals are animals of uniform heat or whose temperature is unvarying. The thermometer if introduced into the rectum of a man, whether he be in the tropics or in the frozen regions of the North, will register about 38° C. The temperature of the surface of his body varies with that of the air—a fact with which all are familiar—but the internal temperature is the same, irrespective of whether it is winter or summer. What is true of man is true also of other mammals and of birds; that is, of those animals commonly denominated warm-blooded.

Poikilothermal animals are animals of varying heat, or whose temperature varies according to that of the medium, air or water, in which they live. The frog's temperature is slightly above that of the water, and if this be warmer the temperature in the frog will rise, to fall again when the temperature of the water is lowered.

Fishes also exhibit this same variation of temperature, so that cold-blooded and poikilothermal are practically interchangeable terms. A study of insects shows that these creatures also produce heat, the thermometer registering, in some experiments on butterflies in active motion, a temperature of 5° C. above that of the air. These insects are poikilothermal. The same power of generating heat is observed also in plants. The amount of heat varies under different circumstances, being especially marked at the time of germination and flowering, sometimes from 5° to 10° C. above the air.

Heat-unit.—The standard of measure of heat is the heat-unit or calorie. It is the amount necessary to raise the temperature of 1 gramme of water 1° C. A kilo-calorie is equal to 1000 calories, and it represents the amount of heat necessary to raise the temperature of 1 kilogramme (litre) 1° C. It is estimated that an average man produces daily 2500 kilo-calories, which is about 100 kilo-calories per hour. During active exercise this amount is greatly increased, even to the amount of 300 kilo-calories hourly, while during sleep it is only 40 kilo-calories.

Sources of Heat.—The sources from which the heat of the body is derived are as follows:

1. The oxidation of the food-stuffs is one of the important sources of vital heat—the production of carbon dioxide (CO_2) by the oxidation of the carbon, and of water (H_2O) from the hydrogen. One gramme of carbon produces 8080 heat-units, and the same amount of hydrogen 34,460 units. The oxygen which thus combines with these elements is derived from the air during the respiratory process, and is an index of the amount of heat produced. That is to say, those animals have the

highest temperature that consume the most oxygen. The oxidation of sulphur and phosphorus, producing sulphuric and phosphoric acids, is also a source of a little heat. While oxidation is one of the principal sources of heat, many of the other chemical processes taking place in the body also result in its production.

2. Besides the chemical causes of heat-production there are physical causes. Every movement which occurs in the body produces some heat; thus, the various muscular contractions contribute largely in this direction. Active exercise always results in an increase of heat-production—a fact which is made use of when the body is chilled from exposure.

3. The changes which take place in glands during their activity are still another source of heat. This is especially noteworthy in the liver, the blood issuing from which has the highest temperature to be found anywhere in the body.

4. A factor which is doubtless of no great importance in contributing to heat-production is the electricity generated in muscles and nerves. This is converted into heat, and in that form of energy leaves the body.

Temperature of Different Parts of the Body.—The temperature of the skin at the middle of the upper arm is 35.4° C., while in the sole of the foot it is but 32.26° C. In the axilla it is about 36.5° C.; under the tongue, 37.19° C.; and in the rectum, 38° C. The mean temperature of the blood may be stated as 39° C. The temperature of the muscles is increased in contraction 1° C. Mental exertion also increases the production of heat. After such exertion the temperature of the body has been found to be 0.3° C. higher than before.

Temperature at Different Ages.—The temperature of

the child just born is 37.86° C. (rectum); in twenty-four hours, 37.45° C. (rectum). From five to nine years of age, it is 37.72° C. (rectum); from twenty-five to thirty, 36.91° C. (axilla); from fifty-one to sixty, 36.83° C. (axilla); and at eighty, 37.46° C. (mouth). The amount of heat produced in old people is less than that in the middle-aged, and they therefore need greater protection from the cold.

Daily Variations in Temperature.—The temperature of an individual is not the same at all times of the day. His lowest temperature is between 2 and 6 o'clock A. M.; it rises during the day, and between 5 and 8 P. M. is at its height, falling again until it reaches the minimum in the early morning. Thus, in one set of observations, at 5 A. M. the thermometer registered 36.6°; at 8 P. M., 37.7° C.; and at 2 A. M. the following day, 36.7° C. If the temperature be taken every hour during a day, the mean of the readings is called the "daily mean," and is about 37.13° C. in the rectum.

Remarkable Instances of High and Low Temperature.—The lowest temperature which the writer has been able to find was 24° C. This was in a drunken person who recovered from his debauch. A case of myxœdema is reported in the London *Lancet* in which, on the day previous to death, the temperature varied from 19° C. to 25° C. In the same journal is recorded a case of shock produced by a fall on the spine in which the temperature fluctuated between 47° C. and 50° C., and for seven weeks did not fall below 42° C.

The following case, recorded in the *Brooklyn Medical Journal*, illustrates the remarkable variations of temperature which may take place in a few hours. The patient was a man aged forty-eight; the diagnosis of the case was intermittent fever. He had been treated two or three months before for delirium tremens. He left the hospital, became partially paralyzed, and then developed fever, his temperature rising to 42° and 45° C.; May 1, at night, it was 44° C.; May 2, in the morning, 37° C.; May 4, 2 A. M., 44° C. He had chills, and was treated for malaria. After May 17 he had no rise of temperature. He was a wreck from alcohol.

Regulation of Temperature.—When the temperature of the muscles is raised to 49° C., they lose their contractility. This figure has been regarded as the highest that can be reached by a living human being; indeed, much below this, 45° C., has long been considered as fatal, although a temperature of nearly 52° C. has been recorded. When the temperature falls to 19° C., a fatal result will follow.

To prevent the body from becoming too hot is one of the functions of the skin. This it accomplishes by radiation, conduction, and evaporation. Of the total heat given off from the body, 73 per cent. is by radiation and conduction from the skin, and 14.5 per cent. is by evaporation. Thus there is carried off by the skin nearly 88 per cent. of the total heat. This topic will again be discussed in the consideration of the skin and its functions.

The prevention of the reduction of the temperature of the body to an extent that would be harmful is accomplished by wearing proper clothing, by the ingestion of food, both solid and liquid, by warming the air which comes in contact with the body, and by increased muscular activity. The use of alcohol for this purpose is, as previously stated, delusive.

5. Circulation of the Blood.

The blood, in carrying nutrition to, and in carrying waste products from, the tissues, makes the circuit of the circulatory apparatus, and this constitutes circulation. The circulatory apparatus consists of (1) the heart; (2) the arteries; (3) the capillaries; and (4) the veins.

The heart (Figs. 26, 27) is a muscular organ whose functions consist in acting as a reservoir and also as a pump, the *auricles* being the reservoir and the *ventricles* being the pump (Pl. 2). The heart has a conical form, its base being above and to the right, and its apex below and to the left. It is divided longitudinally by a partition or septum into a right and left half, which are sometimes denominated the right heart and the left heart. Each half is composed of an auricle and a ventricle; thus there are four cavities—the right auricle, the right ventricle, the left auricle, and the left ventricle.

The *right auricle* (Fig. 26) is somewhat larger than the left, and has the thinnest walls of the four cavities, measuring about 2 mm. in thickness. Discharging into this cavity are the superior and the inferior vena cava, at the mouths of which there are no valves. Within the cavity is the Eustachian valve, which will further be described when discussing the fœtal circulation. This valve is situated between the opening of the inferior vena cava and the auriculo-ventricular orifice.

The *right ventricle* (Fig. 26) has walls whose thickness is greater than that of either auricle, but is less than that of the left ventricle. The cavity of the right ventricle communicates with that of the right auricle by the right auriculo-ventricular orifice, at which is situated the tricuspid valve. It ordinarily contains, when filled, 180 grammes of blood. Connected with this ventricle is the

PLATE II.

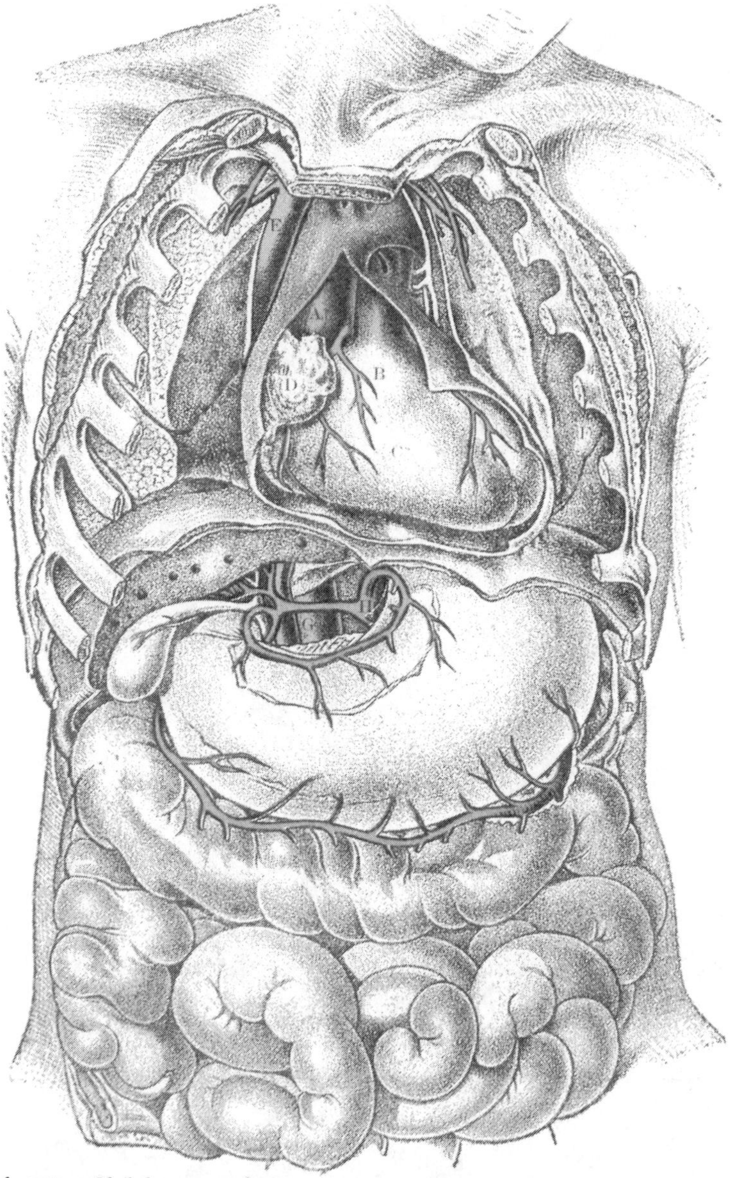

A, aorta, with left vagus and phrenic nerves crossing its transverse arch; *B*, root of pulmonary artery; *C*, right ventricle; *D*, right auricle: *E*, vena cava superior, with right phrenic nerve on its outer border; *F*, *F*, right and left lungs collapsed, and turned outward to show the heart's outline; *G*, inferior vena cava; *H*, cœliac axis, dividing into the gastric, splenic, and hepatic arteries.

pulmonary artery, at whose point of junction with the ventricle is the pulmonary orifice, at which is situated the pulmonary valve.

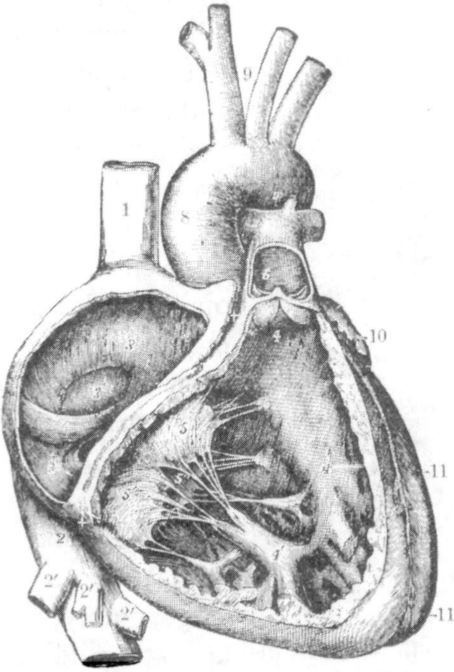

FIG. 26.—Interior of Right Auricle and Ventricle, exposed by the removal of a part of their walls (Allen Thomson): 1, superior vena cava; 2, inferior vena cava; 2′, hepatic veins; 3, 3′, 3″, inner wall of right auricle; 4, 4, cavity of right ventricle; 4′, papillary muscle; 5, 5′, 5″, flaps of tricuspid valve; 6, pulmonary artery, in the wall of which a window has been cut; 7, on aorta near the ductus arteriosus; 8, 9, aorta and its branches; 10, 11, left auricle and ventricle.

The *left auricle* (Fig. 27) is not so large as the right, but its walls are thicker. Discharging into it are the two right and the two left pulmonary veins, the former coming from the right and the latter from the left lung. The left veins sometimes join, and have but a single opening, in which case there would of course be but three openings instead of four. At these openings there are no valves.

The *left ventricle* (Fig. 27) is by far the most powerful of the four subdivisions of the heart. Its walls are three times as thick as those of the right ventricle. The capacity of its cavity is the same as that of the right. The left auricle and ventricle communicate by the left auriculo-ventricular orifice, at which is situated the mitral valve. Connected with this ventricle is the aorta, the opening of communication being the aortic orifice, at which is situated the aortic valve.

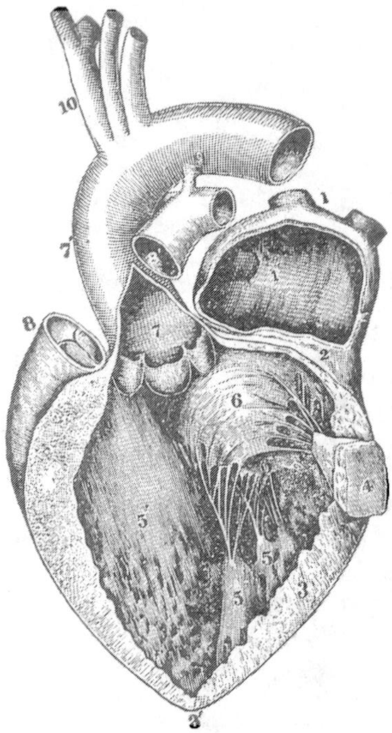

FIG. 27.—Left Auricle and Ventricle, opened and part of their walls removed to show their cavities (Allen Thomson): 1, right pulmonary vein cut short; 1′, cavity of left auricle; 3, 3″, thick wall of left ventricle; 4, portion of the same with papillary muscle attached; 5, the other papillary muscles; 6, 6′, the segments of the mitral valve; 7, in aorta is placed over the semilunar valves; 8, pulmonary artery; 10, aorta and its branches.

On the inner surface of the ventricles the muscular tissue projects, and forms the columnæ carneæ, or fleshy columns; some of these are ridges only, while others are attached at both ends, but are unattached in the middle, while still others project into the cavity and are attached at one extremity only; the latter are the musculi papillares, or papillary muscles.

Cardiac Valves.—There are four sets of valves in the heart: (1) The tricuspid; (2) the pulmonary; (3) the mitral; and (4) the aortic. The *tricuspid valve* (Fig. 28) is situated at the right auriculo-ventricular orifice, and, as its name implies, consists of three cusps or segments.

The bases of these cusps are attached to the opening, while the other edges are free, and to them are attached the chordæ tendineæ, or tendinous cords, the other ends being connected with the free extremities of the musculi papillares above referred to. This valve, when shut, closes the right auriculo-ventricular orifice; when open, the segments are in the cavity of the right ventricle. The tendinous cords prevent these segments from passing into the cavity of the auricle at the time of the valve's closure, while the papillary muscles by their contraction keep the cords taut at the time of the ventricle's contraction, as will be seen later.

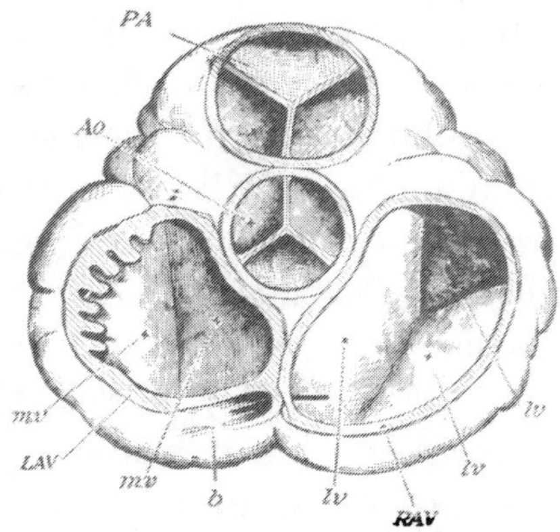

FIG. 28.—Orifices of the Heart, seen from above, both the auricles and the great vessels being removed (Huxley): *PA*, pulmonary artery and its semilunar valves; *AO*, aorta and its valves; *RAV*, tricuspid, and *LAV*, bicuspid valves; *MV*, segments of mitral valve; *LV*, segments of tricuspid valve.

The *pulmonary valve* is sometimes spoken of as the "pulmonary semilunar valve" or valves. It is composed of three, occasionally of two, segments, and is situated at the beginning of the pulmonary artery. These segments are attached at their bases to the wall of the artery, and on the free edge of each is a projection called corpus Arantii. When the valve is open the segments lie against the walls of the artery; when it is shut, they are in contact, and thus close the orifice of the pulmonary artery.

The *mitral valve* is also described as the bicuspid, because it consists of two cusps. The attachments of the segments, the presence of chordæ tendineæ, and the other anatomical points referred to in speaking of the tricuspid valve are to be seen in connection with the mitral. It closes the left auriculo-ventricular orifice.

The *aortic valve* resembles in all essential particulars the pulmonary; it likewise is sometimes called the "semilunar valve," and closes the aortic orifice. The ventricular septum is the partition between the right and the left ventricles. It is at all periods of life closed. The auricular septum, between the auricles, is closed from the tenth day after birth; prior to this time and during fœtal life it has an opening, the foramen ovale, which serves as a means of communication between the right and the left auricles.

The arteries are composed of three coats—an internal, a middle, and an external. The middle coat has a special physiological interest. In the large arteries—that is, those larger than the carotids—this coat is principally yellow elastic tissue, only about one-fourth being muscular tissue. Vessels of this size are therefore characterized by their elasticity. In the arteries of medium size—that is, those between the carotids and those having a diameter of 2 mm.—the amount of muscular tissue is very much increased, while the elastic tissue is also well represented. Such arteries possess, therefore, both contractility and elasticity. In the small arteries—that is, those less than 2 mm. in diameter—the external coat gradually disappears until in the arterioles there remains only muscular tissue, representing the middle coat and the internal coat. These vessels are endowed with the property of contractility.

The capillaries are minute vessels, being, on an average, 16 m.mm. in diameter. In some tissues, as in the brain, they are smaller, while in the skin they are larger. They are composed of endothelial cells joined edge to edge, and are exceedingly thin. From a physiological standpoint this system of vessels is the most important part of the circulatory apparatus.

The Veins.—The structure of the veins is in many respects similar to that of the arteries. They are likewise composed of three coats, but the middle coat is thinner—so much so, indeed, that, while the arteries when cut remain patulous, the veins collapse. This coat contains both elastic and fibrous tissue: the former gives these vessels some elasticity, while to the latter is attributable the greater strength of the veins as compared with the arteries. The greater thickness of the arterial wall would seem calculated to make these vessels the stronger, but, although possessed of thin walls, still the white fibrous tissue which aids in their formation gives the veins greater resisting power. Valves are to be found in most of the veins, but are absent in those whose diameter is less than 2 mm.; also from the venæ cavæ, hepatic, portal, renal, uterine, ovarian, cerebral, spinal, pulmonary, and umbilical veins. The valves are so arranged that they permit the blood to flow in the direction of the heart, but prevent its flow in the opposite direction.

Circulation of the Blood.—The course of the blood, starting from any point, may be traced through the circulatory apparatus. Beginning with the right auricle, the blood flows into this cavity from the venæ cavæ (inferior and superior); thence through the right auriculo-ventricular orifice into the right ventricle; thence into and through the pulmonary artery to the lungs; thence by the pulmonary veins into the left auricle; thence through the left auriculo-ventricular orifice into the left ventricle; thence into and through the aorta and the arterial system to the capillaries; through these vessels to the veins, by which it returns to the right auricle, the place of beginning.

Cardiac Movements.—If the heart be exposed in a living animal—a dog, for example—it will be seen that the ventricles are at one time in motion and at another time at rest. Each period of motion and rest constitutes a "pulsation" or a cardiac cycle, and these pulsations recur very rapidly, so much so that the intervals are recognized with difficulty. These different states of the heart are better detected by the sense of touch than by that of sight. If the ventricles be grasped by the hand, it will be found that, corresponding with the resting stage, the muscular tissue composing them is soft and flaccid, while during the active stage it is hard and resisting. If these movements be studied still more carefully and analyzed, it will be found that the beginning of the cardiac movement, which immediately follows the stage of rest, occurs in the auricles, in the region of the openings of the venæ cavæ on the right side, and in the pulmonary veins on the left; that this movement is propagated along the auricles in the direction of the ventricles; and that by the time it has reached the auriculo-ventricular orifices it has ceased at the orifices of the veins, and the muscular tissue in this region has begun to relax. It is to be noted that the auricles act synchronously, so that whatever is the condition of one auricle as to relaxation or contraction of its muscular tissue, the same condition exists in the other. This contraction of the auricles is spoken of as the "auricular systole," and has something of the peristaltic character, which has already been studied in the stomach and small intestine, although differing very materially in that it is much more rapid.

Up to this time the ventricles have been relaxed, or in a condition of diastole, but as soon as the auricular contraction reaches the ventricles these organs take it up, although in a different manner. For, while in the auricles one portion is contracting while another is relaxing, in the ventricles the whole mass of muscle contracts at once with a degree of suddenness and vigor which might be expected of so large a mass of striped muscular tissue. This contraction is the "ventricular systole," and while it is taking place the auricles are relaxing throughout; this relaxation constitutes the "auricular diastole." Thus the auricular systole and ventricular diastole, and the auricular diastole and ventricular systole, are respectively synchronous. Immediately after the systole of the ventricles these structures relax, and for a brief period the whole heart, both auricles and both ventricles, is in a state of relaxation; this is the "pause" of the heart. The work performed by the ventricles is so much more important than that of the auricles that when the terms *systole* and *diastole* are used reference is always had to these states of the ventricles, the auricles being practically ignored. To designate the corresponding states of the auricles it is always necessary to speak of the auricular systole and diastole.

Movements of Blood during Systole and Diastole.—Before considering other movements of the heart it will be well to study the course of the blood while contraction and relaxation of the muscular tissue of this organ are taking place.

The venous blood, returning from the head and upper

extremities by the superior or descending vena cava, and from the portion of the body below the heart by the inferior or ascending vena cava, flows into and through the right auricle, passing into the right ventricle through the right auriculo-ventricular orifice. The tricuspid valve at this time is open, and offers no obstacle to the passage of the blood. More blood enters the auricles than can at once pass out of them into the ventricles; consequently some blood accumulates in, and gradually fills, the auricles, although at the same time as much blood is flowing into the ventricles as the auriculo-ventricular orifices will permit to pass, nearly filling these cavities, and floating up the segments of the mitral and tricuspid valves until they are nearly closed. This is the condition at the end of the pause. At this moment begins the auricular systole. Near the ends of the veins which discharge into the auricles—that is, the venæ cavæ and pulmonary veins—are muscular fibres: these fibres contract, diminishing the size of the orifices of the veins, thus taking the place of valves, and partially preventing regurgitation or a back-flow of blood into these vessels. Then the muscular fibres of the auricles in contiguity with these fibres contract, the motion spreading to the adjoining fibres until the wave of contraction has reached the ventricles. This auricular contraction forces more blood into the ventricles, and as the fibres relax the blood enters the auricles again from the veins. It will thus be seen that the interval during which the venous flow is arrested is the briefest time possible. The principal office of the auricles is to serve as reservoirs to supply the ventricles; the work they do in completing the filling of these cavities is comparatively unimportant.

The auricular systole is followed by the systole of the

ventricles. These cavities are at this time filled with blood, and the auriculo-ventricular valves are nearly closed, the segments having been raised up by the blood from the auricles. The ventricles, as has been stated, contract *en masse*, and the blood which they contain is compressed with great force. Under the pressure it tends to escape from the ventricles by all outlets—on the right side by the right auriculo-ventricular orifice back into the right auricle, and by the pulmonary orifice into the pulmonary artery; on the left side by the left auriculo-ventricular orifice into the left auricle, and by the aortic orifice into the aorta. The pressure of the blood instantly closes the tricuspid valve, and thus prevents the blood from going back into the right auricle. The same force closes the mitral valve, and the regurgitation of blood into the left auricle is made impossible. The pulmonary and aortic valves, as has been stated, open from the ventricles into the arteries. At the beginning of the ventricular systole the valves are closed, but when this occurs the pressure of the blood forces them open, and the contents of the ventricles, 180 grammes for each, are propelled into the pulmonary artery and the aorta respectively. In accomplishing this injection the ventricles have to overcome the pressure which the blood already in the arteries is exerting on the other side of the valves to keep them closed. This pressure in the aorta is equal to a column of mercury 200 mm. high, and in the pulmonary artery is one-third as much. The amount of work done by the ventricle daily in thus forcing blood into the arteries is equal to that which is performed by an individual weighing 75 kilogrammes in climbing a mountain 806 metres in height.

As soon as the ventricles cease their contraction the

pressure of the blood in the arteries closes the pulmonary and aortic valves, the ventricles begin their diastole, and the pause of the heart commences. As it was at this point that the consideration of the changes which take place was begun, the study of a cardiac cycle, cardiac period, or heart-beat is now completed. If the time occupied by such a period be divided into one hundred parts, it will be found that the auricular systole lasts during nine of the parts, the ventricular systole during thirty, and the pause during sixty-one; or, in other words, the heart is at rest six-tenths and at work four-tenths of the time.

Shortening of the Heart.—At the time of the systole of the heart (ventricular systole) the organ becomes shorter, yet the apex does not change its place, for the lengthening of the aorta which occurs compensates for the shortening, so that while the apex and base approximate the whole heart is lowered, the result being to keep the apex in its original position with reference to the chest-wall.

Cardiac Impulse.—The situation of the heart in the thoracic cavity is such that its apex is against the chest-wall at the fifth intercostal space, the space between the fifth and sixth ribs, and an inch and a half below and half an inch within the left nipple. The apex of the heart is the extreme point of the left ventricle. If the finger be placed in this region during the ventricular systole, there will be felt a *tap* as if something were gently striking it. This tap is known as the "apex-beat." It was so called because it was formerly supposed that during the systole the heart was raised up and so carried forward as to cause the apex to strike against the chest-wall and thus to produce this sensation. A more careful study of the changes which the heart undergoes during systole has, however, demonstrated that the apex of the heart is always in contact with the chest-wall, and that this supposed striking does not take place. Indeed, the tap is not due to the apex at all. The term *apex-beat* is a misnomer: it should rather be called a "cardiac impulse," the sensation being produced by the anterior surface of the contracting ventricles swelling out and hardening. The location at which this impulse is felt most pronouncedly is not over the apex, but higher up. If a long needle were to be introduced deeply at this point, it would penetrate the left ventricle at a point where the middle and lower thirds unite. The cardiac impulse is not always, even in health, detected at the same place: it changes somewhat with respiration and also with changes in the position of the body.

Papillary Muscles.—It has been stated that during the ventricular systole the heart shortens. It is manifest that unless some provision were made this change in the shape of the heart would permit of regurgitation of the blood into the auricles, and thus would result a damming back of the blood in the venæ cavæ and pulmonary veins; for if the chordæ tendineæ were of just the right length at the beginning of the ventricular systole to keep the segments of the mitral and tricuspid valves so exactly in place as not to permit a leakage, then when the ventricles shortened these cords would be too long, and would permit the segments to enter the cavity of the auricles and thus separate, leaving a considerable gap through which the blood could pass. That this does not occur is due to the papillary muscles. As the ventricles shorten these structures contract sufficiently to take up the slack in the cords, and keep them just long enough to maintain the proper approximation of the segments of the valves.

Cardiac Sounds.—When the ear is placed against the chest-wall in the region of the heart, two sounds are heard during each cardiac period. The first of these sounds is heard loudest—that is, at its maximum of intensity—over the apex, and is by some writers called the "apex-sound." For the reason that it is the first sound heard after the pause it is called the "first sound," and because it occurs at the beginning of the systole of the heart (ventricular systole) it is called the "systolic sound." The second sound is heard loudest over the base of the heart, and is therefore sometimes described as the "basic sound;" inasmuch as it occurs during the diastole, it has received the name of the "diastolic sound." More commonly, however, it is spoken of as the "second sound."

Characteristics of the Cardiac Sounds.—The first sound, as compared with the second, is lower in pitch and longer in duration, and has been likened to the sound of the word *lūbb.* The second sound is higher in pitch and shorter in duration than the first, and has been likened to the sound of *dŭp.* These sounds occur successively, without any interval between them; in the pause which follows no sound is heard.

Causes of the Cardiac Sounds.—The cause of the second sound is undoubtedly the closure of the aortic and pulmonary valves. This has been demonstrated by hooking back the segments of the valves, when the sound disappeared, to reappear when the segments were set free. The causation of the first sound is not so simple; indeed, authorities are not at one on this point. The closure of the mitral and tricuspid valves contributes something to it, but the closing of the valves is not the sole factor, for in a heart in which there is no blood the sound may still be heard, although modified, and in such a heart the valves would not close. The contraction of the muscular tissue of the heart gives forth a sound, as does indeed the contraction of other muscles, and this is also an element in producing the first sound. The striking of the apex against the chest-wall, the so-called apex-beat, formerly regarded as one of the factors of the first sound, can take no part in its production, because, as has been pointed out, this action does not take place.

Every student should familiarize himself with the cardiac sounds, not simply by reading about them in books, but by listening to the human chest. A thorough knowledge of their character is essential to a comprehension of the diseases of the heart. It is important to remember that the impulse of the heart, the systole of the ventricles, the first sound, and the closure of the mitral and tricuspid valves are synchronous, and that when the second sound is heard the ventricles are beginning their diastole and the aortic and pulmonary valves have just closed.

Circulation in the Arteries (Fig. 33).—Each time that the ventricles contract they send into the arteries 360 grammes of blood, each ventricle expelling 180 grammes. The arterial system is always over-distended; that is, even when the heart is at rest the amount of blood in the arteries is enough to stretch their walls a little. When an additional amount of blood is forced into them by the muscular contraction of the heart, these vessels are distended still more, for the blood already in them cannot at once flow on in an amount equal to that which comes from the heart. If an artery at this time should be felt with the finger, it would beat against the latter, this beat being the *pulse.* As soon as the systole ceases the elastic coats of the arteries squeeze the blood within them, and this blood tends to flow away from the point of pressure in two directions—back toward the heart and onward toward the capillaries. Its backward flow at once closes the pulmonary and aortic valves, and in this direction, therefore, its progress is barred. The blood then can only go forward. Before the onward flow of the blood has ceased another systole occurs, and again the ventricles are emptied into the arteries, and thus continues this action during the life of the individual. If a cannula be inserted into the cavity of the ventricle, it will be seen that at each systole the blood spurts out in a jet, which ceases at the end of the systole; that is, the flow from the heart is intermittent. If the cannula be inserted into the aorta, the blood will jet out at each systole of the heart, but, instead of ceasing to flow during diastole, it will not entirely cease, but will continue to flow a little under the influence of the elastic force of the aorta. If the cannula be inserted into successive portions of the arterial system farther and farther from the heart, the blood will come out in jets as before under the influence of the heart's contraction, but it will continue to flow in the intervals, the difference between the jet and the continuous flow being less and less marked the greater is the distance of the insertion of the cannula from the heart. In the capillaries the flow is regular and continuous, unaffected by the action of the heart.

Internal Friction.—If the blood be studied as it is flowing through a small artery in the web of a frog's foot, it will be seen that in the centre of the current it is flowing much faster than at the sides; this is the "axial stream," and in it will be observed the red corpuscles. That portion of the current which is between the axial stream and the walls of the vessel moves more slowly, the rate diminishing from the centre outward, until at the walls themselves it is at the minimum. This outer portion is known as the "inert layer." It should be stated that this arrangement of the current is not due to any peculiarity of the blood or of the vessels through which it flows, but is present in every fluid while flowing through a tube. Between the different layers of fluid there is friction, called "internal friction." The smaller the tubes the greater the internal friction, so that the amount of friction in the subdivisions of the aorta and the larger arteries and in the capillaries is very great, and this friction acts as an obstacle to the outflow of the blood, constituting peripheral resistance.

Arterial Pressure.—If a U-tube containing mercury be connected with an artery, the mercury will rise in the distal end under the influence of the pressure on the other end of the blood on the column. This, then, will indicate the arterial pressure; that is, the pressure under which the blood is in the arteries. In the aorta it is equal to a column of mercury 200 mm. in height. At the time of the systole it will be 5 mm. more. In the pulmonary artery the pressure is one-third that in the aorta.

Rate of Flow in the Arteries.—It has been calculated that in the carotid artery of a man the blood flows at the rate of 400 mm. per second. Inasmuch as the capacity of the arterial system increases as the arteries divide, the current in the smaller arteries will be slower than in the larger; in the metatarsal artery one observer found it to be but 56 mm.

Pulse-wave.—The rate at which the blood flows and that at which the pulse-wave moves are two different quantities. In the former case we are dealing, as it were, with the velocity of the same portions of the blood or the same individual corpuscles. In the latter case we are dealing with a wave which starts at the aortic valve and is propagated through the entire mass of arterial blood; manifestly the rate of the latter will be much

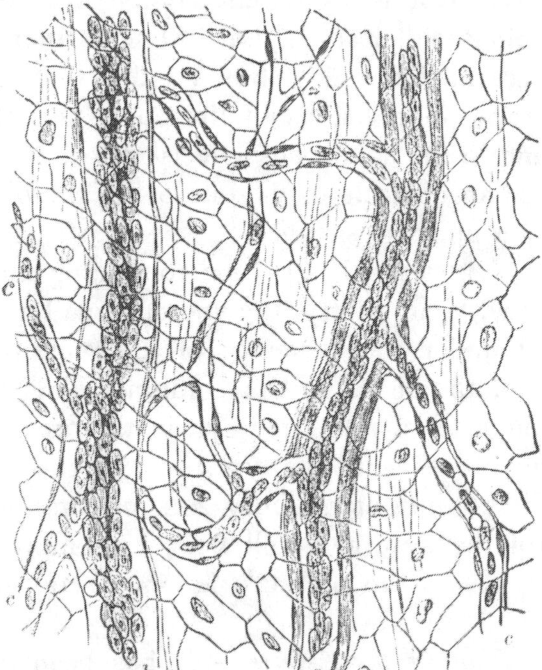

FIG. 29.—Normal Vessels and Blood-stream (Landerer): *a*, artery; *b*, vein; *c*, capillary.

faster. At the commencement of the aorta the wave begins; in 0.159 seconds it will be felt at the wrist, and in 0.193 seconds at the ankle. It travels at the rate of 9 metres per second.

Circulation in the Capillaries (Fig. 29).—The forces which propel the blood through the arteries—namely, the contractile force of the ventricles and the elastic force of the arteries, collectively called the *vis a tergo*—are sufficient to carry the blood on through the capillaries. The sectional area of the capillaries is seven hundred times greater than that of the aorta, so that the blood which flows through this latter vessel at the rate, perhaps, of 500 mm. per second is, when it reaches the capillaries, so widely distributed that its flow is very much reduced in rapidity—only about 1 mm. per second.

It is while passing through the capillary system that the important interchanges take place between the blood and the tissues. It is here that the tissues receive from the blood the materials they require for their nutrition, and in the case of glands for their secretion; and it is likewise here that the blood receives from the tissues their waste products. The thin walls of the capillaries are admirably adapted for this interchange. In fact, it is within bounds to say that the heart, the arteries, and the veins are simply subsidiary to the capillaries, the arteries carrying to these vessels the blood which the heart pumps into them, while the veins return the blood to the heart.

Circulation in the Veins (Fig. 29).—The *vis a tergo* is not exhausted in the capillary system, but is still at work in the veins, and would of itself be sufficient to return the blood to the heart; for, as has been noted, the pressure in the aorta is equal to a column of mercury 200 mm. in height. In the veins this pressure is at most only about 5 mm., and it is sometimes actually negative, so that there is a difference of pressure of 195 mm. of mercury. The *vis a tergo* is, however, in the systemic circulation—that is, that which begins with the left ventricle and ends in the right auricle, aided by two other forces: 1, compression of the veins; 2, aspiration of the thorax.

Compression of the Veins.—It will be remembered that in the veins there are, at different points along their course, valves which are so arranged as to permit the blood to flow in but one direction; that is, toward the heart. Many of these veins are so situated with reference to muscles that when the muscles contract the contiguous veins are compressed. This compression forces the contained blood away from the points of pressure, and as the closure of the valves prevents the blood from flowing backward, it must go forward.

Aspiration of the Thorax.—At each inspiration the cavity of the chest is enlarged and the pressure on its contents is diminished. It has already been stated that one of the results of this inspiration is the inflowing of air. Another result is the inflowing of blood into the venæ cavæ and right auricle, for while the intrathoracic pressure is diminished, that upon the blood-vessels outside remains the same. A similar tendency exists for the blood in the aorta to flow back into the left ventricle, but this is prevented by the aortic valve. Inasmuch as the whole of the pulmonary circulation is within the chest, all parts are alike influenced during the respiratory movements, so that the force of aspiration of the thorax has no effect upon this part of the circulation.

Force of Gravity.—The force of gravity assists in the return of the blood to the heart from the upper portions of the body, but retards its return from the lower portions, so that as a factor in aiding the circulation as a whole it may be ignored. This force may, however, be utilized whenever for any reason there is congestion in a part—as, for instance, in a foot the seat of inflammation. In such a case the elevation of the lower extremity facilitates the flow of blood in the veins and proves beneficial. Also, when by reason of an imperfect performance of its function the heart fails to send enough blood to the brain, and fainting occurs, relief will come more promptly if the patient be at once placed on the back, with the head lower than the heart, thus assisting that organ in sending blood to the anæmic brain.

The average rate of flow in the large veins is about 100 mm. per second. It is slowest in the small veins, and increases as the heart is approached. The length of time required to complete the entire systemic circulation is about twenty-four seconds. It is estimated that the blood occupies but one second in traversing the capillaries.

6. Lymphatic System.

The lymphatic system is composed of lymphatic vessels and lymphatic glands.

Lymphatic Vessels.—The larger lymphatic vessels structurally are like the veins, being composed of three coats, the middle coat containing both muscular and elastic fibres. Unlike the veins, however, muscular fibres are found in the external coat. The smaller vessels have only a connective-tissue coat lined with endothelium. In the lymphatic vessels, as in the veins, are valves opening toward the heart. The origin of these vessels in the tissues, as a rule, is by plexuses or by stomata, as in serous membranes, or by blind extremities, as in the lacteals. They ultimately discharge into the venous system—on the left side through the thoracic duct, and on the right side by the right lymphatic duct.

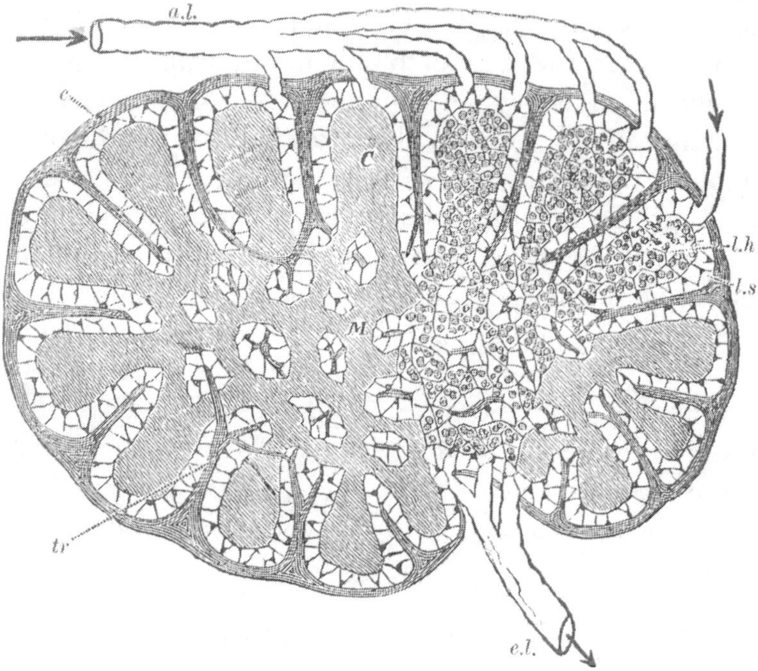

Fig. 30.—Diagram of a Lymphatic Gland (Sharpey), showing afferent (*a.l.*) and efferent (*e.l.*) lymphatic vessels; cortical substance (*C*); medullary substance (*M*); fibrous coat (*c*), sending trabeculæ (*tr*) into the substance of the gland, where they branch, and in the medullary part form a reticulum; the trabeculæ are surrounded by the lymph-path or sinus (*l.s*), which separates them from the adenoid tissue (*l.h*).

Lymphatic Glands.—The lymphatic glands (Fig. 30) are bodies of a pale reddish color, and are oval in shape. Their diameter is from 2 mm. to 20 mm. Lymphatic vessels run into the glands—the afferent; and out of them—the efferent; and through them pass the lymph and the chyle. They consist of capsule, trabeculæ, and alveoli. In the alveoli is the lymphoid tissue containing the lymph-corpuscles or leucocytes. In passing through these glands poisonous matter which has been absorbed by the lymph may be deposited, and thus its entrance into the blood may be prevented.

The lymph and its source, having already been discussed, need not again be referred to. It is taken up by the lymphatic capillaries in the tissues by endosmosis, and, as it accumulates there, gradually fills the larger vessels, and, as it is readily discharged into the venous system, there is set up a current which is the lymphatic circulation. It is to be noted, however, that there is no true circulation, as in the case of the blood. The blood goes out from the heart and returns again, completing a circuit, but here the flow is always in one direction, toward the heart.

Additional aids to the endosmotic force in producing the movement of the lymph are the contractions of the muscles of the body, by which, as in the veins, the lymphatics are compressed, and the lymph, being prevented by the valves from flowing back, is propelled toward the heart. The pressure exerted by the walls of the aorta in its pulsations compresses the thoracic duct in a similar manner, and, as this possesses valves, the onflow of the lymph and chyle is favored. The force of aspiration of the thorax is also a factor in the movement of the lymph, acting as was stated in the case of the venous blood. It has been estimated that the amount of lymph absorbed daily in a human adult is about 2000 grammes, and of lymph and chyle together 3000 grammes.

7. Ductless Glands.

This term includes the spleen, the thymus and thyroid glands, the suprarenal capsules, the pineal gland, and the pituitary body. They have received this name because they lack excretory ducts. For the reason that they are believed to have important relations to the blood they are sometimes described as "blood-glands" or "vascular glands."

Spleen.—The weight of the spleen varies at different periods of life, being at birth to the entire body as 1 is to 350; in adult life, as 1 to 320 and 400; and in old age, as 1 to 700, while in certain diseased conditions, such as ague, syphilis, or heart disease, it may be enormously increased, in some cases as much as 1 to 7 or 9 kilogrammes, the average normal weight being about 170 grammes. The size of the spleen is greatest during digestion and least during starvation. The splenic substance is made up of fibrous bands or trabeculæ, vessels, nerves, Malpighian bodies, and a dark-brown soft mass called the "spleen-pulp." In the latter are cells and free nuclei, together with blood-corpuscles both white and red, many of the red corpuscles being in various stages of disintegration. The large size of the splenic artery and its tortuosity are noteworthy.

Functions of the Spleen.—The large size of the splenic artery suggests that under some circumstances a very considerable amount of blood may be carried to this organ. This has suggested the view that the spleen might serve as a reservoir for the blood when it was not needed in the other abdominal organs. This view may or may not be correct, but this function is certainly not essential, as is shown by the fact that after the removal of the spleen, so far as can be seen, no interference with the functions of these organs occurs.

Authorities are in general united in the belief that the connection of the spleen with the blood is intimate. Some of them incline to the theory that the red corpuscles are here formed from the white; other authorities maintain that here the red corpuscles undergo disintegration; while still others attribute to the spleen the formation of leucocytes. This last it certainly does to a very great extent in cases of leukæmia.

Whatever its functions may be—for it is possible that they may be several—this organ is one which is not essential to life either in animals or in man. From the dog it has repeatedly been removed, and the results have been an increase of appetite and of ferocity, although in some instances even this was not observed. Besides these changes the red corpuscles are diminished and the white corpuscles are increased, but, as has already been stated, the marrow of bones has blood-making powers, and this marrow probably soon takes up the work formerly performed by the spleen in making red corpuscles, and the normal proportions are soon reproduced.

The congenital absence of the spleen has occurred in the human subject without the corresponding loss of any functions of the body so far as known. The human spleen has also been removed, with the result of lessening the number of red, and increasing the white, corpuscles, but this, as in the dog, has not been permanent. The spleen has been extirpated after injuries, and also in the condition known as "floating spleen" and in enlargement of the organ, but the fatal results which have followed have caused the practice to be abandoned.

Thymus Gland.—This organ belongs to fœtal life and to that of early childhood, forming at the third month of intra-uterine life and reaching its maximum of growth at the end of the second year, at which time it diminishes, and disappears at puberty. It is regarded by some as a producer of red blood-corpuscles, while others consider it a former of leucocytes, pointing in confirmation of this to the fact that in reptiles, where lymphatic glands are not found, the thymus does not atrophy, but is a permanent organ.

Thyroid Gland.—The function of the thyroid gland is unknown, although it is regarded by some authorities as a blood-forming gland. The effect of its removal would seem to indicate that it has something to do with regulating the amount of mucin formed in the body. After this operation a condition known as "myxœdema" is observed, in which the connective tissues become infiltrated with a mucin-containing material. A similar condition may result from disease of the thyroid. Another result of the removal of the thyroid is cretinism, a disease common in the Alps, in which there is a condition of the intellectual faculties approaching idiocy. Associated with it, in the Alps, there is usually goitre, an enlargement of the thyroid. Goitre may, however, exist without cretinism.

Suprarenal Capsules.—The fact that in some cases of Addison's disease (characterized by a bronzing of the skin) the suprarenal capsules have been found diseased has led some authors to entertain the opinion that they were in some way related to the coloration of the skin. Some authorities think that they are concerned in preventing the production of too much blood-coloring substance, but as a matter of fact nothing definite is known about them. They may be removed without producing any marked results.

Pituitary Body and Pineal Gland.—These small bodies are situated at the base of the brain. Their functions are unknown, but, being vascular, they are regarded as belonging to the vascular ductless glands.

8. The Skin.

The skin is composed of a deep portion, the corium, derma, or true skin, and of a superficial portion, the epidermis or cuticle.

Corium.—The corium makes up by far the greater part

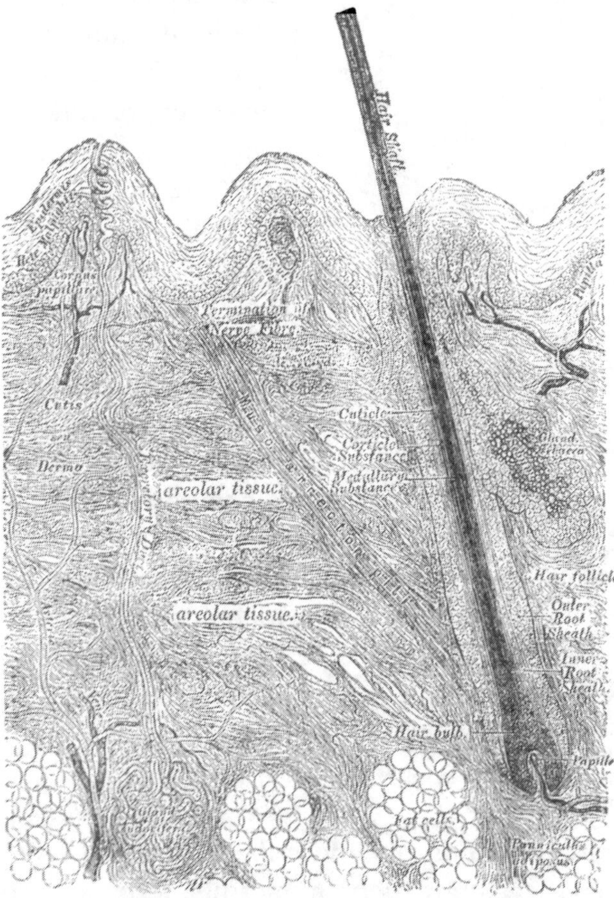

Fig. 31.—Vertical Section of the Skin, diagrammatic (after Heitzmann).

of the skin, and within it are the perspiratory glands, the sebaceous glands, the hairs, together with both blood-

and lymphatic vessels. The upper surface, where it joins the epidermis, is irregular, being composed of elevations—papillæ—and intervening depressions. In some of these papillæ are the tactile corpuscles, in which nerve-fibres end.

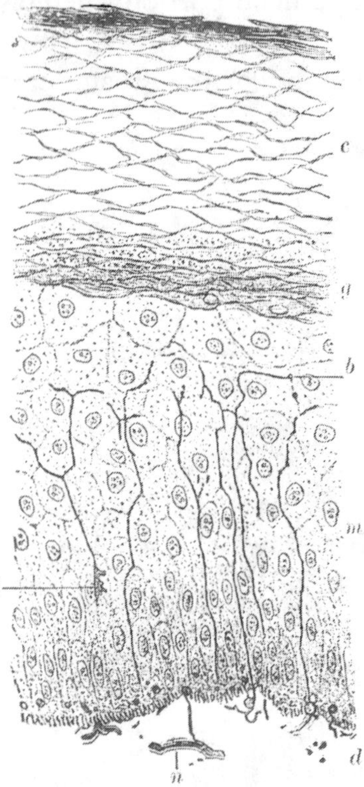

FIG. 32.—*c*, corneous (horny) layer; *g*, granular layer; *m*, mucous layer (rete Malpighii). The stratum lucidum is the layer just above the granular layer. Nerve-terminations: *n*, afferent nerve; *b*, terminal nerve-bulbs; *l*, cell of Langerhaus (after Ranvier).

Epidermis.—The epidermis is made up of a deep and a superficial layer. The deep layer (rete mucosum or rete Malpighii) covers the papillæ of the corium and fills the depressions between them. It is composed of cells, round or of different shapes due to pressure of contiguous cells, the material of which they are composed yielding readily. It is in this layer that the pigment is deposited which characterizes the dark races. The superficial layer of the epidermis is composed of cells which are flat and dry or horny.

Perspiratory Glands.—The perspiratory glands, also described as sweat- and sudoriparous glands, are very numerous, it being estimated that in the entire skin there are not less than 2,400,000. They are more abundant in some parts of the body than in others: in the palm of the hand there are 42 to the square centimetre; on the forehead, 190; and on the cheek, 85. If all these glands in the body were straightened out and put end to end, they would extend a distance of 4 kilometres.

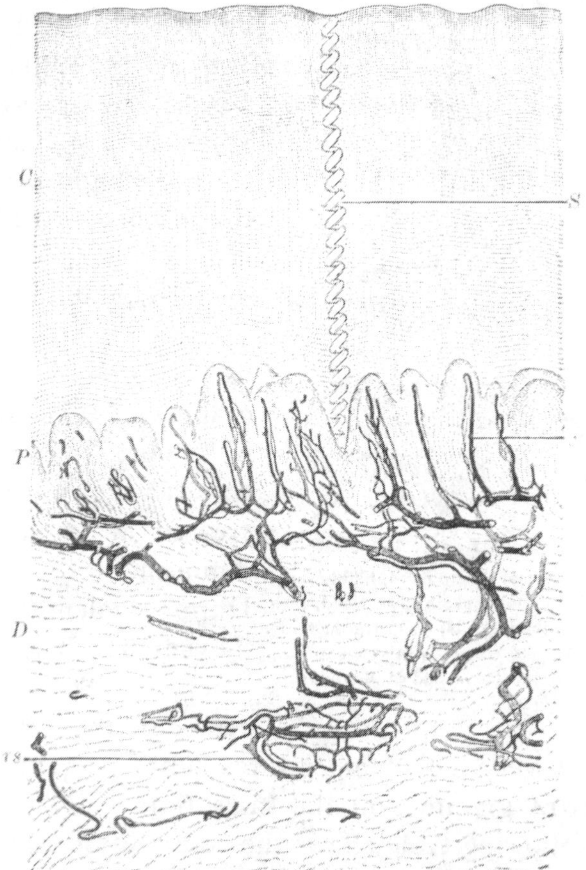

FIG. 33.—*C*, epidermis; *D*, corium; *P*, papillæ; *S*, sweat-gland duct; *v*, arterial and venous capillaries (superficial or papillary plexus) of the papillæ (deep plexus is partly shown at lower margin of the diagram); *vs*, an intermediate plexus, an outgrowth from the deep plexus, supplying sweat-glands and giving a loop to hair-papilla (after Ranvier).

This brief consideration of the perspiratory glands suggests that their function must be very important.

They are constantly at work pouring out their secretions upon the surface of the skin. Ordinarily this secretion is not perceptible, and it is then called "insensible perspiration." Upon active exercise or when the temperature of the air is high this secretion becomes visible, and it is then called "sweat" or "perspiration." The average total amount daily formed is 900 grammes. This amount is subject to considerable variations, being increased in summer and diminished in winter. During violent exercise the amount may be as much as 380 grammes per hour, and during exposure to very high temperatures it has been known to reach 1814 grammes in the same time.

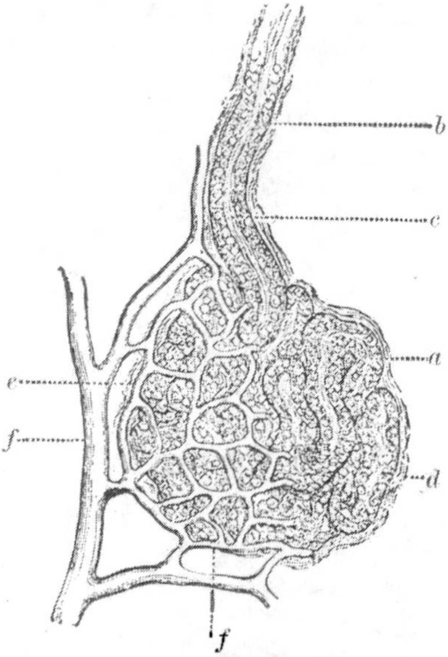

FIG. 34.—A Normal Sweat-gland, highly magnified (after Neumann): *a*, sweat-coil, with secreting epithelial cells; *b*, sweat-duct; *c*, lumen of duct; *d*, connective-tissue capsule; *e* and *f*, arterial trunk and capillaries supplying the gland.

The following table shows the composition of sweat:

Water	99.00	per cent.
Urea	.15	" "
Neutral fats, fatty acids, cholesterin, sodium and potassium chloride and other salts . .	.85	" "
	100.00	

Sweat has a salty taste, a specific gravity of 1003 to 1005, and is acid in reaction. It is claimed by some writers that its true reaction is alkaline, and that its acidity is in reality due to the presence of fatty acids resulting from the decomposition of the sebum. In uræmia the amount of urea may be so great as to crystallize on the skin; in diabetes sugar may be found in the sweat; and in cases of gout uric acid has been detected.

Office of Perspiration.—One of the important means of regulating the temperature of the body is the perspiration. Without it exposure to high temperatures would be injurious, and in some cases would even be fatal. An external temperature of 52° C. is not infrequently met with in the southern part of the United States: to this heat human beings are exposed without suffering from its effects. The evaporation of the perspiration abstracts heat from the body. Of the heat given off from the body, 88 per cent. passes off by the skin; of this amount, 73 per cent. is by radiation and conduction, and 14.5 per cent. by evaporation.

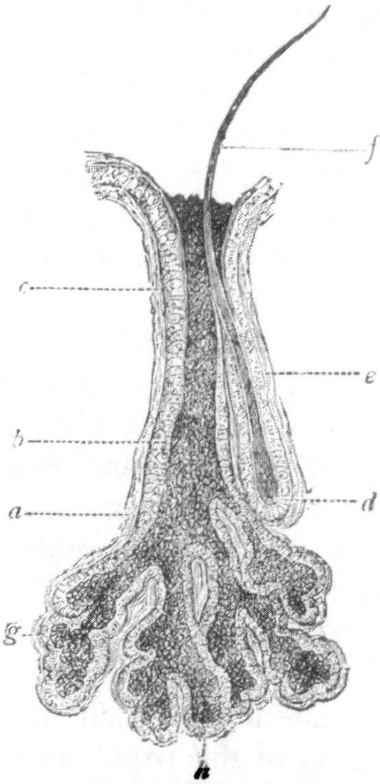

FIG. 35.—A Normal Sebaceous Gland in connection with a lanugo hair; greatly magnified (after Neumann): *a*, connective-tissue capsule; *b*, fatty secretion; *c*, *h*, fat-secreting cells; *d*, root of a lanugo hair; *e*, hair-sac; *f*, hair-shaft; *g*, acini of sebaceous gland.

Sebaceous Glands.—The sebaceous glands are racemose glands, and discharge their product—sebum—into the hair-follicles of large hairs, as upon the scalp, while in other portions of the body, as the forehead, where the hairs are small, the hair projects from the mouth of the sebaceous gland, and is more like an appendage than a separate structure.

Composition of Sebum.—The sebum, or sebaceous matter, is of an oily nature. It contains albumin, fat, and cholesterin. The *vernix caseosa* which covers the infant during the latter part of fœtal life is of the same character, consisting principally of fat with epithelium. At the temperature of the body the sebum is fluid, but it solidifies on the surface of the skin. Its office is mainly to keep the skin and the hairs soft and pliable. Besides this it is probably excrementitious to a certain extent.

Cerumen, commonly called "ear-wax," is the product of the sebaceous and perspiratory glands of the external auditory meatus, and is composed principally of fat with some soap. It is a reddish substance having a sweetish-bitter taste.

Hairs and Nails.—These structures are modified epidermis. The hair grows from the hair-papilla, in the interior of which there is a blood-vessel. The integrity of this papilla is essential to the existence of the hair; when destroyed the hair can never be reproduced. It should be noted that the hair-papillæ and the papillæ already described in connection with the corium are very different structures, and they should not be confounded. It has been estimated that there are, on an average, 120,000 hairs in the scalp. As a rule, the lighter the color of hair the finer it is; in the female it is coarser than in the male.

Functions of the Skin.—The functions of the skin are numerous and very important.

(1) *Protection.*—The tissues which lie beneath the skin are delicate and sensitive, and are protected from injury by it. The epidermis, by reason of its hard and tough

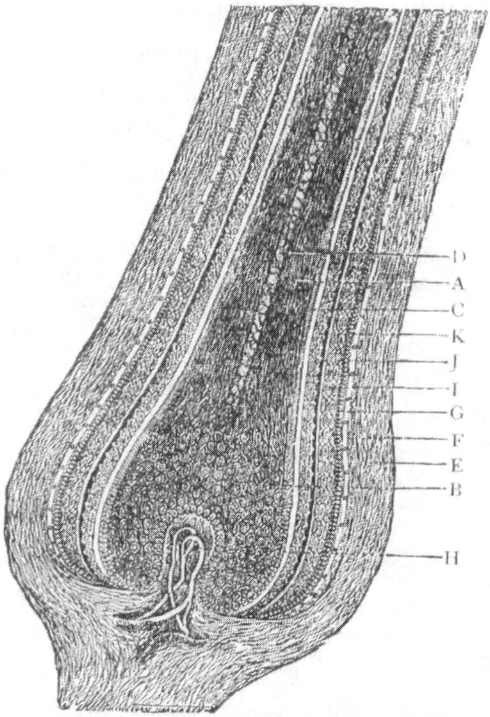

Fig. 36.—A, shaft of the hair; B, root of the hair; C, cuticle of the hair; D, medullary substance of the hair; E, external layer of the hair-follicle: F, middle layer of the hair-follicle: G, internal layer of the hair-follicle; H, papilla of the hair; I, external root-sheath; J, outer layer of the internal root-sheath; K, internal layer of the internal root-sheath (after Duhring).

character, especially in the palms of the hands and on the soles of the feet, is peculiarly adapted to this end.

(2) *Excretion.*—It has already been noted that by the skin a litre of fluid is daily eliminated from the body. In this fluid are dissolved materials representing the waste of the tissues. There is a reciprocal relation between the skin and the kidneys: in summer, when

the skin is active, the amount of fluid passed off by the kidneys is reduced, while in winter, when the skin is inactive, the work of the kidneys is much increased. In diseased conditions of the kidneys, when these organs are incapacitated for the performance of their function, the retention in the blood of poisonous materials which are eliminated in health is prevented by causing the perspiratory glands of the skin to assume the task.

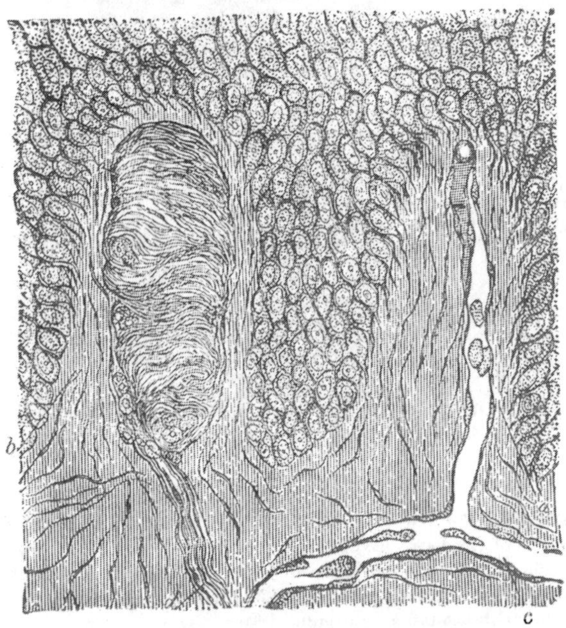

FIG. 37.—*a*, a vascular papilla; *b*, a nervous papilla; *c*, a blood-vessel; *d*, a nerve-fibre; *e*, a tactile corpuscle (after Biesiadecki).

(3) *Sensation.*—The skin, especially at the tips of the fingers, being very sensitive, gives knowledge of the consistency of objects, whether they are rough or smooth, sharp or dull, hard or soft, etc. This subject of general sensibility will be fully discussed in connection with the Nervous Functions.

(4) *Respiration.*—Interchanges are constantly taking place in the skin analogous to those which take place in the lungs, although to a much less extent. Oxygen is absorbed from the air by the blood in the cutaneous blood-vessels, and at the same time carbon dioxide is given off. In frogs these interchanges are much more extensive than in man.

(5) *Regulation of temperature,* which has already been discussed.

Care of the Skin.—That the skin may perform its functions properly it must be taken care of. The orifices of the ducts of the perspiratory and sebaceous glands must be kept free, so that they may not become clogged. If the skin of an animal be covered with varnish, it speedily dies. This is not due to the retention of waste materials, which act as poisons, but to the great loss of heat, in the rabbit the temperature falling to 20° C. Experiment has shown that if an animal that has been varnished be packed in cotton and kept in a temperature of 30° C., it will survive.

The skin requires both friction and bathing to maintain it in a physiological condition. The process of rubbing removes the useless epidermic scales and any obstructions which tend to clog the mouths of the glands. The oily nature of the sebaceous matter, which is always present and which retains the dust and dirt coming in contact with it, requires that the skin be washed with water and soap. But the soap must be free from irritating ingredients, such as rancid fat, and from too large an amount of alkali and coloring matter, and from drugs of various kinds. If the skin be diseased, medication by means of soap may be needed, but it should be prescribed by a physician. If the skin be not diseased, medicated soaps are harmful. Old white castile soap meets all the indications in health.

Baths.—Baths may be classified as follows:

Cold bath	0° to 24° C.
Temperate bath	24° to 26° C.
Tepid bath	26° to 32° C.
Warm "	32° to 37° C.
Hot "	37° to 44° C.

As a rule, hot baths are relaxing, and should not, therefore, be indulged in too frequently; indeed, in persons suffering with disease of the heart they may actually endanger life. The Turkish bath, taken under competent medical supervision, is often of great benefit, and many persons take it weekly, and even oftener, with the effect of toning up the system and of making them more competent to endure both physical and mental fatigue. Cold baths, except for the very robust, are also to be taken with great caution. If afterward there be reaction and if the skin become warm and pink, they are beneficial, but if the skin become cold and blue, they are injurious. In fact, this should be the test for each individual to apply to his own case. Bathing, except a sponge- or plunge-bath, should not be practised when the vital powers are low, as early in the morning, nor after a long fast, nor should it be indulged in too soon after eating; eleven o'clock in the morning is, for the average person, a proper time for a bath of considerable duration.

9. Kidneys.

The kidneys are situated in the lumbar region of the abdominal cavity, one on each side of the spinal

PLATE III.

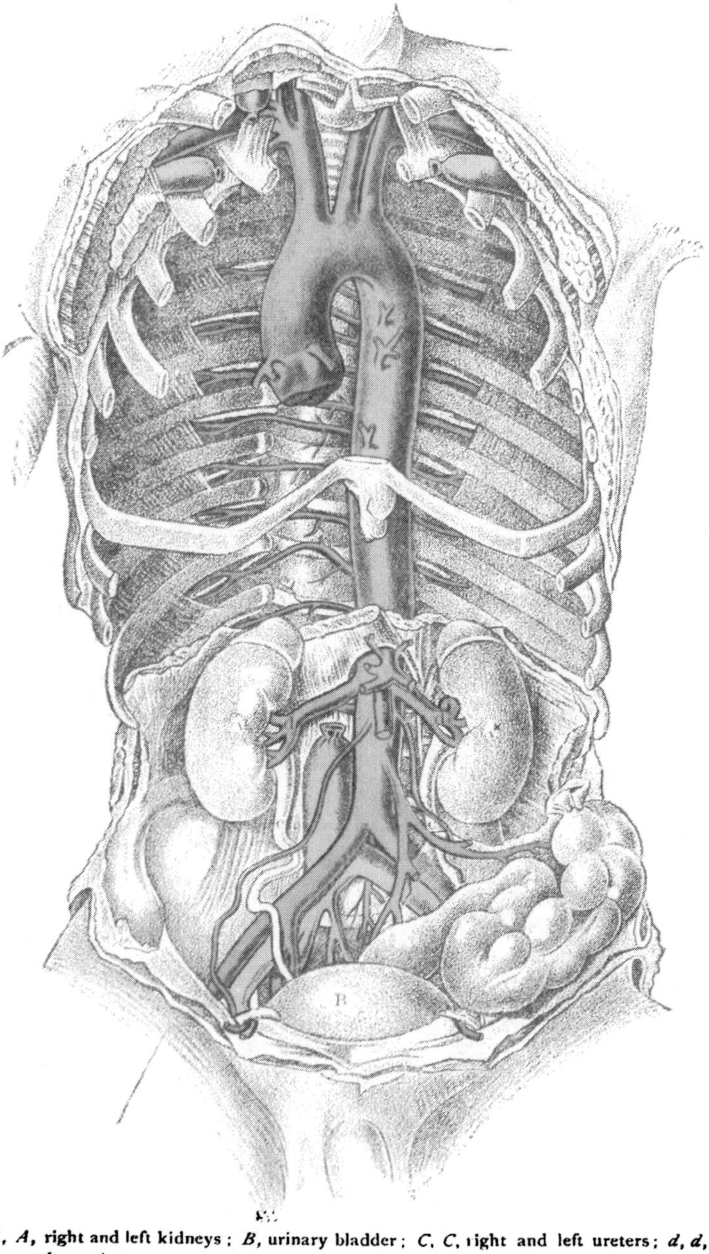

A, A, right and left kidneys; *B,* urinary bladder; *C, C,* right and left ureters; *d, d,* renal arteries.

column. The shape of the kidney is like that of a bean, the internal border being concave and presenting a fissure—the hilum—at which the vessels, the nerves, and the ureter enter the organ. When the kidney is

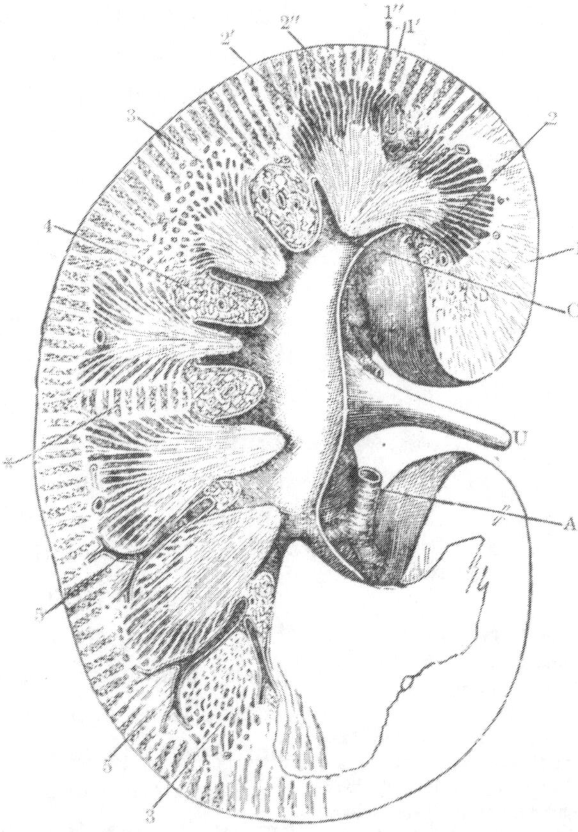

FIG. 38.—Longitudinal Section through the Kidney (after Tyson and Henle): 1, cortex; 1′, medullary rays; 1″, labyrinth; 2, medulla; 2′, papillary portion of medulla; 2″, boundary layer of medulla; 3, transverse section of tubules in the boundary layer; 4, fat of renal sinus; 5, artery; *, transverse medullary rays; *A*, branch of renal artery; *C*, renal calyx; *U*, ureter.

longitudinally cut in two, it is seen to be made up of an external or cortical portion—cortex—and an internal or medullary portion. The medullary portion is made up of numerous pyramids (those of Malpighi), from eight to eighteen in number, and, dipping down between them, as well as forming the outer part of the kidney, is the cortical portion. Each pyramid terminates in a papilla projecting into a calyx, which, with the calices of other pyramids, forms the pelvis, the upper dilated cavity of the ureter.

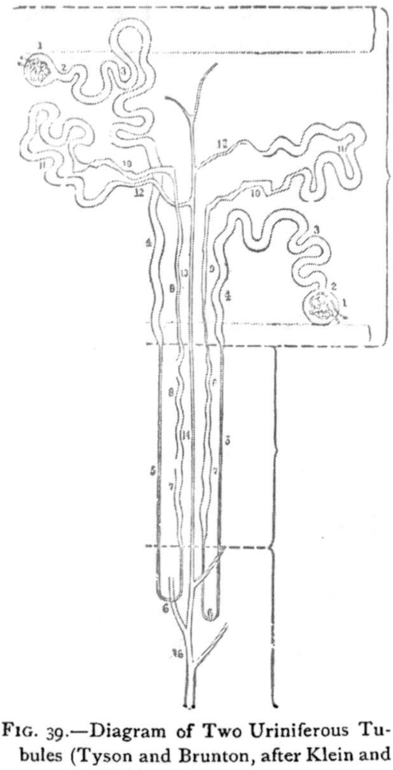

FIG. 39.—Diagram of Two Uriniferous Tubules (Tyson and Brunton, after Klein and Noble Smith): 1, Malpighian tuft surrounded by Bowman's capsule; 2, constriction, or neck; 3, proximal convoluted tubule; 4, spiral tubule; 5, descending limb of Henle's loop; 6, Henle's loop; 7 and 8, ascending limb of Henle's loop; 9, wavy part of ascending limb of Henle's loop; 10, irregular tubule; 11, distal convoluted tubule; 12, first part of collecting tube; 13 and 14, straight part of collecting tube; 15, excretory duct of Bellini.

At each papilla there open about twenty uriniferous tubules, which can be traced to the base of the pyramid. Each tubule continues into the cortical portion of the kidney, where it is larger and becomes convoluted, narrowing again and entering the pyramid, in which it again becomes straight, forms a loop, and re-enters the cortical portion, again becomes convoluted, and finally terminates in a spherical body, the Malpighian capsule or capsule of Bowman.

This complicated structure may, perhaps, be traced more easily in the opposite direction. Beginning with the Malpighian capsule in the cortical portion, there is next the convoluted tubule, which, as it passes into the medullary portion, becomes straight and is known as the "descending limb of Henle's loop." This bends on itself, forming the ascending limb, likewise straight, passes back into the cortex, becomes convoluted, and enters a straight collecting tube which opens at the apex of a pyramid.

The Malpighian capsule is lined by a layer of squamous epithelium which is reflected over the glomerulus it contains. Between these two layers of cells there is a cavity continuous with the uriniferous tubule. The tubule throughout its entire length is lined by epithelium, which, however, varies in character in different portions.

The renal artery enters the kidney at its hilum, and its branches, after pursuing a peculiar course, terminate in afferent vessels, each of which penetrates the wall of a Malpighian capsule, forming the glomerulus. The vessels coming from the capsules—efferent vessels—pass out through their walls and form a venous plexus around the uriniferous tubules, ultimately taking part in the formation of the renal vein, which emerges from the kidney at the hilum and discharges into the inferior vena cava.

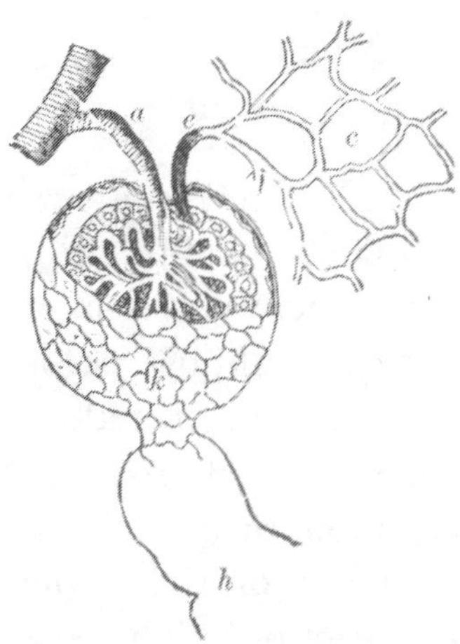

FIG. 40.—Bowman's Capsule and Glomerulus (after Landois): *a*, vas afferens; *e*, vas efferens; *c*, capillary network of the cortex; *k*, endothelial structure of the capsule; *h*, origin of convoluted tubule.

Urine.—The function of the kidney is to form the urine, which is a yellow or amber-colored fluid, acid in reaction, and having a specific gravity of about 1020 in the adult; in the new-born child, of about 1005. The quantity of urine voided in twenty-four hours is about 1500 grammes. Water constitutes 95.2 per cent., and the solids 4.8 per cent., of which 2.2 per cent., nearly one-half, is urea. The following table shows the composition of urine:

	Percentages.	Daily amount.
Water	96.0	1450. grammes.
Urea	2.0	30. "
Uric acid	.05	0.75 "
Hippuric acid	.04	0.75 "
Creatinin	.11	1.5 "
Phosphates		3. "
Chlorides	1.5	7.5 "
Sulphates		3. "
Mucus and other ingredients	.3	

The general characteristics of the urine and its composition are subject to considerable variation in a condition of health. It may, when its specific gravity is low (1002), be almost colorless, while when concentrated its color will be a reddish-brown. Its reaction, although generally acid, may be alkaline, as at the beginning of digestion, or its acidity may be increased, as during the afternoon or the night. The kind of food also affects the reaction. Thus in the carnivora the urine is acid, while in the herbivora it is alkaline. If vegetables be fed to a carnivorous animal and flesh to an herbivorous, the reaction of the urine will be the opposite to that of the urine when each is consuming its normal food The feeding of flesh to the herbivorous animal is practically accomplished by giving it no food, under which circumstances it lives upon its own tissues. The acidity of urine is usually attributed to acid sodium phosphate, but several organic acids or organic salts are probably involved.

Water.—The amount of water excreted daily is on an average 1450 grammes, and constitutes 96 per cent. of the urine. It is separated from the blood by the epithelial cells covering the glomerulus, and not by filtration due to blood-pressure. It is true that as blood-pressure in the glomerulus increases the amount of water eliminated also increases, but this is not due to the simple increase of pressure, but is due to the fact that with increased pressure more blood flows through the glomerulus; consequently there is more material from which the cells can separate water.

Urea.—Of all the ingredients of the urine, urea is the most important. It represents to a great extent the nitrogenous waste of the tissues. The amount of urea daily excreted is in the male about 30 grammes; it is less in the female. The actual amount eliminated in children is less, but, proportional to the weight of the body, the child excretes more urea than does the adult.

Source of Urea.—The ingredient urea is not *formed* by the kidney: it exists in the blood when this fluid reaches the kidney, and this organ separates it from the blood. The separation is brought about by the epithelium of those portions of the uriniferous tubules about which is entwined the venous plexus already referred to; that is, the convoluted tubules and the ascending limb of Henle's loop. The source of urea is threefold: 1, the proteids of the food; 2, the proteids of the tissues; and 3, the proteids of the blood and lymph.

1. *Urea from the Proteids of the Food.*—The greater the amount of proteids absorbed, the greater is the amount of urea excreted. Thus if large quantities of

meat be eaten, the amount of urea in the urine will be very large, whereas if food without nitrogen in its composition be taken, the urea will be present in a minimum amount. It might be thought that the increased amount of urea excreted under these circumstances is derived from the tissues, but it appears in so short a time (an hour or two) that this cannot be the case. In discussing intestinal digestion it was stated that when an excess of proteid food was taken the overplus of the peptones was changed into leucin and tyrosin by the action of the trypsin. These two substances are absorbed by the blood-vessels and carried by the portal vein to the liver, where they are probably converted into urea. There is no direct proof of this conversion, but the hypothesis is a reasonable one, for so far as is known the liver is the only gland which contains urea, and, further, it has been shown that when leucin is fed to animals it reappears as urea.

2. *Urea from the Proteids of the Tissues.*—The muscles contain creatin to the amount of from 0.2 to 0.4 per cent. Creatin is recognized as a substance intermediate between proteids and urea, and it exists also in the brain and nervous system generally, in the spleen, and in various glands. Creatin in all probability is one of the sources of urea, but where the conversion takes place is unknown; possibly it is accomplished by the epithelium of the tubules of the kidney.

3. *Urea from the Proteids of the Blood and Lymph.*—All the proteids present in the blood and lymph do not become integral parts of the tissues, so that there is a certain amount of the proteids constantly circulating. The circulating proteids are not permanent, but, like other proteids, undergo conversion into urea. It is not to be assumed from this statement of the origin of urea that

the proteids are converted directly into that substance. It has already been seen that there are some intermediate stages—for example, leucin, tyrosin, and creatin—and there are doubtless others of which nothing is known.

Uric Acid.—Besides being an ingredient of the urine, uric acid has also been detected in the spleen, the heart, the liver, and the brain. In the blood it is also present, especially in gout. In the urine the amount of uric acid under ordinary circumstances does not exceed 0.75 grammes per diem. The amount will be still less if the diet be vegetable, but if it be animal and abundant the quantity may be as much as 2 grammes. It is less in attacks of gout, during which the quantity in the blood is increased. In febrile conditions the amount is also increased. Uric acid is not free in the urine, but is combined with sodium, ammonium, potassium, calcium, and magnesium to form urates, the

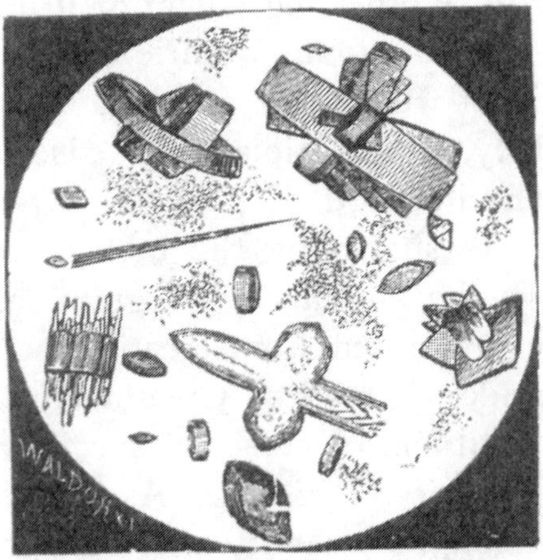

FIG. 41.—Uric Acid and Urates (Funke).

sodium and ammonium urates being the most abundant. Under ordinary circumstances it remains in combination, but when the urine is very acid it appears in the form of crystals (Fig. 41).

Source of Uric Acid.—Uric acid is regarded by some writers as being an intermediate product in the formation of urea. These believe that the process of oxidation of the nitrogenous materials has for some reason, as from an insufficient supply of oxygen, been arrested before the stage of urea is reached; but this theory of the formation of uric acid has not been substantiated. From the evidence now at our disposal it must be regarded as one of the final products of oxidation, as is the case with urea. There is some evidence that uric acid is formed in the spleen of man, the quantity eliminated being increased when the spleen is enlarged, and being diminished when this organ is reduced in size. There is no reliable evidence that the human liver produces this acid, although it is doubtless formed in the liver of birds.

Hippuric acid, another ingredient of urine, is excreted in about the same amount as uric acid. A vegetable diet, especially of fruits, may increase this excretion to 2 grammes daily. Hippuric acid has also been found in perspiration and in blood.

Creatinin.—As shown by the table, creatinin is excreted daily to the amount of 1.5 grammes. It is considered as being formed from creatin, and is spoken of as the anhydride of creatin. Creatin, it will be remembered, is a constituent of muscles especially, although it is found also in nervous tissue. As would be expected from its derivation, the quantity in urine will be increased under a diet of flesh.

Inorganic Constituents of Urine.—The inorganic constituents of urine are principally phosphates, chlorides, and sulphates. The phosphates especially worthy of mention are those of sodium, both neutral and acid. To the latter is attributed the acidity of the urine. The

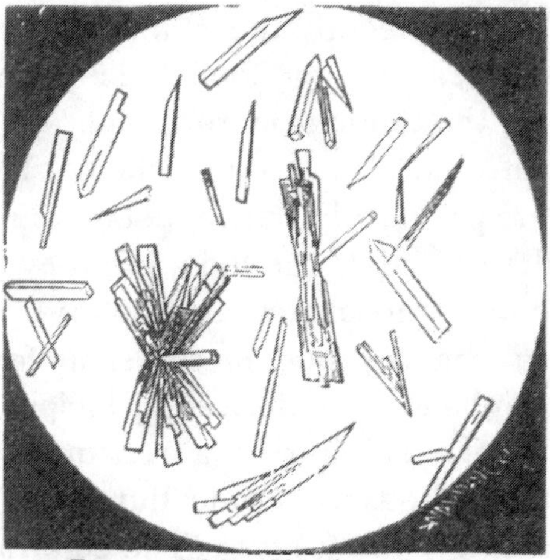

FIG. 42.—Calcium Phosphate (Laache).

phosphates of the urine are derived from the phosphates of the food, and there is no foundation for the theory that

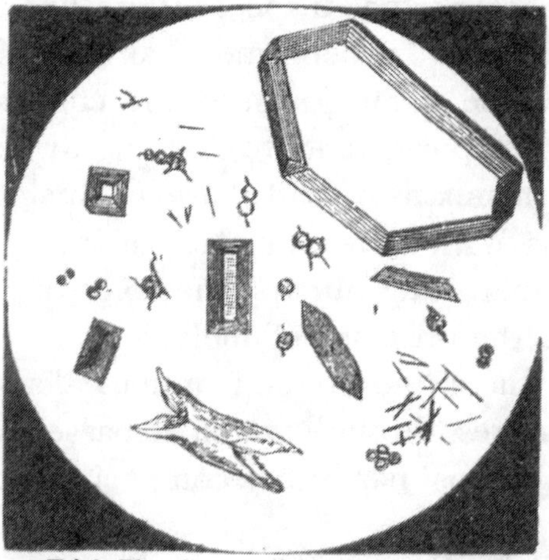

FIG. 43.—Triple Phosphates and Ammonium Urate (Laache).

they are increased by mental exertion and represent the waste of nerve-tissue. The amount of phosphates excreted is increased in fevers and in diseases of the bones, and is diminished during pregnancy. The chlorides are mainly represented by the chloride of sodium, and, as they are derived from the food, the amount eliminated depends upon the amount in the food. In pneumonia the amount of chlorides is diminished. The sulphates in the urine are principally salts of potassium and sodium, which are derived from the food, but they differ in this respect from the phosphates and chlorides, that while the latter exist in the food in the same form as in the urine, the sulphates are derived principally from the proteids, of which sulphur is a constituent, while the sulphates of the food contribute but little.

Coloring-matter of the Urine.—The coloring-matter of the urine is not ordinarily abundant. It probably does not consist of one substance alone, but of several, the best known of which is urobilin. Some writers, however, hold that normal urine contains but one pigment, to which the name "urochrome" has been given. "Uroerythrin" is the name given to the coloring-matter in pink urinary deposits and to the highly-colored urine present in rheumatism, and "urinary melanin" to that found in the dark-brown or black urine of persons suffering from melanotic tumors, the color of which is very dark, due to the presence of melanin.

Mucus.—The urine contains mucus, derived from the various passages through which it passes, which under normal conditions has no decomposing action on the urea.

Gases of the Urine.—Oxygen, nitrogen, and carbon dioxide are present in the urine, the latter gas being the most abundant, the quantity being increased after active muscular exertion.

III. NERVOUS FUNCTIONS.

1. General Considerations.

There is a most intimate relationship existing between the different organs of the body—so intimate, indeed, that not one of the whole number can be said to be entirely independent. Many illustrations of this dependency might be given, but one will suffice.

The respirations of an individual at rest are not far from sixteen per minute, and the pulsations of the radial artery are, in the same condition, about seventy. If, now, he exercise violently—running around the block, for instance—the respirations will be found to have greatly increased, amounting perhaps to thirty per minute, while at the same time the pulsations of the artery will have reached one hundred and twenty per minute. Is this change from the quiescent condition a mere coincidence, or is there a reason for it? If the latter, how has the change been brought about?

During a resting condition the muscles of the body do not make much demand upon the blood, and with the heart beating seventy times per minute the muscles, as well as the other tissues, are receiving all the material they need for the performance of their functions. The sixteen respirations a minute are also sufficient to supply the blood with all the oxygen required and to remove from it the necessary amount of carbon dioxide. When, however, the muscles are called upon for the increased exertion above referred to, they must have a greater supply of the necessary materials, to furnish which a larger amount of blood must be sent to them. Then, too, as a result of the extra work, more muscular tissue is wasted, and the waste must be taken away rapidly to the organs whose duty it is to eliminate it. To send the larger supply of blood the heart must beat faster, and to provide the increased oxygen and to remove the additional carbon dioxide the respiratory movements must be more rapid. The muscles of the body have not the power within themselves to increase their activity, but when acted upon properly from without they have. Neither has the heart-muscle the power to beat more quickly until stimulated thereto by some influence outside itself. Equally powerless are the agencies which produce the respiratory movements. These outside influences, by which the muscles contract and by which the heart and the respiratory apparatus act in harmony, are derived from the nervous system, a collection of organs one of whose functions is to cause the different organs to act harmoniously. The effect of a want of harmony under the circumstances just supposed would be most disastrous. If the nervous force were not at command to make the muscles respond when their increased action was desired, there would be a condition of paralysis, or if, when the muscles attempted to perform this added task, the heart should fail to respond, the effort would be fruitless, and equally unavailing would be the attempt if at the crucial moment the lungs and other respiratory organs should be unresponsive. As was said, many illustrations of the interdependence of the organs might be given, but a little reflection will suggest them almost *ad infinitum*.

The simplest movements that are made require for their performance the conjoint action of several, often many, muscles, and were it not for the exciting and controlling power of the nervous system, instead of the harmony which is everywhere and at all times apparent there would result the utmost confusion.

In what has been said thus far reference has been had only to the individual, as if he were alone on the face of the earth and interested only in himself; but there are other human beings with whom he is constantly brought into relation, and a world of other animate objects as well as an infinite amount of inanimate matter. This relationship is also accomplished through the nervous system, principally by means of the special senses. It will, therefore, be seen that the nervous functions are those which bring the different organs of the body into harmonious relations with one another, and, in addition, bring the individual, through the special senses, sight, hearing, etc., into relation with the world outside him.

The nervous system is made up of collections of nervous tissue, which is composed of two kinds of matter—cellular or vesicular, and fibrous.

Cellular or vesicular nervous matter is found in the external portions of the brain, the internal portions of the spinal cord, and in ganglia generally, a ganglion being a collection of nerve-cells. Such a collection of nerve-cells is also spoken of as a "nerve-centre," being so called for the reason that it is composed of nerve-cells or vesicles (Fig. 44). From its grayish color it is also known as *gray nervous matter*, and, because of its ashy appearance, as *cineritious* nervous matter. When examined under the microscope it is seen to be made up of nerve-cells or ganglion-corpuscles, which are the characteristic elements, together with nerve-fibres and blood-vessels, all imbedded in neuroglia, a form of connective tissue.

Nerve-cells vary in size, from 10 m.mm. in the sympathetic ganglia to 135 m.mm. in the anterior cornua of the spinal cord. These bodies vary also somewhat in shape, some being spherical and others ovoid, while still others are exceedingly angular. They possess very prominent nuclei and nucleoli, and they have processes varying in number and giving rise to a nomenclature by which they are distinguished. Cells with one process or pole are

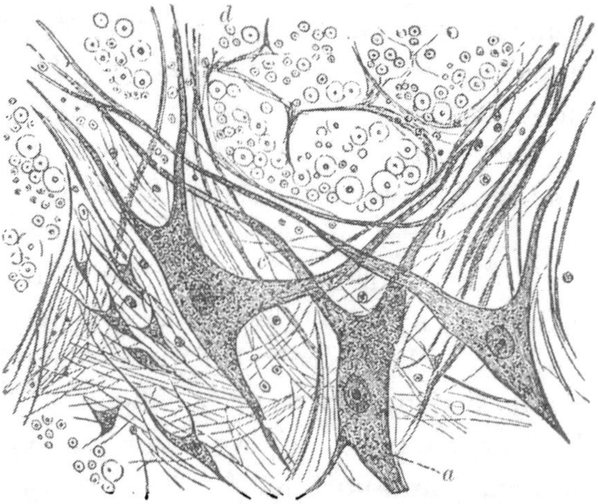

FIG. 44.—Multipolar Nerve-cells: *a*, from the anterior gray column of the spinal cord of the dog-fish lying on a texture of fibrils, *c*; *b*, prolongation from cells; *d*, nerve-fibres cut across (Cadiat).

unipolar; with two poles, *bipolar*; with three or more poles, *multipolar*. Sometimes cells are found having no process; to such the term *apolar* has been given. It is doubtful, however, whether there are such cells, except as the result of accident by which a process has been broken off. In the spinal ganglia unipolar cells exist, while in the cord cells are found the number of whose processes is as many as eight. Frequently the processes may be seen to be branched, the branches themselves subdividing again and again. Often, however, one process may be traced for a considerable distance from the nerve-cell in which it originated without any branch being discovered. Such a process is continuous with the axis-cylinder of a nerve-fibre, and is therefore called the "axis-cylinder prolongation." The branched processes disappear in the nervous tissue: they probably connect with processes from other nerve-cells.

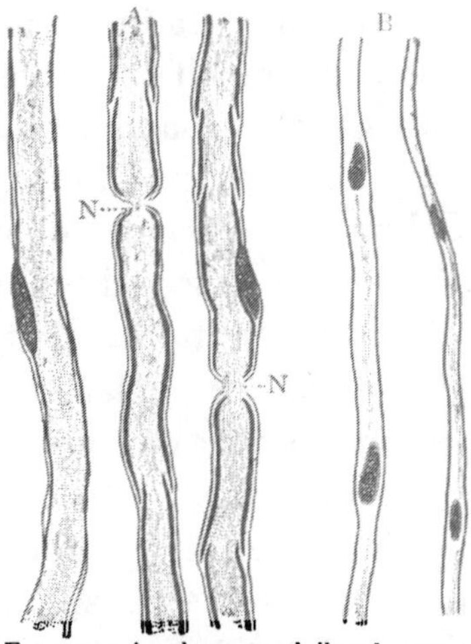

FIG. 45.—A, three medullated nerve-fibres, the medullary sheath of which is stained dark with osmic acid; N, nodes of Ranvier; B, two non-medullated nerve-fibres, with nuclei in the primitive sheath.

Fibrous nervous matter, which is the material composing nerve-fibres, is of two kinds: (1) medullated, and (2) non-medullated.

(1) *Medullated fibres,* which are called also "white fibres" by reason of their color, make up the white portion of the brain and the spinal cord, and, with few exceptions, the cerebro-spinal nerves—namely, those having their origin in the brain and spinal cord. A medullated fibre is composed of the axis-cylinder, the most central portion, the white substance of Schwann, which envelops it, and the primitive sheath, sometimes called "neurilemma," a delicate external membrane (Fig. 45). Of all these structures the axis-cylinder is the most important; indeed, it is an essential, as without it the nerve could not perform its functions. The neurilemma and the white substance are not always present in all portions of a medullated nerve. At the commencement and at the termination they are absent. The size of the medullated fibres is very variable. In the gray substance of the spinal cord they may be found,

having a diameter of 2 m.mm., while in the peripheral nerves this may be as much as 18 m.mm.

(2) *Non-medullated fibres*, which are known also as "gray and gelatinous fibres" and "fibres of Remak," compose the olfactory nerve and the sympathetic nerves, and are also found elsewhere. As their name implies, they have none of the medullary or white substance of Schwann. They are composed of fibrillæ within a sheath, the former being the axis-cylinder, the latter the neurilemma. Scattered along the fibre between these two structures are nuclei.

Termination of Nerve-fibres.—Nerve-fibres terminate in various ways. In voluntary muscles they terminate in end-plates, fibres from which, doubtless representing the axis-cylinders, are connected with the contractile tissue of the muscular fibres. In involuntary muscular

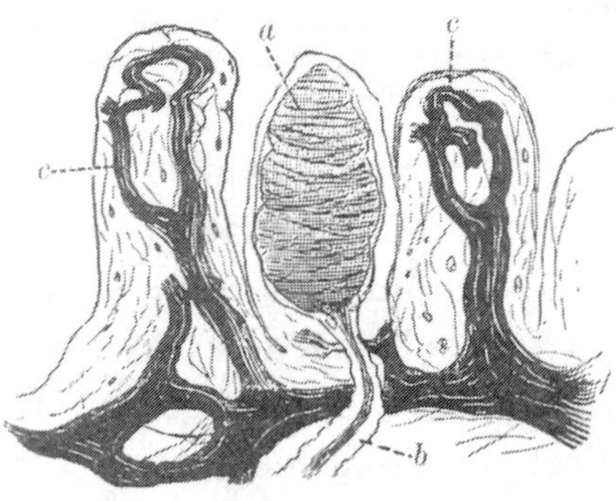

FIG. 46.—Drawing from a Section of Injected Skin, showing three papillæ, the central one containing a tactile corpuscle (*a*), connected with a medullated nerve, and that at each side (*c*) occupied by vessels (Cadiat).

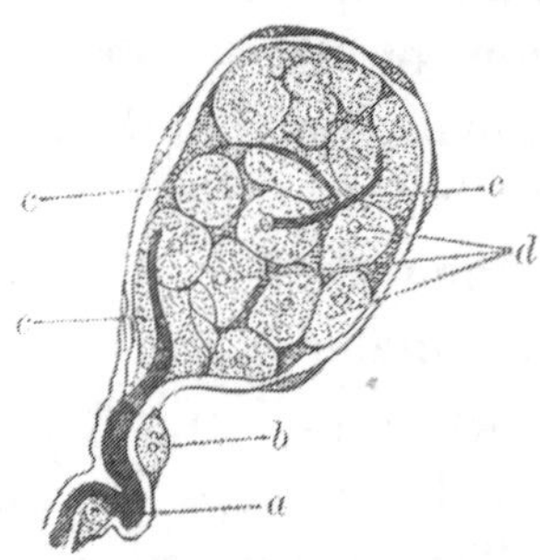

FIG. 47.—End-bulb from Human Conjunctiva, treated with osmic acid, showing cells of core (Longworth): *a*, nerve-fibre; *b*, nucleus of sheath; *c*, nerve-fibre within core; *d*, cells of core.

tissue the nerve-fibres form a plexus from which are given off smaller fibres that are ultimately distributed to the nucleoli. In glands the nerve-fibres end in secreting cells; in the skin some terminate in the hair-follicles and others in the epithelium. Besides these nerve-fibres there are three kinds of corpuscles in and beneath the skin with which nerves are connected—namely:

(1) *The corpuscles of Pacini*, which are constantly found in the subcutaneous tissue of the palms of the hands and the soles of the feet, and are sometimes found also in other situations, such as the dorsal surface of the hands and feet, and the nipples;

(2) *The tactile corpuscles* (Fig. 46), which are present in about one in four of the papillæ of the skin of the third phalanx of the index finger, are found also in other papillæ, but not in such great proportion. As a rule they are most abundant on the plantar surface of the feet;

(3) *The end-bulbs* (Fig. 47), which occur in the conjunctiva, the mouth, the tongue, the glans penis, and the clitoris.

Chemistry of Nervous Matter.—The chemical composition of nervous matter is by no means thoroughly understood. Among its constituents are cholesterin, lecithin, cerebrin, protagon, and neuro-keratin.

Functions of Nerve-cells and Nerve-fibres.—The nerve-cells receive and generate impulses, while nerve-fibres have the power only to conduct the impulses.

Classification of Nerve-centres.—A collection of nerve-cells, whether it be large or small, is a nerve-centre or ganglion. In such a centre there are, besides the cells, blood-vessels, nerve-fibres, and neuroglia, but the cells are the characteristic element upon which the function of a centre depends. These centres may be divided into (1) conscious; (2) reflex; (3) automatic; (4) relay; and (5) junction.

Conscious nerve-centres are located in the brain. In them the sensation of pain is produced, and out from them go the impulses which result in voluntary movements.

Reflex Nerve-centres.—The gray matter of the spinal cord is an admirable example of a purely reflex centre. Impressions reaching it by the sensory roots of the spinal nerves excite impulses which travel out along motor nerves to muscles, and cause them to contract. In this there is no consciousness; indeed, in an animal that is decapitated the same action takes place. Reflex centres are found also in the brain.

Automatic nerve-centres do not require to be excited to action by impulses coming to them through afferent nerves, as is the case with the reflex centres, but they send out impulses without such excitation. The cardio-inhibitory centre in the medulla oblongata, in which centre originate the impulses that have already been spoken of as being sent to the heart through the pneumogastric, is one of these.

Relay Nerve-centres.—When a feeble impulse reaches a relay centre, that centre is excited, and from it may go out very powerful impulses, just as a feeble current of electricity may bring into play a local battery which will have much greater power than the current which brought it into action.

Junction nerve-centres are those which are so connected with other centres that an impulse exciting one may also excite the other, and thus impulses may be sent to several regions of the body.

Classification of Nerve-fibres.—Nerve-fibres conduct impulses from within outward and from without inward. Whether it is the function of a given nerve to do the one or the other does not depend upon anything in the nerve itself, but upon its relations; and there is every reason to believe that were it possible to separate a nerve from its anatomical connections and attach it to different structures, it would be just as capable of acting in its new relations as it did in the old; just as a copper wire will equally well carry a current of electricity to ring a bell or to supply a motor or to turn a hand on a dial: the result depends not upon the wire, but upon the mechanism with which it is in connection.

Studying nerves, then, as they are actually found in the body, it will be found that there are some which carry impulses outward from nerve-centres; these are efferent nerves. Inasmuch as the impulse is going away from the centre, they are also called "centrifugal nerves;" those which carry impulses from the periphery to the centres are called "afferent" or "centripetal nerves;" while a third class comprise those which connect nerve-centres with one another, and are called "intercentral nerves."

Efferent nerves were formerly spoken of as motor nerves, and indeed even now some writers use the terms *efferent* and *motor* as synonyms. All motor nerves are efferent, for they carry impulses outward, but all efferent nerves are not motor nerves. A nerve which carries an impulse to a muscle, and thus brings about motion, is properly called a "motor nerve;" but one that conducts an impulse to a gland, the result of which is the activity of its cells and the production of a secretion, is improperly named a motor nerve, although it is unquestionably an efferent nerve. *Secretory* is a much more expressive name. Efferent nerves may be divided as follows: (1)

motor; (2) vaso-motor; (3) secretory; (4) trophic; and (5) inhibitory.

Motor nerves terminate in muscles, and convey to them impulses which cause and regulate their contraction.

Vaso-motor nerves, although distributed to the muscular tissue of blood-vessels, and thus act as motor nerves, regulate the amount of blood supplied to a part, and it seems wise to separate them from the purely motor nerves and put them in a class by themselves.

Secretory Nerves.—The impulses which these nerves carry to glands bring about their secretion. The chorda tympani is a striking example.

Trophic nerves are supposed by some to govern the nutrition of the structures to which they are distributed entirely independently of the regulation of the blood-supply. It is still a mooted question whether such nerves exist. The subject will be again discussed in the consideration of the functions of the fifth pair of cranial nerves.

Efferent inhibitory nerves carry outward impulses which restrain or inhibit the action of the organs to which they are distributed. The pneumogastric, so far as the heart is concerned, is such a nerve. Without its restraining influence the heart would beat much faster.

Afferent nerves in some physiological works are called "sensory nerves," but there is the same impropriety in using these terms synonymously as in the case of efferent and motor nerves. All sensory nerves are afferent, but all afferent nerves are not sensory. Afferent nerves may be divided as follows, although the distinction is by no means so well marked as in the efferent nerves: (1) sensory; (2) nerves of special sense; (3) thermic nerves; (4) excito-reflex; and (5) inhibitory.

(1) *Sensory Nerves.*—When these nerves are stimulated an impulse is carried to the brain, which there gives rise to a conscious sensation that may amount to pain.

(2) *Nerves of Special Sense.*—The impulses carried by these nerves do not give rise to pain, but with each nerve is connected a special sensation: with the olfactory, the sense of smell; with the optic, the sense of light; and with the auditory, the sense of hearing.

(3) *Thermic Nerves.*—It is believed by some writers that these are special nerves which convey the sense of temperature only, but this is still an unsettled question.

(4) *Excito-reflex Nerves.*—In these nerves there is an impulse carried to a nerve-centre without producing a conscious sensation: this centre is excited, and from it or from another centre with which it is in communication there goes out an impulse that, if it be a gland to which it is distributed, produces secretion. Such a nerve would be an excito-secretory nerve; or if it be distributed to a muscle it produces motion, and would in that case be considered an excito-motor nerve.

(5) *Afferent Inhibitory Nerves.*—The afferent inhibitory nerves are also called "centro-inhibitory" to distinguish them from the efferent inhibitory nerves. The centro-inhibitory nerves carry impulses to nerve-centres, which are so affected as to prevent them from sending out impulses. A familiar instance is that of pinching the lip to prevent sneezing. It is, however, doubtful whether there exists a separate class of nerves performing this function, rather than ordinary sensory fibres which act in this peculiar manner for the moment.

Intercentral Nerves.—The nerve-centres are intimately connected with one another by nerves which are neither afferent nor efferent, and which are called "intercentral fibres." As has already been said, even the simplest movements of the body bring into action several, and sometimes many, muscles; of course this action is more obvious in complex movements. To accomplish this various nerve-centres must be at work, and that they may act harmoniously and produce co-ordinated movements they are required to be in intimate relationship. Study for a moment the intricate mechanism brought into play in the ordinary act of picking up a pin from the floor, and it will be readily understood how essential it is that the nerve-centres responsible for these movements should act in the most perfect harmony, sending to each muscle just the right amount of nerve-force and at exactly the right moment; otherwise the act could not be accomplished in the perfect manner that it is.

Nerve-stimuli.—Nerve-fibres have no power of receiving or generating impulses: they are simply conductors. It is extremely difficult to define a nerve-impulse. If certain nerves are acted on in the proper manner at their peripheral extremities, there is produced in the nerve a certain change which manifests itself at the distal extremities: the something which acts upon these nerves is called a "stimulus," and that which travels along the nerve is called a "nervous impulse." It has been assumed that this is a molecular change in the axis-cylinder. Stimuli may excite nerve-centres from which impulses travel outward along efferent nerves, or they may excite the end-organs of nerves, and the impulses they generate may travel inward along afferent fibres to the centres. Besides, a nerve may be stimulated at any point between its ends. A current of electricity applied to a motor nerve at any such point will cause contraction of the muscles to which it is distributed, as if the stimulus had been applied to its origin. In the same way, if a sensitive nerve were to be stimulated, the sensation would be felt as if the stimulus had been applied to its end. Thus, if the ends of the nerves in a stump resulting from an amputation of the arm, for instance, be pressed upon by the scar-tissue which forms, it will seem to the individual affected that the pain is in the fingers, the sensation being referred to the parts in which the nerves originally terminated.

Classification of Nerve-stimuli.—Nerve-stimuli are *general* and *special*. The former excite all nerves, while the latter excite only special nerves.

General nerve-stimuli are electrical, chemical, mechanical, and thermal. A current of electricity in the form of a shock will stimulate a nerve; a blow will do the same; so also will some chemical substances. Heat or cold suddenly applied will produce a similar effect.

Special Nerve-stimuli.—Light affects only the optic nerve, and sound only the auditory nerve; hence light and sound are special nerve-stimuli. Other special stimuli excite the nerves of smell and taste.

The rate at which impulses travel along the human motor nerves is about 33 metres per second.

2. General Arrangement of the Nervous System.

The nervous system is divided into two subdivisions: (1) the cerebro-spinal system, and (2) the sympathetic system.

The cerebro-spinal system includes the brain and spinal cord, which together form the cerebro-spinal axis, and the nerves which come from them—namely, the cranial and spinal nerves.

Spinal Cord.—The spinal cord is situated in the vertebral canal, and is covered by three membranes—the dura mater, arachnoid, and pia mater. It is about 0.43 metres in length, and, in general, is of a cylindrical shape; it weighs 42.5 grammes.

Enlargements of the Spinal Cord.—Two enlargements along the course of the spinal cord are noteworthy. The cervical enlargement extends from the third cervical to the first or the second dorsal vertebra, and the lumbar enlargement is at the eleventh and twelfth dorsal vertebræ. From the cervical enlargement go off the nerves which supply the upper, and from the lumbar those which supply the lower, extremities.

Fissures.—On the anterior surface of the spinal cord is a groove, the anterior median fissure, which extends to the anterior white commissure. On the posterior surface is also a fissure, the posterior median fissure, which is not so wide as the anterior, but is deeper, extending to the posterior gray commissure. It will thus be seen that the anterior and posterior fissures nearly divide the cord into two symmetrical halves, which are connected by the commissure.

At a little distance from the anterior median fissure on each side is the antero-lateral fissure. Strictly speaking, this is not a fissure, being rather a line of small openings at which emerge the anterior roots of the spinal nerves. Between the antero-lateral fissure and the anterior median fissure the white matter of the cord is called the "anterior column." In front of the posterior median fissure and on either side is the postero-lateral fissure. Here emerge the posterior roots of the nerves. The white matter between the origins of the two sets of roots is called the "lateral column." The anterior and lateral columns are together sometimes denominated "antero-lateral." Between the postero-lateral and posterior me-

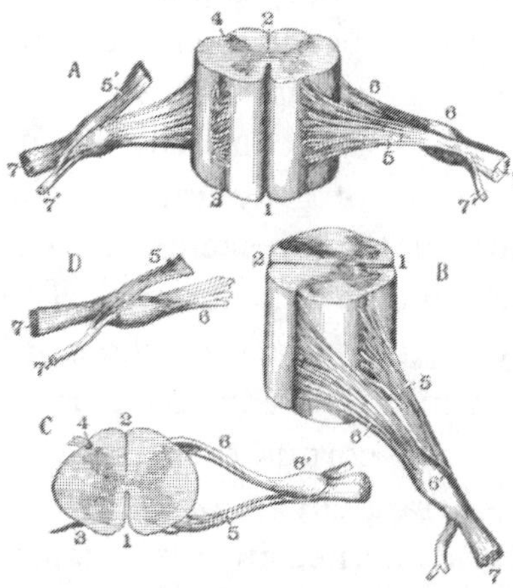

FIG. 48.—Different Views of a Portion of the Spinal Cord from the cervical region, with the roots of the nerves. In *A* the anterior surface of the specimen is shown, the anterior nerve-root of its right side being divided; in *B* a view of the right side is given; in *C* the upper surface is shown; in *D* the nerve-roots and ganglion are shown from below: 1, the anterior median fissure; 2, posterior median fissure; 3, anterior lateral depression, over which the anterior nerve-roots are seen to spread; 4, posterior lateral groove, into which the posterior roots are seen to sink; 5, anterior roots passing the ganglion: 5′, in *A*, the anterior root divided; 6, the posterior roots, the fibres of which pass into the ganglion, 6; 7, the united or compound nerve; 7′, the posterior primary branch, seen in *A* and *D* to be derived in part from the anterior and in part from the posterior root (Allen Thomson).

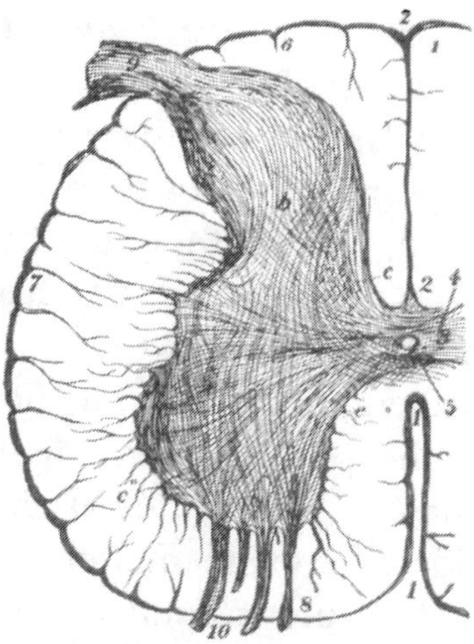

FIG. 49.—Transverse Section of Half the Spinal Cord, in the lumbar enlargement (semi-diagrammatic): 1, anterior median fissure; 2, posterior median fissure; 3, central canal lined with epithelium; 4, posterior commissure; 5, anterior commissure; 6, posterior column; 7, lateral column: 8, anterior column (the white substance is traversed by radiating trabeculæ of pia mater); 9, fasciculus of posterior nerve-root, entering in one bundle; 10, fasciculi of anterior roots, entering in four spreading bundles of fibres: *b*, in the cervix cornu, decussating fibres from the nerve-roots and posterior commissure; *c*, posterior vesicular columns. About halfway between the central canal and 7 are seen the group of nerve-cells forming the tractus intermedio-lateralis; *e*, *e*, fibres of anterior roots; *e′*, fibres of anterior roots which decussate in anterior commissure (Allen Thomson).

dian fissure is the posterior column. A subdivision of this column is indicated by a slight groove, giving rise to the designation of that portion between this groove and the fissure as the posterior median column.

Section of the Spinal Cord.—A cross-section of the spinal cord shows a central gray substance and an external white substance. The gray matter presents the appearance of two crescents, with the concavities outward, joined together by a band of gray matter, the gray commissure. The points of the crescents are the horns or cornua, two anterior and two posterior. The posterior cornua come nearly to the surface of the cord at the postero-lateral fissure, while between the surface and the extremities of the anterior cornua there is considerable white matter. The arrangement of the white matter into columns is readily discerned in this section. In the gray commissure is a small canal—the central canal—which is only of interest in connection with the development of the cord. That portion of the commissure in front of the canal is the anterior gray, and that behind the posterior gray, commissure. Sections of the cord at different levels show that the white substance is most abundant in the upper part, and gradually becomes less abundant as the examination is made down the cord. The cervical and lumbar enlargements are due to the increased amount of gray matter at these points.

Minute Structure of the Cord.—Neuroglia supports both the white and gray matter of the spinal cord. The white matter is composed of medullated nerve-fibres, together with blood-vessels, running longitudinally, except that in the white commissure they run transversely, and when traced are seen to pass from the anterior horn of one side to the anterior column of the other side, the fibres from each side crossing those from the other, forming a decussation. By this means each anterior column is connected with the gray matter of the opposite side. There are also fibres passing in a more or less transverse direction from the gray matter to the roots of the nerves, and from the gray matter to the columns, into which they enter and probably become longitudinal.

Tracts in the Cord.—The columns of the spinal cord have been shown to be made up of separate collections of fibres called "tracts," and there is every reason to believe that each of these tracts has its own peculiar function. These tracts are as follows:

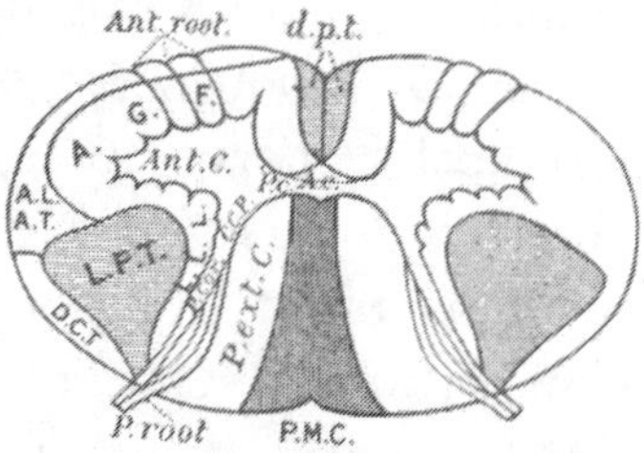

FIG. 50.—Diagram of the Spinal Cord, at the lower cervical region, to show the track of fibres; *d. p. t.*, direct pyramidal tract; *D. C. T.*, direct cerebellar tract; *P. M. C.*, posterior median column; *A. G. F.*, anterior ground fibres; *A. c.*, anterior commissure; *P. c.*, posterior commissure; *A. L. A. T.*, antero-lateral ascending tract; *Ant. C.*, anterior cornu; *P. Cor.*, posterior cornu; *C. C. P.*, intermediate gray substance; *L. L. L.*, lateral limiting layer (after Gowers).

1. The direct pyramidal tract, or fasciculus of Türck, is the anterior portion of the anterior column, next the anterior median fissure, and is continuous with the fibres of the pyramid of the medulla oblongata on the same side. This tract gradually becomes smaller and disappears in the middle of the dorsal region of the cord.

2. The fundamental fasciculus is the remaining portion of the anterior column;

3. The anterior radicular zone;

4. The mixed lateral column;

5. The crossed pyramidal fasciculus;

6. The cerebellar column. The last four tracts compose the lateral column. The fibres of the crossed pyramidal fasciculus, as the name implies, are continuous with the

decussating fibres of the pyramid of the medulla, while those of the cerebellar column connect with the cerebellum.

7. The column of Goll, which is a part of the posterior column, is situated next to the posterior median fissure. Outside of this, and making up the rest of the posterior column, is

8. The column of Burdach, or cuneate fasciculus. Columns 7 and 8 can both be traced into the medulla.

The gray matter of the spinal cord is composed of nerve-cells, nerve-fibres, neuroglia, and blood-vessels. The large nerve-cells are multipolar, some having as many as eight processes, and they are aggregated to form groups. One of these groups, situated in the anterior horn, is the vesicular column of the anterior cornu. It is in reality two groups—one in the middle near the anterior column, and the other laterally situated near the lateral column. Another, Clarke's posterior vesicular column, is situated at the base of the posterior column toward the inner side. A third collection of cells is the intermedio-lateral tract at the external part of the gray matter, where the anterior and posterior cornua join. The small nerve-cells are found throughout the gray matter, and not in groups as are the larger cells.

The nerve-fibres of the gray matter are, as a rule, smaller than those in the columns. In the posterior cornua they form Gerlach's nerve-network, very small fibres together with larger ones. The fibres of this network can be traced to the fibres of the posterior nerve-roots, and also to the processes of nerve-cells occupying an intermediate position. In the anterior cornua some of the processes of the nerve-cells communicate directly with the fibres of the anterior nerve-roots, and others with the nerve-network of Gerlach. The neuroglia at the tip of the posterior cornu is, from its gelatinous character, called "substantia gelatinosa."

Spinal Nerves.—From the spinal cord pass off thirty-one pairs of spinal nerves, which are distributed to the neck, the trunk, and the extremities. Each nerve is made up of an anterior (small) and a posterior (large) nerve-root. The latter is characterized anatomically by having upon it a ganglion. Beyond the ganglion the roots unite, forming a mixed nerve.

Functions of Spinal Nerves.—Stimulation of an anterior root causes contraction in the muscle to which it is distributed, while its division is followed by a loss of motion in the same muscle. In neither instance is sensation affected. If after the division the distal portion of the nerve be stimulated, muscular contraction will follow, while stimulation of the proximal end, that which is in connection with the cord, will produce no effect. The anterior roots are therefore efferent and motor, and are distributed to muscles.

Stimulation of a posterior root causes a sensation of pain in the part to which the nerve is distributed. Division of the root causes a loss of sensation in that part. If after division the distal portion of the nerve be stimulated, no effect is produced, while stimulation of the proximal portion produces sensation. The posterior roots are therefore afferent and sensory, and are distributed to the skin. The two roots uniting form a mixed nerve; that is, one in which there are both motor and sensory fibres.

Recurrent Sensibility.—When the distal end of a divided anterior root is stimulated, besides the muscular contraction which follows there is also some pain produced. If the trunk of the nerve beyond the ganglion be divided, and then the anterior root be stimulated, no muscular contraction results, but the pain is felt as before. If, however, the posterior root be divided, no sensation is produced. The sensation experienced when the anterior root is stimulated is accounted for by the presence in this root of some sensory fibres which pass up into it for a short distance and form a loop, returning to the junction of the two roots, and then pursuing their course in the posterior root. These are called "recurrent sensory fibres." The impulse passes down these fibres to the point of junction of the two roots, and then along the posterior root to the nerve-centre.

Function of the Spinal Ganglia.—As has already been stated, upon each posterior root of a spinal nerve is a ganglion. When examined under the microscope the root-fibres spread out, passing between groups of large cells having prominent nuclei and a diameter of about 100 m.mm. With one of these ganglion-cells a root-fibre is in communication, and the function of these cells is doubtless to regulate the nutrition of the fibres connected with them. They are true trophic centres, if any such are to be found in the body, a matter still in dispute.

Connection of the Nerve-roots with the Cord: Anterior or Motor Roots.—The fibres of the anterior root may be traced through the fibres of the antero-lateral column into the anterior cornu, where they separate. (1) Some pass through the anterior commissure to the opposite side, where they terminate in the axis-cylinder processes of the large multipolar cells of the anterior cornua; (2) others end in the middle group of cells in the anterior column of the same side; (3) others are traced to the axis-cylinder processes of the cells of the lateral group of the vesicular column of the anterior cornu; (4) others pass through the gray matter, and emerge from it to enter the lateral column, where they become longitudinal fibres; (5) others pass backward to become connected with the axis-cylinders of the cells of Clarke's column at the base of the posterior cornu.

Posterior or Sensory Root.—These fibres enter the posterior cornua: (1) Some become vertical, while (2) others cross over to the other side through the posterior commissure, and (3) others pass into the anterior cornu of the same side.

Functions of the Spinal Cord as a Conductor of Impulses.—The spinal cord is the principal channel through which all impulses from the trunk and the extremities pass to the brain, and all impulses to the trunk and extremities pass from the brain. If through disease or injury the cord be disorganized at any point, all power to produce voluntary motion in the parts below the injury is lost, and conscious sensation in these parts is from that moment abolished. The cord therefore acts as a conductor of impulses, both motor and sensory, between the brain and the trunk and the extremities. From the description already given of the course the motor and sensory fibres take in the cord, it would naturally be inferred that the different kinds of impulse which they carry follow different paths in the cord.

Methods of Examination.—The identity in the structure of nerves, whether motor or sensory, and the vast number of nerves in the cord, make it impossible to trace with the eye, even aided by the microscope and the most careful dissection, the course of nerve-fibres for any distance. Several methods have been developed by patient investigators which have done much toward solving this most difficult problem of the position which the different fibres occupy. The most important is the degenerative method.

Degenerative Method.—When a nerve is divided the first result is a loss of its function. Afterward the nerve undergoes degeneration, which results in changes in its structure that can readily be seen. Thus the course of a nerve or a collection of nerves may be traced throughout its entire extent. These changes are believed to be due to the severance of the nerve from its trophic centre. If an anterior root of a spinal nerve be divided, the distal end, being separated from the gray matter of the cord which is its centre of nutrition, undergoes degeneration, while the end which remains connected with the cord retains its integrity. If a posterior root be divided between the cord and the ganglion, the degeneration takes place between the cord and the ganglion, while if divided below the ganglion, the degeneration takes place in that portion separated from the ganglion, showing that the ganglion is the nutritive centre for the posterior root.

This same method is used to study the course of the fibres of the cord, and as a result it has been found that they degenerate in the direction in which the impulses travel—namely, that if those fibres which carry impulses downward be divided, the degeneration takes place in the same direction, while the reverse is true for those which carry impulses upward.

Conducting-paths in the Cord.—The paths by which voluntary motor impulses traverse the cord are fairly well ascertained. These impulses originate in the brain and pass through the pyramids in the medulla, crossing principally at the decussation of the pyramids, and to a less degree in the upper part of the cord, to the opposite side, whence they follow the course of the pyramidal tracts, direct and crossed, terminating in the cells of the anterior cornua, from which the anterior roots arise to be distributed to the muscles.

The course pursued by the sensory impulses is not so well understood; indeed, opinions differ very materially. It was formerly held by many of the best investigators that the sensory impulses crossed in the cord, but at the present time the evidence is accumulating that, as with motor impulses, so sensory impulses cross mainly in the medulla and to a less degree in the cord. That both motor and sensory impulses do cross is shown by the fact that whenever there is a lesion of the brain resulting in paralysis either of motion or of sensation, the paralysis is on the side of the body opposite to that of the lesion.

In reference to the routes taken by the various sensory impulses, as those of pain, temperature, touch, etc., the evidence is so conflicting that it would be confusing to give it. Besides the function which the cord performs as a conductor of motor and sensory impulses by virtue of its nerve-fibres, it also acts as a nerve-centre in which, by virtue of its nerve-cells, afferent impulses are received and motor impulses are generated.

The Spinal Cord as a Nerve-centre.—Voluntary motion in the extremities, which motion originates in the brain, is abolished when the cord is divided and its anatomical connection with the brain cut off, but there still remains the power of exciting muscular contractions in these muscles, due to the cells of the cord itself.

Reflex Action.—If a frog be decapitated, it has no

longer the power of producing voluntary movements, but if the skin of a foot be irritated by pinching, the foot is pulled away from the source of irritation. A slight pinch will cause only the one foot to be withdrawn, but if it be stronger the other foot may also be withdrawn. This is an instance of reflex action. Such movements are not spontaneous, but they require the application of a stimulus for their production. The irritation does not act upon the muscles directly, but through the medium of nerves, an afferent nerve carrying the sensory impulse inward to the cord, and an efferent nerve conducting a motor impulse outward to the muscles. If either of these nerves be divided, the action does not take place, nor does it if the gray matter be broken up. For the performance of a reflex act, therefore, three things are necessary—an afferent nerve, a nerve-centre, and an efferent nerve, all in a physiological condition.

In the human subject, when the cord is injured or diseased at any point, so as to cut off communication between the brain and extremities, but is still intact below this point, tickling of the soles of the feet will be followed by their withdrawal, although the individual will be entirely unconscious of any sensation. This is also an instance of reflex action. As in the frog, so in man, the three structures mentioned must exist in a state of integrity for the performance of this act.

It is not essential that the cord be diseased in order to have it manifest reflex action. Thus if the hand come in contact with a flame, it is immediately withdrawn. This is not a voluntary act, for the act of withdrawal takes place before the sensation of pain is felt in the brain. It is a purely reflex act, in which the gray matter of the cord, after being stimulated by an impulse carried to it by an afferent nerve, generates an impulse which is conveyed by an efferent nerve to the muscles concerned in withdrawing the arm. If the attention were fixed upon the subject at the time the burn was received, it might be possible to prevent the withdrawal. This would be an instance of inhibition of reflex action. During sleep there take place many reflex acts which do not occur in a waking condition. Thus tickling the feet during sleep may result in their withdrawal; when the tickling is practised during wakefulness the reflex act can, by the influence of the will, be inhibited.

This power of the spinal cord to respond to afferent impulses independently of the will is of great advantage in preserving the body from injury. The closing of the eye when moving objects are liable to injure it, the attempt to retain one's equilibrium after slipping on the sidewalk, the raising of the arms in front of the face to ward off an unexpected blow, are all instances of this action.

Walking, playing on musical instruments, and similar acts are all performed under the influence of the gray matter of the cord. To start them requires the action of the brain, but when once they are begun their continuance is accomplished by the cord, and the brain can be busy about other things without interfering in the slightest degree with the perfection of their performance. Indeed, any attempt to control them is more apt to hinder than to help them. Thus in coming rapidly down a flight of steps, if the spinal cord be permitted to take entire charge of the act the descent will be made with ease and safety, but if each step be made as the result of volition, the chances of stumbling or of tripping are very much increased.

The reflex action of the cord may be diminished by shock to the nervous system; thus in the frog immediately after decapitation the reflex power cannot be excited, but after a short time it manifests itself under the influence of a stimulus. A similar diminution of the reflex power of the cord may be caused by opium, by chloroform, and by some other substances, while the reflex action is increased by strychnine. If under the skin of the decapitated frog a solution of strychnine be injected, the cord in a short time becomes so irritable that a stimulus which before would have had no effect will now produce the most marked results, a slight blow upon the skin sufficing to throw the animal into a convulsive state. In tetanus the same irritable condition of the cord exists, and in this state the patient may be thrown into convulsions by the simple opening and closing of a door.

Special Centres in the Cord.—It is the practice to speak of certain centres as existing in the spinal cord; that is, of definite collections of cells which preside over definite functions. Among these centres the following have been described: Musculo-tonic, respiratory, cardio-accelerator, vaso-motor, sudorific, cilio-spinal, genito-spinal, ano-spinal, vesico-spinal, trophic, for erection of the penis, for parturition, and others.

Musculo-tonic Centre.—This centre is continually discharging impulses which keep the muscular system in a condition of slight contraction: this is called "muscular tone." It is questionable whether this condition is to be attributed to any special centre rather than to the action of all those cells whose function it is to send out motor impulses.

Respiratory Centre.—The principal respiratory centre

is in the medulla, but experiments in which this structure has been destroyed while some respiratory movements persisted demonstrate that to a certain extent, doubtless very slight, the spinal cord controls the respiratory processes.

Cardio-accelerator Centre.—The spinal cord through the cardiac nerves and plexus sends impulses to the heart, causing it to beat more rapidly; that is, they accelerate its movements. These impulses are not constantly emitted, as are the inhibitory impulses which travel by the pneumogastric.

Vaso-motor Centre.—The vaso-motor centre in the cord is entirely subsidiary to that in the medulla.

Sudorific Centre.—The existence of special nerves controlling the secretion of sweat seems to be demonstrated. These nerves come from the spinal cord, being a part of the anterior roots.

Cilio-spinal Centre.—Nerve-fibres pass from this centre to the iris, and they are concerned in the dilatation of the pupil. These fibres come out from the cord through the anterior roots of the spinal nerves, from the fifth cervical to the fifth thoracic, and join the cervical sympathetic.

Genito-spinal Centre.—The genito-spinal is the centre which governs the emission of semen, and is situated in the lumbar region of the cord. Sensory impulses from the glans penis reach this centre through afferent nerves and stimulate it, and from it go out efferent impulses which cause contraction of the muscular fibres of the vasa deferentia, seminal vesicles, and accelerator urinæ, the result of which is to produce an ejection of semen.

Ano-spinal Centre.—The act of defecation is governed by the ano-spinal centre. The mucous membrane and muscular coat of the rectum are supplied with nerves from the several plexuses of spinal nerves. Fæces do not ordinarily pass into the rectum until about the time of evacuation, when they are expelled from the sigmoid flexure into the rectum. At this time the sphincter ani is in a state of contraction, which is its usual condition, kept so by the impulses that come from the spinal cord. This contraction keeps the anus closed even during sleep, and it is entirely independent of the action of the brain; it is an involuntary act. When, however, fæces enter the rectum, the nerves of its mucous membrane become stimulated, and these impulses are conveyed by afferent nerves to the ano-spinal centre in the lumbar enlargement of the cord, and from this are reflected impulses which, conveyed to the sphincter, cause its relaxation. Under the influence of similar impulses which pass to the levator ani this muscle contracts and draws upward the edges of the anus, causing it to open, while at the same time the muscular fibres of the rectum contract and expel the fæces. If the stimulation be very pronounced, the abdominal muscles may also be called into action, irrespective of the will, but when the stimulus is slight they may only respond when called upon by the brain. The connection between the brain and the ano-spinal centre is very close, so that the action of the latter may for a time be inhibited, but if the rectum become very much distended the impulses may be so strong that, despite the will, defecation will take place.

Involuntary Discharges.—In some forms of disease the irritability of the ano-spinal centre is so great that when the rectum is only partially filled defecation takes place, and there is no power to retard it. Discharges under these circumstances are said to be involuntary.

Involuntary and Unconscious Discharges.—If by reason of disease or of injury the middle or the upper portions of the cord become so disorganized as to cut off communication with the brain, while at the same time the lower portion is in normal condition, the act of defecation takes place when the rectum becomes sufficiently distended to stimulate the ano-spinal centre to action; but there is no power to retard it nor is there any consciousness of it, since the connection with the brain is severed. Under these circumstances the discharges are involuntary and unconscious. If the lumbar portion of the cord be the seat of injury or of disease to such an extent as to destroy this centre, the sphincter is permanently relaxed, and the fæces are discharged as fast as they reach the anus.

Vesico-spinal Centre.—The act of micturition is under the influence of the vesico-spinal centre. Like the genito-spinal, this is situated also in the lumbar enlargement. The urine formed in the kidneys passes into the ureters, and thence, under the influence of the peristaltic action of the muscular coat of the walls of these vessels, into the bladder. This contraction lasts about one-third of a second, and takes place alternately in the ureters, so that the urine does not flow into the bladder from both kidneys at the same time. It accumulates in the bladder until such time as it is voided.

The bladder, like the rectum, is supplied with nerve-fibres which have their origin in the vesico-spinal centre. The urine is retained within the bladder by the tonic contraction of the sphincter vesicæ in the same manner as fæces are retained in the rectum by the sphincter ani. The pressure of the urine when the bladder is full is only equal to 1 cm. of mercury, while it takes a pressure of at least 3 cm. to overcome the elasticity of the sphincter.

When the bladder is about to be emptied a voluntary impulse transmitted to the sphincter vesicæ causes its relaxation. At the same time the muscular coat of the bladder and the abdominal muscles contract, and the urine begins to flow. The pressure which is thus exerted equals 10 cm. of mercury. Although the starting of the act is voluntary, when once it has begun it continues under the influence of the vesico-spinal centre alone until the bladder is empty.

Up to a certain point the brain is able to inhibit the centre and postpone the evacuation of the bladder, but after a time, if too long delayed, the resistance of the sphincter is overcome and urine will flow. It is more difficult to stop the act after it has once begun than to delay its beginning, for the urine, flowing over the mucous membrane of the urethra, stimulates the vesico-spinal centre, and the efferent impulses to the contracting muscles are increased.

If the mucous membrane of the bladder be inflamed, as in cystitis, the stimulation of the centre may be so great as to prevent the brain from inhibiting the evacuation, and evacuation may occur when only a small quantity of urine has accumulated. Or it may happen that the spinal cord is injured or is diseased in the upper or middle portion, and thus all sensation caused by a full bladder may be abolished. Under these circumstances the bladder, when full, will be emptied by the reflex action of the vesico-spinal centre. Or, again, if the lesion of the cord be such as to disorganize this centre, then there will be no reflex action of the cord, and the elasticity of the tissues about the neck of the bladder will keep the urine in that viscus until it is overcome by the distention, when it will flow in drops as fast as it comes from the kidneys, but the organ will not empty itself. Inexperienced persons are often deceived by this dribbling of the urine, thinking that its discharge is evidence that the bladder is performing its duty, while the fact is that it is evidence of paralysis and retention.

Trophic Centres.—It has already been seen that when nerve-fibres are divided they undergo degeneration, and that this is explained by the fact that under these circumstances their connection with certain nerve-cells is severed, and that they are thus deprived of the nutritive influence which such centres exert. Such centres are called "trophic centres," and the cells of the anterior cornua of the cord and the ganglia on the posterior roots of the spinal nerves are familiar illustrations. That these are true trophic centres for nerves seems to be beyond dispute, but this is an entirely different question from that which deals with trophic nerves as regulating the nutrition of tissues other than nerves. About the existence of such nerves there is considerable doubt.

Other Centres.—Some writers describe a centre for erection of the penis, and locate it in the lumbar enlargement. The afferent nerves from the penis cause this centre to send out efferent impulses by which the blood-vessels are dilated and the muscles are compressed, thus preventing the return of the venous blood from the penis and bringing about erection. A centre for parturition is also located in the lumbar region of the cord, above the centres already mentioned, under the influence of which the muscular tissue of the uterus contracts at the proper time and expels the fœtus. Other reflex centres are described, but the tendency to extend the number of such centres seems to be beyond what the actual facts warrant. However, enough has been said to show the great importance of the spinal cord as a nervous centre, independently of its function as a conductor of nervous impulses to and from the brain.

THE BRAIN.

The brain, or encephalon, is that part of the cerebro-spinal axis situated within the cranium or skull. Its divisions are sometimes described as the *fore-brain*, including the hemispheres, with the olfactory lobe, the corpora striata, and the optic thalami; the *mid-brain*, being the corpora quadrigemina and the crura cerebri; and the *hind-brain*—that is, the cerebellum, the pons Varolii, and the medulla oblongata.

In the adult male the brain weighs, on an average, 1415 grammes avoirdupois: in the female, 1245 grammes. In 278 cases of males in which the brain was weighed the maximum was 1841 grammes and the minimum 963 grammes. In 191 cases of females the maximum was 1586 grammes and the minimum 878 grammes. The brain of Cuvier, the great naturalist, weighed 1815 grammes; that of an idiot weighed 651 grammes. The brain of a mulatto not remarkable for intelligence weighed 1927 grammes. The fore-brain weighs about 1245 grammes in the adult male.

The gray matter of the brain is in some parts on the surface, as in the convolutions of the cerebrum; in other parts it is deeply situated, as in the basal ganglia, the corpora striata, and the optic thalami; while in still other parts it is scattered about without any fixed arrangement, as in the pons Varolii. The white matter is made up of fibres which come from the spinal cord; of fibres having their origin in the gray matter, and which, escaping from the skull, go to their points of distribution as the cranial nerves; and of still other fibres connecting the ganglia with one another and forming commissures.

The Medulla Oblongata.—The medulla oblongata, or bulb, is a continuation of the spinal cord, and is about 2.5 cm. long, 2 cm. broad, and 1.2 cm. thick. It is composed of gray and white matter. The gray matter, which in the cord has the characteristic double crescentic shape, approaches more and more the posterior surface of the cord as the region of the medulla is reached and the posterior cornua become more and more external, the whole mass of gray matter flattening out, until in the medulla it forms a layer the outer portions of which represent the posterior horns and the middle portions the anterior. The posterior columns separate in the medulla, the central canal coming to the surface posteriorly and ending in the fourth ventricle, the floor of which is the gray matter above referred to, which is, however, not limited to this site, but is present about the aque-

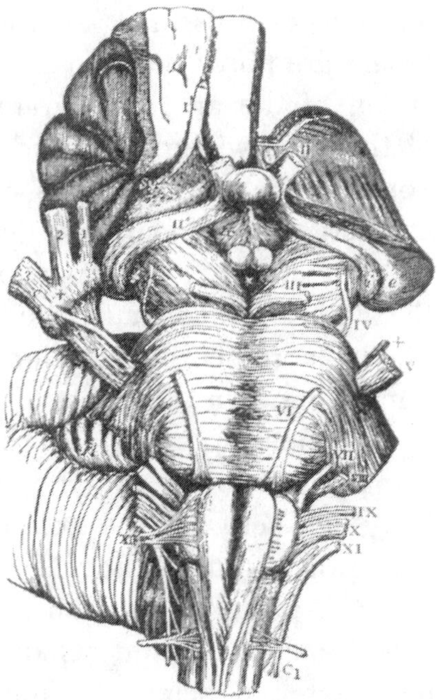

FIG. 51.—View, from below, of the Connection of the Principal Nerves with the Brain: I', the right olfactory tract; II, the left optic nerve; II', the right optic tract (the left tract is seen passing back into *i* and *e*, the internal and external corpora geniculata); III, the left oculo-motor nerve; IV, the trochlear; V,V, the large roots of the trifacial nerves; + +, the lesser roots (the + of the right side is placed on the Gasserian ganglion); 1, the ophthalmic; 2, the superior maxillary; and 3, the inferior maxillary divisions; VI, the left abducens nerve; VII, VIII, the facial and auditory nerves; IX–XI, the glosso-pharyngeal, pneumogastric, and spinal accessory nerves; XII, the right hypoglossal nerve; C_1, the left suboccipital or first cervical nerve (Nancrede).

duct of Sylvius. From this gray matter arise all the cranial nerves excepting the olfactory and optic.

The medulla, like the cord, has an anterior and a posterior median fissure. At the lower part of the anterior fissure are fibres that cross from side to side, the decussation of the anterior pyramids. The posterior fissure of the cord widens out and forms the fourth ventricle. Some of the cranial nerves come out from the medulla, and serve as boundaries to describe the different portions of the medulla. That portion of white matter between the anterior median fissure and the roots of the hypoglossal nerve is the anterior pyramid. The lateral column is between the roots of the hypoglossal and those of the glossò-pharyngeal, the pneumogastric, and the spinal accessory. At the upper portion the olivary body lies between the column and the pyramid. The posterior column is between the lateral column or tract and the posterior median fissure. It is composed of three smaller columns separated by shallow grooves, the most external being the funiculus of Rolando, next the funiculus cuneatus, and the most internal the funiculus gracilis, the first two being joined in the upper part of the medulla to form the restiform body. The outer portion of the pyramid is derived from the direct pyramidal tracts of the same side, while the decussation consists of the fibres of the crossed pyramidal tract of the lateral column.

In the restiform bodies are to be found, besides the funiculus of Rolando and the funiculus cuneatus, fibres of the direct cerebellar tract of the lateral column. These bodies form the inferior peduncles of the cerebellum. The funiculus of Rolando is the enlarged head of the posterior cornu of the cord, and is therefore gray matter.

The funiculus cuneatus is the continuation of Burdach's column of the cord, and the funiculus gracilis is the continuation of Goll's column.

Functions of the Medulla Oblongata.—*Conduction.*—All the impulses, whether afferent or efferent, passing between the brain and the cord must pass through the medulla.

Nerve-centres.—Experiments have demonstrated that all the brain above the medulla and all the spinal cord may be removed and yet life be maintained, provided that the origin of the phrenic nerves be left intact, while if all these structures be undisturbed and the medulla be broken up death will result. The centres in the medulla are both reflex and automatic.

Reflex Centres.—One of the most important of these centres is that which presides over deglutition. As has already been seen in discussing this process, the first stage of the act is voluntary, but as soon as the food has passed into the pharynx the act becomes involuntary. The mucous membrane of the pharynx is stimulated by the food, and the afferent fibres of the glosso-pharyngeal transmit the impulse to the medulla, in which a motor impulse is generated, and out along the efferent fibres comes the impulse to the constrictors of the pharynx. Centres for vomiting, coughing, sucking, and for other movements are described by some writers.

Vomiting.—When the act of vomiting takes place there is first an inspiration; after this the glottis is closed and so remains. The lungs being filled with air and the glottis being closed, no air can escape, and the diaphragm therefore remains fixed as it is at the end of an inspiration. The abdominal muscles then compress the stomach against the fixed diaphragm, and the circular fibres at the cardiac orifice of the stomach (the cardiac sphincter) being relaxed, this orifice opens, and, as at the same time the pyloric orifice is closed, the stomach is emptied of its contents into the œsophagus. The muscular coat of this tube by reversed peristalsis carries the material to the pharynx and the mouth, where it is expelled. Whether the muscular coat of the stomach takes any part in the evacuation is questioned by some authors, on the ground that the stomach may be replaced by a bag whose contents will be expelled by the contractions of the abdominal muscles alone; but the probability is that the gastric muscular fibres also contract. Whether these contribute much toward expelling the contents in the adult is not determined, but they are probably the only agency in the infant.

The act of vomiting is a reflex one, in which the fibres of the pneumogastric serve as afferent fibres, the impulses stimulating the centre in the medulla from which emanate motor impulses to the respiratory and other muscles concerned in the act. If the act of vomiting be brought on by stimulating the pharynx with a feather or with a finger, the glosso-pharyngeal is the carrier of the afferent impulses. Afferent impulses producing vomiting may also come from other organs, such as the kidneys, or the testicles when injured.

Central Vomiting.—In central vomiting the centre is stimulated by impulses which come from the brain.

Rumination.—The power to ruminate, by virtue of which animals chew the cud, is possessed by some human individuals, who can regurgitate the food whenever they feel so disposed, and chew it again.

Automatic Centres.—Besides reflex centres, which require a stimulus from without to bring them into action, the medulla possesses automatic centres which generate and emit impulses independently of stimuli from without.

Respiratory Centre.—This centre is situated in the floor of the fourth ventricle, and when injured respiration ceases immediately. Some authorities place it among the reflex centres. As will be seen, it may be excited reflexly, but there are reasons for believing it to possess automatic powers as well. If the spinal cord be divided below the medulla, although the respiratory movements of the thorax cease, those of the nose and larynx continue. Under these circumstances no afferent impulses can be transmitted through the spinal nerves, and the only channel is the cranial nerves; but if, while the medulla and cord are left undisturbed, the cranial nerves be cut, respiration continues. These two series of experiments show that respiration will continue without the reception of any impulses from without; that is, automatically.

The principal nerves that transmit the impulses producing the respiratory movements are the intercostals, and the phrenics to the diaphragm. The respiratory centre is double, so that one side may act after the other is divided. Division of one phrenic paralyzes only the side of the diaphragm to which it is distributed. The respiratory centre may also be excited reflexly. The afferent fibres under these circumstances are those of the pneumogastric.

Resistance Theory of Respiration.—If a pair of bellows be connected with the trachea of an animal, and air thereby be supplied to its lungs, there will be no respiratory movements made by the animal itself, but if the supply of air be discontinued, after a time respiratory efforts will be made, and they will be rhythmic in character. The explanation of this fact is by no means certain, but the following theory has been advanced:

In the respiratory centre of the medulla certain chemical changes are constantly taking place, the result of which is the production of a substance which is a stimulant to the nerve-cells composing this centre, and these cells when stimulated send out impulses to the inspiratory muscles, causing them to contract, thus producing an inspiration. This substance is destroyed by oxygen when the amount in the blood reaches a certain point. This point is reached when air is supplied by the bellows in the experiment above referred to; but the blood, which, under normal conditions, is supplied to the medulla, is not rich enough in oxygen to completely destroy this substance, and therefore it accumulates and stimulates the nerve-cells, bringing about the inspiratory act. When the blood is venous this substance accumulates more rapidly and the respiratory acts are more frequent.

The rhythmic character of respiration is accounted for by supposing that the nervous energy from the cells, passing over the respiratory nerves to the muscles, meets with such resistance that the discharge can only take place after the impulses have accumulated to a certain extent in the centre, and that when this occurs the discharge takes place and the inspiration follows; then there is a period of rest, during which time the accumulation is again taking place, and when the proper point is reached another discharge occurs, to be followed by the inspiratory act. It is of course to be understood that this theory is provisional only. Whether such a substance exists or not is undetermined.

Asphyxia.—This condition may be appropriately described at this place, now that the relation between the lungs and the nervous system is understood. The term literally means "pulselessness," and is especially applicable to the fourth stage. If by any means the supply of air to an animal be prevented, death results within a very few minutes by asphyxia. The animal before the fatal termination arrives passes through four stages—namely, (1) dyspnœa; (2) convulsion; (3) exhaustion; and (4) inspiratory spasm.

(1) *Dyspnœa.*—As soon as the air is cut off the blood becomes more and more venous; that is, loses more and more of its oxygen. The respiratory centre becomes more stimulated, and efferent impulses call into play the extraordinary muscles of respiration—the sterno-mastoid, the serratus magnus, the pectoralis, and the trapezius. This dyspnœic stage, or stage of difficult or labored breathing, continues for about one minute.

(2) *Convulsion.*—In the second stage the movements of inspiration become feebler, while those of expiration become stronger, and at length the muscles of the whole body are thrown into a state of convulsion. This stage is very brief.

(3) *Exhaustion.*—The expiratory muscles being exhausted, the animal becomes quiescent, only a few slight attempts at inspiration being perceptible. After a time these become deeper, but only occur at comparatively long intervals. The third stage is longer than the first or the second.

(4) *Inspiratory Spasm.*—The intervals between the inspirations have in this stage greatly increased, and apparently ceased, but they recur occasionally. The pupils are dilated and the pulse is less and less perceptible; finally a last inspiration occurs and the animal is dead.

Cardio-inhibitory Centre.—In the cardio-inhibitory centre are generated those impulses which, travelling to the heart by the pneumogastric nerve, inhibit or restrain the action of that organ. This subject will be more fully discussed in connection with the functions of the pneumogastric nerve. The accelerator nerves of the heart have their origin in the spinal cord, and are distributed to that organ through the sympathetic ganglia. Whether they have any origin in the medulla is doubtful. They are antagonistic to the pneumogastric, and carry impulses to the heart which hasten its action.

Vaso-motor Centre.—The exact location of the vaso-motor centre in the medulla of man is not definitely settled, but it is probably in the floor of the fourth ventricle. From this centre go impulses over the vaso-constrictor nerves, which impulses tend to constrict the arteries; hence it has been suggested that it should be called the "vaso-constrictor centre."

The muscular coat of the arteries is innervated first by fibres which arise in ganglion-cells situated either in the walls of the vessels or very near them. These ganglia are called "intrinsic ganglia," and the nerves coming from them are called "intrinsic nerves." They are constantly generating and emitting impulses which keep the muscular fibres in a state of slight but generally constant contraction, called "muscular tone." The second source of innervation of the muscular coat of the arteries is the vaso-constrictor nerves just described. These nerves are spoken of as "extrinsic," and the impulses which they transmit cause the vessels to be more constricted than they would be by the impulses coming from the intrinsic ganglia. The vaso-constrictor fibres come from the sympathetic, but their real origin is in the medulla, from which they pass down the cord, and emerge as constituent parts of the anterior roots of some of the spinal nerves, joining the sympathetic system subsequently.

Although the vaso-motor centre is here classified among the automatic centres, it may also be excited reflexly. The sensory nerves of the body are for the most part connected with it, and when severe pain is experienced the centre may be stimulated, and as a result the impulses generated may constrict the arteries, and thus by increasing the resistance of the blood-current increase arterial pressure.

Depressor Nerve-fibres.—Between the heart and the medulla are nerve-fibres which carry impulses from the heart to the vaso-motor nerve-centre, which impulses inhibit the centre, and thus diminish the impulses to the muscular coat of the arteries, thereby causing the arteries to dilate and reducing arterial pressure. In the rabbit these fibres are together and form the depressor nerve, but in most animals they are joined with the fibres of the pneumogastric. By means of these fibres the nerve-centre can be inhibited and arterial pressure be lessened, thus reducing the work of the heart.

Pons Varolii.—The pons Varolii (tuber annulare or mesocephalon) is situated just above the medulla, and is made up of three sets of fibres and of some gray matter. The first set is composed of superficial transverse fibres which cross the upper part of the medulla and connect the two hemispheres of the cerebellum, forming at the sides the crura cerebelli or middle peduncles. The second set is made up of longitudinal fibres which come from the pyramids of the medulla and pass on to help form the crura cerebri. The third set is also transverse and is deeply situated, connecting the middle peduncles of the cerebellum. Among its fibres are collections of gray matter.

Functions of the Pons Varolii.—The anatomical relations of the pons show that it must serve as a conductor of impulses both to and from the centres above. As to the function of its gray matter comparatively little is known, save that from a portion of it some of the cranial nerves arise. If it be stimulated or divided, pain and spasms are produced. When a lesion is situated in the lower half of the pons, there result facial paralysis on the same side as the lesion, and motor and sensory paralysis of the opposite side of the body. This is called alternate paralysis. If the lesion be in the upper half of the pons, the facial paralysis and that of the body are on the same side. When the pons is suddenly and extensively injured, a condition of hyperpyrexia is often produced, the temperature rising rapidly within an hour. This is probably due to the influence of the gray matter in the floor of the fourth ventricle, or possibly to the involvement of some special heat-regulating centre.

Cerebellum.—The cerebellum is composed externally of gray matter, which also penetrates into the substance of the organ, forming with the white matter the *laminæ*. In the central part of the cerebellum is white matter in which is imbedded a collection of gray matter, the *corpus dentatum*. The cerebellum is connected with the rest of the encephalon by the superior, the middle, and the inferior peduncles. The superior peduncles (*processus e cerebello ad testes*) connect the cerebellum with the cerebrum; the middle peduncles (*crura cerebelli*) connect the two cerebellar hemispheres; the inferior (*pro-*

cessus ad medullam) connect the cerebellum and medulla oblongata.

The gray matter, as has been said, is upon the surface and in the interior: that upon the surface, called the "cortex," is made up of two layers—an external gray, consisting of neuroglia, fibres, and cells, and an internal rust-colored layer. In the gray are peculiar cells, the corpuscles of Purkinje, which are flask-shaped, and which give off from the side toward the internal layer processes that terminate in axis-cylinders of medullated nerve-fibres. From the other side pass off processes which branch in the external layer, some of them at least joining with the cells in this layer. The gray matter in the interior is the corpus dentatum and the "roof-nuclei" of Stilling.

Functions of the Cerebellum.—If the surface of the cerebellum be irritated, no muscular movements are produced nor is there any evidence of sensation; if, however, the irritation be applied near the medulla or inferior peduncles, both pain and muscular contraction result. If the cerebellum be removed wholly or partially, sensation is not diminished in the part of the body below, nor is there any impairment of the power of producing muscular movements, nor of the special senses, nor of the intelligence; but there is a marked want of harmony in the muscular movements, a lack of co-ordination. Attention has already been called to the fact that even the simplest movements that are made require the harmonious action of different muscles, and when these movements are more complex they require different sets of muscles. If these movements do not occur at just the right time and are not produced in the right manner, the result is disorder instead of harmony;

or, as it is expressed, there is a want of co-ordination. This is the effect of removing the cerebellum. Thus, if the cerebellum of the pigeon be removed, and an attempt be then made by it to fly, it is unsuccessful, for this act requires the consentaneous action of both wings, which action is absent. In walking the bird reels like a person intoxicated, and cannot go to the spot for which it apparently set out. It should be borne in mind that there is no paralysis either of motion or of sensation in this condition, but the voluntary movements which originate in the cerebrum, and which are in the normal condition co-ordinated by the cerebellum, pass to the muscles without this regulating influence, and the result is a series of disordered movements.

It is interesting to know that in animals that produce complex movements the cerebellum is considerably developed, while in those animals whose movements are simple, such as the frog, this organ is exceedingly small.

Cerebrum.—The cerebrum, which in man makes up about four-fifths of the encephalon, is divided into two hemispheres which are separated by the great longitudinal fissure (Fig. 52), but are connected by a white commissure, the *corpus callosum* (Fig. 54). The surface presents depressions, called "fissures" and "sulci," and prominences, termed "convolutions" or "gyri." The external portion of the hemispheres is gray nervous matter about 3 mm. in thickness, beneath which is white matter. The fissures are not numerous, but are quite constant; they are folds of the brain-matter both gray and white. The sulci are depressions of the gray matter alone; they are very numerous and inconstant. As gray matter is present on both sides of the fissures and sulci, this arrangement permits of a larger amount of gray matter than could exist were it only upon the surface of the convolutions. In a brain, therefore, where the sulci are deep and numerous the amount of gray matter exceeds that in a brain where they are more shallow and less abundant. This gray matter is called the "cortical substance."

Fissures of the Cerebrum.—The fissures serve as land-

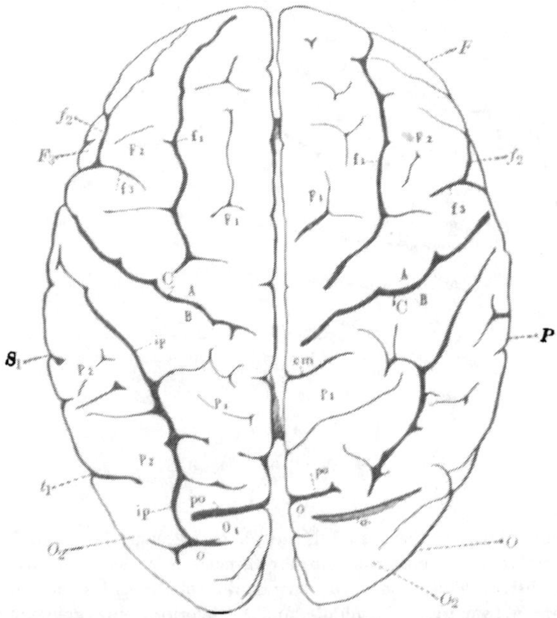

Fig. 52.—View of the Brain from above: *A*, anterior central or ascending frontal convolution; *B*, posterior central or ascending parietal convolution; *C*, central fissure, or fissure of Rolando; *cm*, calloso-marginal sulcus; *F*, frontal lobe; F_1, upper, F_2, middle, F_3, lower frontal convolution; f_1, superior frontal sulcus; f_2, inferior frontal sulcus; f_3, vertical fissure (sulcus præcentralis); *ip*, interparietal sulcus; *O*, occipital lobe; *o*, sulcus occipitalis transversus; O_1, first occipital convolution; O_2, second occipital convolution; *P*, parietal lobe; *po*, parieto-occipital fissure; P_1, upper or postero-parietal lobule; P_2, lower parietal lobule, constituted by P_2, gyrus supramarginalis; P_2', gyrus angularis; S_1, end of the horizontal branch of the fissura Sylvii; t_1, upper temporal fissure.

marks in the description of the different parts of the hemispheres. Besides the great longitudinal fissure, there are (1) the fissure of Sylvius; (2) that of Rolando; and (3) the parieto-occipital fissure (Fig. 53). These fissures divide each hemisphere into five lobes.

(1) *The fissure of Sylvius* is, next to the great longitudinal fissure, the most important. It is found in all animals whose brains have any fissures. It exists in

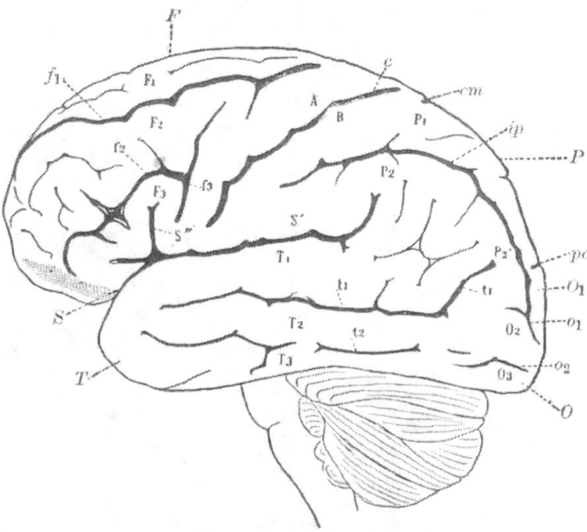

FIG. 53.—Outer Surface of the Left Hemisphere: *A*, anterior central or ascending frontal convolution; *B*, posterior central or ascending parietal convolution; *c*, sulcus centralis or fissure of Rolando; *cm*, termination of the calloso-marginal fissure; *F*, frontal lobe; F_1, superior, F_2, middle, and F_3, inferior frontal convolution; f_1, superior, and f_2, inferior frontal sulcus; f_3, sulcus præcentralis; *ip*, sulcus intraparietalis; *O*, occipital lobe; O_1, first, O_2, second. O_3, third occipital convolutions; o_1, sulcus occipitalis transversus; o_2, sulcus occipitalis longitudinalis inferior; *P*, parietal lobe; *po*, parieto-occipital fissure; P_1, superior parietal or postero-parietal lobule; P_2, inferior parietal lobule—viz. P_2, gyrus supramarginalis; P_2', gyrus angularis; *S*, fissure of Sylvius; *S'*, horizontal, *S''*, ascending ramus of the same; *T*, temporo-sphenoidal lobe; T_1, first, T_2, second, T_3, third temporo-sphenoidal convolutions; t_1, first, t_2, second temporo-sphenoidal fissures.

the human brain in the third month of intra-uterine life. It commences at the base of the brain, and runs outward, backward, and upward, giving off a short anterior branch or limb. The continuation of the fissure backward from where this branch is given off is called the "posterior branch" or horizontal limb, which ends in the parietal lobe. The fissure of Sylvius is the boundary between the frontal and parietal lobes on the one hand and the temporo-sphenoidal on the other. At the middle and anterior part of this fissure, deeply situated, is the island of Reil, or insula, or central lobe (Fig. 53).

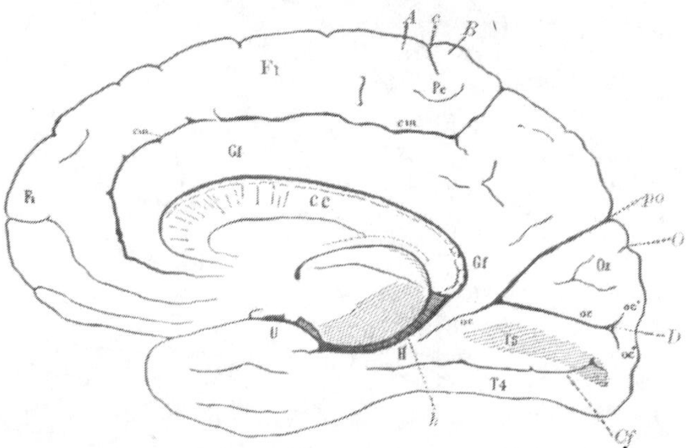

Fig. 54.—Inner Surface of Right Hemisphere: *A*, ascending frontal; *B*, ascending parietal convolution; *c*, terminal portion of the sulcus centralis, or fissure of Rolando; *CC*, corpus callosum, longitudinally divided; *Cf*, collateral or occipito-temporal fissure (Ecker); *cm*, sulcus calloso-marginalis; *D*, gyrus descendens; F_1, median aspect of the first frontal convolution; *Gf*, gyrus fornicatus; *H*, gyrus hippocampi; *h*, sulcus hippocampi, or dentate fissure; *O*, sulcus occipitalis transversus; *oc*, calcarine fissure; *oc'*, superior, *oc''*, inferior ramus of the same; *Oz*, cuneus; *po*, parieto-occipital fissure; P_1'', precuneus; T_4, gyrus occipito-temporalis lateralis (lobulus fusiformis); T_5, gyrus occipito-temporalis medialis (lobulus lingualis); *U*, uncinate gyrus.

(2) *The fissure of Rolando* starts near the median line, and runs downward and forward nearly to the fissure of Sylvius (Fig. 53). It is the boundary between the frontal and parietal lobes.

(3) *The parieto-occipital fissure* is about halfway between the fissure of Rolando and the posterior extremity of the brain, and is the boundary between the parietal and occipital lobes (Fig. 54).

Lobes of the Cerebrum.—The lobes of the cerebrum are (1) the frontal, (2) the parietal, (3) the occipital, (4)

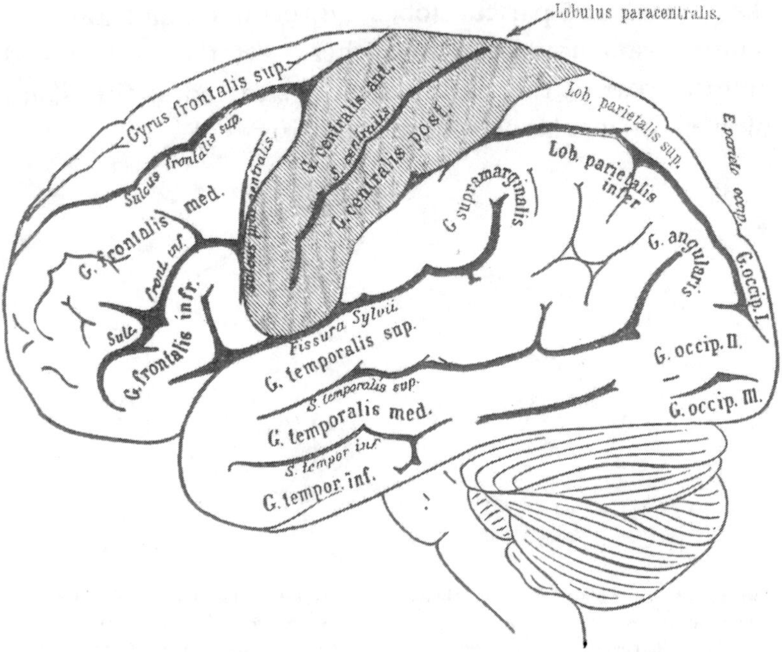

FIG. 55.—Lateral View of the Brain (combined from Ecker): gyri and lobuli marked with antique type, the sulci and fissures with italic type.

the temporo-sphenoidal, and (5) the central, or island of Reil (Figs. 53 and 55).

(1) *The frontal lobe* is above the fissure of Sylvius and in front of the fissure of Rolando. It is divided into four convolutions by three sulci, or fissures as they are sometimes called. The præcentral fissure or sulcus is in front of the fissure of Rolando, and the convolution between the two is the ascending frontal. From the upper extremity of this sulcus the superior frontal sulcus runs downward and forward between the superior and middle frontal convolutions, while from the lower extremity runs off the inferior frontal sulcus, separating

the middle and inferior frontal convolutions. Thus the frontal lobe is divided into the ascending, superior, middle, and inferior frontal convolutions.

(2) *The parietal lobe* is behind the frontal and in front of the occipital lobe, the fissure of Rolando being its anterior, and the parieto-occipital fissure its posterior, boundary. Its inferior boundary is the fissure of Sylvius and the imaginary continuation of it to the superior occipital sulcus. It has two sulci, the intraparietal and the post-central, and three convolutions, the ascending, superior, and inferior parietal.

(3) *The occipital lobe* is posterior to the parietal, and has two sulci, the superior and middle, and three convolutions, the superior, middle, and inferior occipital, the latter being subdivided into the supramarginal and the angular.

(4) *The Temporo-sphenoidal Lobe.*—The fissure of Sylvius forms the anterior and superior boundaries of this lobe, while its posterior boundary is the imaginary continuation of the occipito-parietal fissure. It presents two sulci, the superior tempero-sphenoidal or parallel, and the middle temporo-sphenoidal. Its convolutions are three, the superior, middle, and inferior temporo-sphenoidal.

(5) *The central lobe, or island of Reil,* is situated at the base of the brain, in the fissure of Sylvius. It consists of six convolutions, the *gyri operti.*

Crura cerebri, also called the "peduncles of the cerebrum," are made up of white matter, nerves which are continuous with those already studied in the medulla and pons, together with nerves from the cerebellum, the superior peduncles. Between the superficial fibres of the crura, the crusta, and the deeper ones, the tegmentum, is the locus niger, a collection of gray matter. The fibres of the crura on their way upward to the gray matter of the hemispheres pass through the corpora striata and the optic thalami.

Basal Ganglia.—At the base of the hemisphere are certain bodies, the basal ganglia, which are the corpora striata, the optic thalami, the tubercula quadrigemina or corpora quadrigemina, the corpora geniculata, and the locus niger.

Corpora striata, with the optic thalami, are called the "cerebral ganglia." The corpora striata present a striped appearance, which is due to a mixture of gray and white matter, the latter being bundles of fibres which have come from below and within. Although at the lowest part each corpus striatum is a single body, at the upper part it is divided into two portions called the "caudate nucleus" and "lenticular nucleus." The lenticular nucleus, the more posterior, is separated from the optic thalamus by white matter, the internal capsule, which is the continuation of the crus cerebri. Outside the lenticular nucleus is white matter, the external capsule, beyond which is a layer of gray matter, the claustrum, and external to all these structures is the "island of Reil." The cortical substance is at this point very near the gray matter of the basal ganglia.

Optic Thalami.—These bodies are behind and between the corpora striata. The internal portion is gray matter, and the external white.

Tubercula or *corpora quadrigemina* are sometimes spoken of as the "optic lobes." They are four in number, as their name indicates, the anterior pair being the nates, the posterior the testes. In fishes and birds there are but two of these bodies which are known as the optic lobes. The processus ad testes, superior peduncle of the cerebellum, connects the latter structure with the testes. Its fibres pass through the tegmentum to the optic thalami.

Microscopical Structure of Hemispheres.—*Gray Matter.*—The gray matter on the external surface of the cerebrum, forming the cortex, is divisible into five layers. The first or most superficial layer consists of neuroglia, a few small ganglion-cells, and a nerve-fibre network; the second is made up of small pyramidal nerve-cells having a diameter of about 10 mmm.; the third is similar to the second, except that the cells are larger, their diameter being from 25 to 40 mmm., and it is the broadest of all the layers. The fourth layer consists of small, triangular or elongated cells, and the fifth of spindle-shaped cells. The pyramidal cell or nerve-corpuscle above mentioned is regarded as the most important of all the structures in the gray matter of the cortex. These cells possess no cell-wall; they have nuclei and give off processes. One of these processes is branched and is termed the process of the apex; its direction is toward the surface, and it is continuous with the nerve-fibre network in the first layer. Another process, the process of the centre of the base, is opposite that of the apex; it does not branch, and is the axis-cylinder process. This process receives a medullary sheath and forms a nerve-fibre which passes into the white matter of the brain. From the sides of these pyramidal cells are given off other processes, the processes of the basal angle, which terminate in a network of fine nerve-fibres.

The above description applies in general to the whole cortical substance, but the structure differs in some particulars in special parts, as, for instance, at the posterior portion of the occipital lobe, where there are eight layers.

The gray matter of the corpora striata consists of large and small multipolar nerve-cells. Some of the white matter of the corpora striata is probably nerve-fibres originating in these cells. The gray matter of the optic thalami is composed of multipolar and spindle-shaped nerve-cells. The testes consist almost entirely of gray matter covered by a small amount of white. The nerve-cells are small and multipolar. The structure of the nates differs somewhat from that of the testes, the gray matter being in strata; besides which there is white matter. The cells are similar to those in the testes. The gray matter of the corpora geniculata is continuous with that of the optic thalami. In some of the cells of one of these bodies, the corpus geniculatum externum, there is pigment which gives them a dark color. The locus niger, a collection of gray matter in the crura cerebri, contains also pigmented multipolar cells. From its dark color, due to the pigment, it has received its name.

When the brain is developed during fœtal life the development takes place about a tube, which remains in the adult as the aqueduct of Sylvius and the third and fourth ventricles. This tube is continuous with the central canal of the spinal cord, and is lined with gray matter, so that gray matter exists in the aqueduct of Sylvius, on the inner wall of the optic thalami, where it forms the gray commissure of the third ventricle, on the floor of the third ventricle, and in the tegmentum of the crus. It forms the posterior perforated space, lamina cinerea, tuber cinereum, and infundibulum. The gray matter which has been mentioned as lining the aqueduct of

Sylvius contains multipolar cells which are not isolated, but form collections called "nuclei;" from one of these originates the third, and from another the fourth, cranial nerve. From this description it will be seen that the gray matter of the cerebrum is arranged in three groups: (1) that which forms the cortex; (2) that which is found in the basal ganglia; and (3) that which is in the central portions.

White Matter.—The white matter of the cerebrum, consisting of medullated nerve-fibres, may be divided into three groups:

1. Those fibres that connect the cerebrum with the medulla oblongata, pons Varolii, and spinal cord. These are the crura cerebri or cerebral peduncles; hence the group is described as the peduncular fibres. It will be remembered that the crura cerebri consist of the crusta and tegmentum. The fibres which come from the pyramids of the medulla and are continued through the pons aid in forming the crusta. To these fibres are added others which originate in the gray matter of the aqueduct of Sylvius and in the locus niger.

After forming the crura cerebri the fibres pass upward: some of them go directly to the gray matter of the cortex: these form the corona radiata; others go to the internal capsule, and thence to the corpora striata, where they terminate; while some of the others continue on, receiving fibres from these bodies, and together they assist in forming the corona radiata. More fibres come from the corpora striata than end there, so that the number of those which emerge is greater than the number of those which enter.

The tegmentum of the crus is made up of fibres from the anterior and lateral columns of the cord, the olivary body, funiculus cuneatus, funiculus gracilis, corpora quadrigemina, corpora geniculata, and superior peduncles of the cerebellum. These fibres pass into the optic thalami, some terminating there, while others pass through. To these latter are added fibres having their origin in the optic thalami, and together they assist in forming the corona radiata, being traced to the cells in the cortical substance of the temporo-sphenoidal and occipital lobes.

2. The second group of fibres in the cerebrum consists of those which connect the hemispheres and the basal ganglia, and are the transverse commissural fibres. They compose the corpus callosum and anterior and posterior commissures. The fibres of the corpus callosum connect the hemispheres, being traced into the convolutions and intersecting those of the corona radiata. The anterior commissure connects the corpora striata, and then passes through these bodies into the temporo-sphenoidal lobe. Some of the fibres of the posterior commissure connect the optic thalami, while some come from the tegmentum of one side, traverse the optic thalamus, and terminate in the white matter of the temporo-sphenoidal lobe of the other side.

3. The third group consists of fibres called "arcuate" or association fibres, and those called "longitudinal" or "collateral" fibres. The arcuate fibres, which connect adjacent convolutions, are situated just beneath the cortical substance. As representatives of the longitudinal group there may be mentioned the tænia semicircularis and the fornix.

Functions of the Cerebrum.—That the cerebrum is not essential to life has been demonstrated experimentally many times in birds, fishes, rabbits, rats, and other animals. Of course the same kind of proof is not available in man, but there are instances on record in which the destruction of brain-tissue has been so great as to warrant the statement that in man, as well as in lower animals, life may be maintained without the influence of the cerebrum. Perhaps the most remarkable instance is that of a man whose skull is now in the Warren Anatomical Museum. This man was injured by a premature blast, the iron bar, one inch in diameter, which was used in tamping being driven through the skull and brain. Although delirious and unconscious for several weeks, he finally recovered, with but the loss of one eye. He lived more than twenty years after the injury and performed the work of a coachman and farm-laborer.

The cerebrum is undoubtedly the seat of the intellectual faculties. A study of the lower animals reveals the fact that according as the hemispheres are developed the signs of intelligence are increased: when these structures are destroyed there is an absence of these manifestations.

When the hemispheres are removed there is no spontaneous action. In studying the reflex action of the spinal cord in a decapitated frog it was seen that the animal made no attempt to move or change its position unless some stimulus was applied, and that as soon as this stimulus was withdrawn it lapsed into its original position, remaining therein until again disturbed. If the hemispheres be removed from a pigeon, it will act very much as does the frog. If disturbed it may fly for a short distance, but at once lapses into a state of apparent unconsciousness, with eyes closed. When the foot is pinched it will be withdrawn. If a pistol be discharged, the bird will open its eyes and show unmistakably that the report was heard, but the discharge seems to produce no other effect. The fact that there is danger is not appreciated. It seems, therefore, that the faculty is absent by which the bird in health associates danger with such sounds. When the human brain is diseased or injured, something of the same kind is witnessed, and in idiots, whose brains are imperfectly developed, the intellectual faculties are very deficient. Human intelligence is manifested through memory, reason, and judgment.

Memory is the basis for the action of the other two faculties; without it there could be neither reason nor judgment. It is the faculty of the mind by which it retains the knowledge of previous thoughts or events, the actual and distinct retention and recognition of past ideas in the mind. Afferent impulses are continually reaching the cells of the cortex of the brain, and these impulses produce impressions more or less permanent. If they were evanescent, passing away almost as soon as received, memory would be impossible, but it is this retention which constitutes memory. If the ideas produced by these impulses come again into existence spontaneously and without effort, this is *remembrance*; if it require an effort, this is *recollection*, a re-collecting of the impressions originally produced on the cells by the afferent impulses.

Reason is that faculty of the mind by which is appreciated the nature of nervous impulses, and by which they are referred to their external source—by which an effect is referred to its cause. This reference an idiot cannot make; hence he is said to be "un-reasonable."

Judgment is the faculty of the mind by which a selection is made of the proper means to be used in the attainment of a particular end. Thus if one select inadequate means for the accomplishment of a given object, it is said that one "lacks judgment."

The cerebrum is the seat of conscious sensation, as opposed to sensation alone. The gray matter of the spinal cord is said to be sensitive; that is, it responds to stimuli. If the finger be burned, the afferent impulse is received by the gray matter of the cord and a motor impulse passes out to the muscles. But if the impulse travel no farther than the cord, there is no *conscious* sensation. To excite this sensation it must proceed to the gray matter of the cerebral cortex. It is in the cells of the cortex also that volitional impulses have their origin. The gray matter, then, is the seat of the will as well as the conscious centre, and when largely diseased or destroyed the only movements made are involuntary, depending on other nerve-centres.

Cerebral Localization.—Although the study of the intellectual faculties is both difficult and abstruse, much advance has in late years been made in the knowledge of the physiology of the cerebrum, so far as it relates to the production of voluntary movements. Observations upon both man and the lower animals lead one to believe that the power of producing certain movements is limited to certain restricted areas of the brain. This power is known as *cerebral localization.*

These observations had their beginning in 1870. It was found that when galvanic currents were applied to certain parts of the cerebral convolutions movements of particular muscles followed, and that in order to excite these muscles these parts or areas must be stimulated. Although the dog was first experimented upon, other animals (cat, rabbit, and monkey) have furnished like results. In the application of these experiments the animal is put under ether, the skull is trephined, and the poles of a galvanic battery are applied to the convolutions. When on such application to a given spot or area contractions of certain muscles or groups of muscles follow, such spot or area is said to be the centre of motion for these muscles.

The following statement may be said to summarize what is established with reference to cerebral localization:

In general the motor area is the region of the convolutions in the neighborhood of the fissure of Rolando.

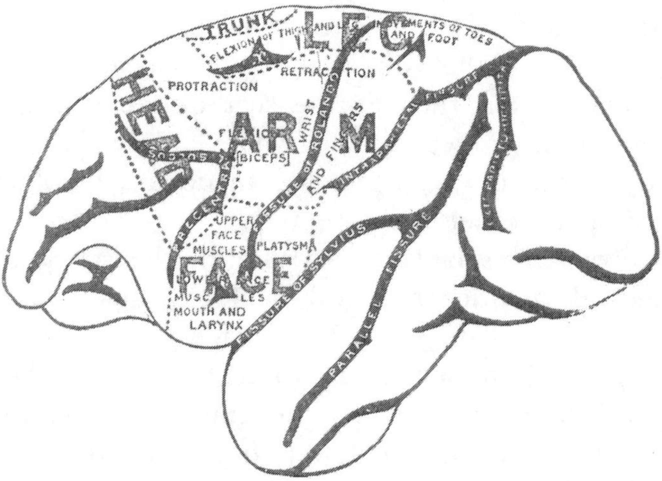

Fig. 56.—The Motor Areas on the Outer Surface of the Braiu.

In this area are centres of motion for the movements of the arms and legs (Figs. 56, 57), as in swimming, for extension forward of the arm and hand, for supination of the hand, and for flexion of the forearm. Around the lower part of this fissure are the centres for the movements of the mouth and tongue. The destruction of these convolutions or the presence in them of lesions results in paralysis of motion in these parts. Of course the action is in all cases crossed; that is, excitation of one side of the cerebrum causes the movements spoken

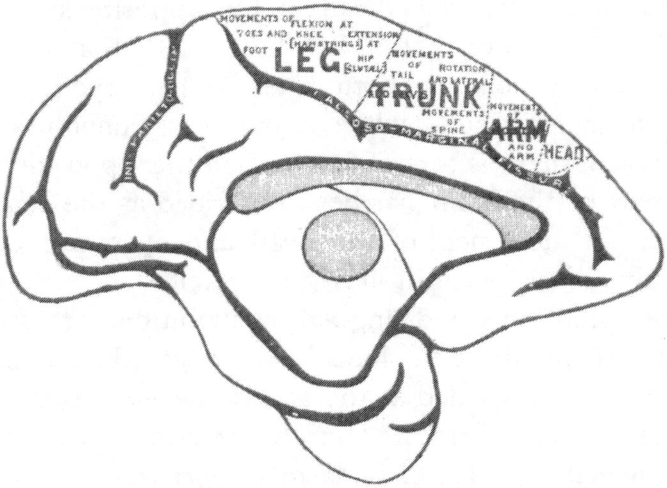

FIG. 57.—The Motor Areas on the Median Surface of the Brain.

of on the opposite side of the body, and the same is true of the paralysis which follows disease or injury.

Centre for Speech.—Articulate speech requires the exercise of memory and the power of producing certain voluntary movements. Inability to produce articulate speech is known as *aphasia.* If the memory of words be absent while the power to produce the movements remains, it is called "amnesic aphasia," and if the reverse condition exist, it is termed "ataxic aphasia." It is believed that the centre which presides over language is in the frontal lobe on the left side. Some localize it in the third frontal convolution; others regard it as being more diffused, and locate the centre in the convolutions surrounding the lower end of the fissure of Sylvius.

Sensory Areas.—While the motor areas appear to be localized, the same is not true for those areas that are sensory. If the superior temporo-sphenoidal convolution be stimulated in its posterior part, the animal pricks up its ear and turns its head to the opposite side, suggestive of the idea that it has heard with that ear. If these convolutions on both sides be destroyed, permanent deafness results, while if only one convolution be destroyed, there is loss of hearing on the opposite side: this part of the brain has been described as the *auditory centre*. A movement of the head and eyes, suggesting that the sense of sight has been excited, occurs when the occipital lobes and angular convolutions are stimulated. If one occipital lobe be destroyed, hemiopia results: this is regarded as the *visual* or *optic centre*. The *olfactory centre* is located in the anterior extremity of the uncinate gyrus. The taste or *gustatory centre* has not been localized.

Functions of Corpora Quadrigemina.—The corpora quadrigemina are the centres for visual sensations. If they be destroyed, the sense of sight is lost; if they become seriously diseased, blindness results. They are regarded also as the centres which govern the movements of the iris: when they are stimulated the pupil contracts, while it dilates if they are removed. In them is also the centre for the co-ordination of the movements of the eyes.

Functions of Corpora Striata and Optic Thalami.—The corpora striata have been spoken of as the great motor ganglia at the base of the brain, probably because lesions of them produce hemiplegia, but this is due to pressure on the internal capsule. The optic thalami have also been regarded as great sensory centres, but if lesions of them produce loss of sensation, it is due to an interference with the posterior limb of the internal capsule. In general it may be said that the functions of these basal ganglia are not understood.

Cranial Nerves.—The cranial nerves have their origin in the gray matter at the base of the brain, and they

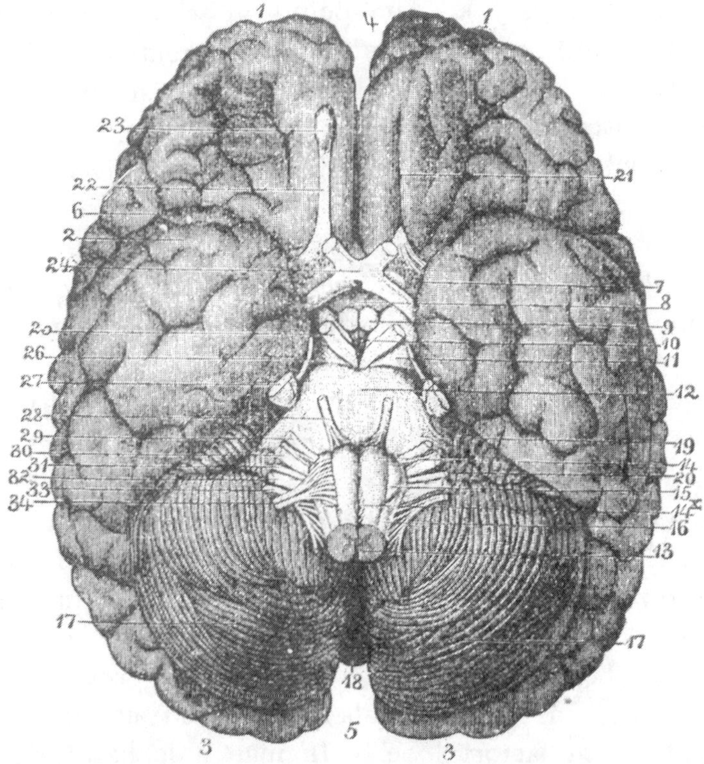

FIG. 58.—Base of Brain: 1, 2, 3, cerebrum; 4 and 5, longitudinal fissure; 6, fissure of Sylvius; 7, anterior perforated spaces; 8, infundibulum; 9, corpora albicantia; 10, posterior perforated space; 11, crura cerebri; 12, pons Varolii; 13, junction of spinal cord and medulla oblongata; 14, anterior pyramid; 14*, decussation of anterior pyramid; 15, olivary body; 16, restiform body; 17, cerebellum; 19, crura cerebelli; 21, olfactory sulcus; 22, olfactory tract; 23, olfactory bulbs; 24, optic commissure; 25, motor oculi nerve; 26, patheticus nerve; 27, trigeminus nerve; 28, abducens nerve; 29, facial nerve; 30, auditory nerve; 31, glosso-pharyngeal nerve; 32, pneumogastric nerve; 33, spinal accessory nerve; 34, hypoglossal nerve.

escape from the skull by various openings, called "foramina," to reach the parts to which they are distributed.

The only exception to this is the spinal accessory, a part of which arises from the gray matter of the cord. Among the cranial nerves are those of special sense, of motion, and nerves having both motor and sensory properties (Fig. 58). The points at which they leave the brain are spoken of as their "apparent origin," but this is only apparent, for they can be traced into the brain-substance, to collections of nerve-cells, nerve-centres, to which the name "nuclei" has been given. The nucleus of a nerve is its real origin.

Of cranial nerves there are twelve pairs, the *number* indicating the order from before backward in which they escape from the cavity of the cranium: 1, Olfactory; 2, Optic; 3, Motor oculi communis; 4, Patheticus; 5, Trigeminus; 6, Abducens; 7, Facial; 8, Auditory; 9, Glosso-pharyngeal; 10, Pneumogastric; 11, Spinal accessory; 12, Hypoglossal.

1. Olfactory Nerve.—The olfactory nerve is a term formerly applied to what is more properly the olfactory *tract*. This tract is a part of the brain lying in a groove, the olfactory sulcus, on the under surface of the frontal lobe, and it may be considered as a process from that lobe. In some animals it is of such size that it is called the "olfactory lobe." In man it is hardly large enough to merit this title. It is composed principally of gray matter, with some white. At the central or posterior extremity the tract is connected with the rest of the brain by three roots, the real origin of which is as yet undetermined. At the anterior extremity the tract expands to form the olfactory bulb, which lies upon the cribriform plate of the ethmoid bone, and which contains nerve-cells. From the under surface of the bulb are given off the true olfactory nerves, from fifteen to twenty in number. These nerves are composed of non-medullated fibres, axis-cylinders with a sheath, but with no white substance of Schwann. They pass out from the cavity of the cranium through the cribriform foramina, and are distributed to the olfactory membrane; that is, that portion of the mucous membrane of the nose (Schneiderian membrane) which covers the superior and middle turbinated bones and the upper part of the septum nasi. The Schneiderian membrane lines the nasal fossæ. Before the time of Schneider, from whom the membrane was named, it was thought that the secretion it forms came from the brain: he demonstrated that it came from the membrane itself. It is covered by epithelium, which, near the orifice of the nostril in the vestibule, is pavement, but elsewhere, except on the olfactory membrane, this epithelium is columnar and ciliated. On the olfactory membrane the cells are columnar, but in general not ciliated. Between these cells are the olfactory cells of Schultze, with which the olfactory nerves, after forming a plexus, are believed to be in communication.

Function of the Olfactory Nerve.—The function of the olfactory nerve is to preside over the sense of smell, which will be discussed in the consideration of the senses.

2. Optic Nerve.—The optic nerve is distributed to the eyeball. Followed backward, the nerves from both eyes are seen to unite to form the optic commissure, from which goes off on each side an optic tract. The optic tract just before its connection with the brain divides into two parts. One of these divisions or bands has its origin in the corpora quadrigemina, and the other in the optic thalamus, the latter receiving fibres from the inner corpus geniculatum.

The structure of the commissure, or chiasma, is quite complex. It consists of nerve-fibres which pass (1) from one retina to the other, inter-retinal fibres; (2) from one side of the brain to the other, intercerebral fibres; (3) from the brain to the retina of the same side; (4) from one side of the brain to the retina of the other side.

Function of the Optic Nerve.—The optic nerve is the special nerve of the sense of sight. Its sole function is to convey to the brain the impulses received from the retina, produced there by the luminous rays falling upon them. These impulses when they reach the brain cause the sensation of light. If the optic nerves be divided, blindness results. The optic nerve is also intimately connected with the movements of the iris, which movements result in changes of the size of the pupil. This is a reflex act in which the optic serves as the afferent nerve. The modus operandi will be better understood after a description of the motor oculi. (For a further discussion of this nerve and its function the reader is referred to the discussion of the sense of Sight.)

3. Motor Oculi.—The third nerve (motor oculi, motor oculi communis, or oculo-motorius) leaves the surface of the brain at the inner surface of the crus cerebri, just in front of the pons Varolii. Its real origin is, however, a nucleus in the floor of the aqueduct of Sylvius. It escapes from the cranium through the sphenoidal fissure, and is distributed to the superior, internal, and inferior recti and to the inferior oblique. It also supplies the levator palpebræ superioris, and sends a branch to the ophthalmic, lenticular, or ciliary ganglion. Another way to describe its distribution is to say that it supplies the levator palpebræ and all the muscles that move the eyeball, except the superior oblique and external rectus.

The action of these muscles is largely indicated by their names. The levator palpebræ by its contraction raises the upper eyelid. The internal rectus turns the eyeball inward toward the nose, and the external rectus turns it outward. The direction and the point of attachment of the superior rectus are such that when it contracts the eyeball is not only turned upward, but it is also slightly rotated inward; this is corrected by the action of the inferior oblique, so that the two acting together produce a movement directly upward. The same deviation inward follows when the eye is turned downward by the inferior rectus, and a similar correction is made by the action of the superior oblique. If the external and superior recti act together, the movement of the eyeball is in the direction of the diagonal—that is, outward and upward; the conjoint action of the external and inferior recti causes the eyeball to move outward and downward, and a corresponding action results when the other adjacent recti are brought into play. If the recti act alternately, the eyeball will be rotated completely, as in looking around a room from one side to the other and back again, from the floor to the ceiling. The motor oculi is purely a motor nerve. When stimulated, contraction is produced in the muscles to which it is distributed; when the nerve is divided, these muscles are paralyzed.

Paralysis of the Motor Oculi.—When the motor oculi is paralyzed the following are the results:

(*a*) *External strabismus*, which consists in a turning of the eye outward. The retention of the eye in its normal position requires the conjoint action of the internal and external recti. In paralysis of the motor oculi the internal rectus has lost its innervation, and therefore its power to contract, and the external rectus, which receives its nervous supply from another nerve (the abducens), having lost its antagonist, turns the eye outward.

(*b*) *Luscitas.*—After external strabismus has been produced the eye remains in that condition, for the muscles which could move it in any other direction have been paralyzed. This immobility is called "luscitas."

(*c*) *Ptosis.*—The levator palpebræ superioris is also paralyzed, and the upper eyelid droops, constituting *ptosis.* The ability to close the eye still remains, as this is the act of the orbicularis palpebrarum, which is not innervated by the third but by the seventh nerve.

(*d*) *Mydriasis.*—A branch of the motor oculi goes to the ciliary ganglion, which gives off the ciliary nerves that supply the iris. Accompanying the manifestations of paralysis of the motor oculi already mentioned there is in addition a dilatation of the pupil, or *mydriasis.* The diminution of the size of the pupil following the action of light upon the retina does not take place when this nerve is paralyzed. The contraction of the pupil is a reflex act requiring the integrity of the optic nerve, which serves as a carrier of the luminous impressions to the brain, and the motor oculi, which is the efferent nerve in this act.

(*e*) *Inability to Focus.*—The muscle concerned in focusing the eye for short distances is the ciliary. The power to focus is lost in paralysis of the motor oculi. This paralysis in human beings may be due to disease of the brain or to pressure on the nerves. If the trunk of the nerve be affected, all the physical signs mentioned may be observed, while if a single branch only be involved, the effect will be seen only in the part to which that branch is distributed.

4. Trochlearis.—The apparent origin of the trochlearis or patheticus is on the outer side of the crus cerebri, in front of the pons, and its real origin is a nucleus continuous with that of the motor oculi. The trochlearis leaves the cranium by the sphenoidal fissure, and is distributed to but one muscle, the superior oblique. When this nerve is paralyzed, the patient cannot turn the eye outward and downward, the action of the superior oblique is, therefore, to turn the eye outward and downward. If the head be not turned toward either side when this nerve is paralyzed, the only thing observable is that the patient sees double when he looks downward, and the image perceived by the affected eye is oblique and below that seen by the eye that is unaffected.

5. Trigeminus.—This nerve, which is also called "trifacial," has received its names from the fact that it has three subdivisions, and is distributed in the main to the parts about the face. It arises by two roots, anterior and posterior. The anterior root, the smaller, is purely motor; the posterior root, the larger, is sensory, and is characterized anatomically by having upon it the Gasserian ganglion. The nerve leaves the brain at the side of the pons Varolii. The real origin of the motor root is a nucleus in the floor of the fourth ventricle; the sensory root arises from a nucleus on a level with the middle of the superior peduncle of the cerebellum, just internal to the margin of the fourth ventricle. Some authorities give it a more extensive origin, from the pons through the medulla and as far as the posterior cornua of the gray matter of the spinal cord.

The motor root passes beneath the Gasserian ganglion, and takes no part in the formation.

Beyond the ganglion the fifth nerve divides into three

parts: (1) ophthalmic; (2) superior maxillary; and (3) inferior maxillary.

(1) *Ophthalmic Division.*—This division, which leaves the cranium by the sphenoidal fissure, is distributed to

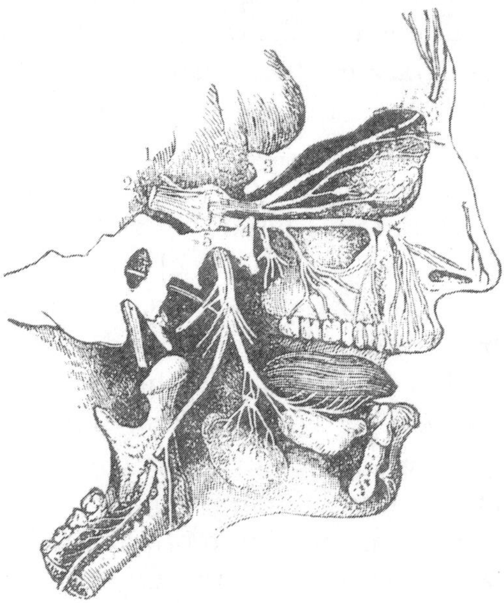

FIG. 59.—General Plan of the Branches of the Fifth Pair: 1, lesser root of the fifth pair; 2, greater root, passing forward into the Gasserian ganglion; 3, placed on the bone above the ophthalmic divison, which is seen dividing into the supraorbital, lachrymal, and nasal branches, the latter connected with the ophthalmic ganglion; 4, placed on the bone close to the foramen rotundum, marks the superior maxillary division; 5, placed on the bone over the foramen ovale, marks the inferior maxillary division (after a sketch by Charles Bell).

the tentorium cerebelli, the eyeball, the Schneiderian membrane, the lachrymal gland, and the skin about the forehead and nose. It also supplies branches to the ciliary ganglion, and contains only fibres from the posterior root, none from the anterior.

(2) *Superior Maxillary Division.*—This division of the fifth pair leaves the cranial cavity by the foramen rotun-

dum. It is distributed to the dura mater, the spheno-palatine ganglion (Meckel's), the skin of the temple and cheek, the teeth, the gums, and the mucous membrane of the upper jaw and upper lip, the mucous membrane of the lower part of the nasal passages, the skin of the lower eyelid, side of nose, and upper lip. There are no fibres of the anterior root in this division.

(3) *Inferior Maxillary Division.*—As has already been stated, there is no anatomical connection between the motor root of the fifth nerve and the Gasserian ganglion. From this ganglion are given off nerve-fibres which join the motor root, together making the inferior maxillary division, which escapes through the foramen ovale. It is distributed to the dura mater, the otic ganglion, the mucous membrane of the cheek, skin, and mucous membrane of the lower lip, the anterior wall of the external auditory meatus, the front of the external ear and the skin of the adjacent temporal region, the sub-maxillary gland and ganglion, the mucous membrane of the mouth and tongue; and to the papillæ at the tip, the edges, and anterior two-thirds of the tongue, the teeth and gums of the lower jaw. It also supplies the following muscles: temporal, masseter, pterygoid, mylo-hyoid, and anterior belly of the digastric.

Physiological Properties of the Trigeminus.—The trigeminus is the largest of the cranial nerves, and its functions are many and important. It supplies the parts to which it is distributed with the general sensibility they possess. If it be divided, there is complete absence of sensation (anæsthesia) of the face on the corresponding side (Fig. 59). So pronounced is this anæsthesia that no amount of irritation applied to such ordinarily sensitive parts as the cornea will produce any effect. An animal thus experimented upon seems entirely oblivious of the irritation. Experimenters have gone so far as to exsect the eyeball and apply

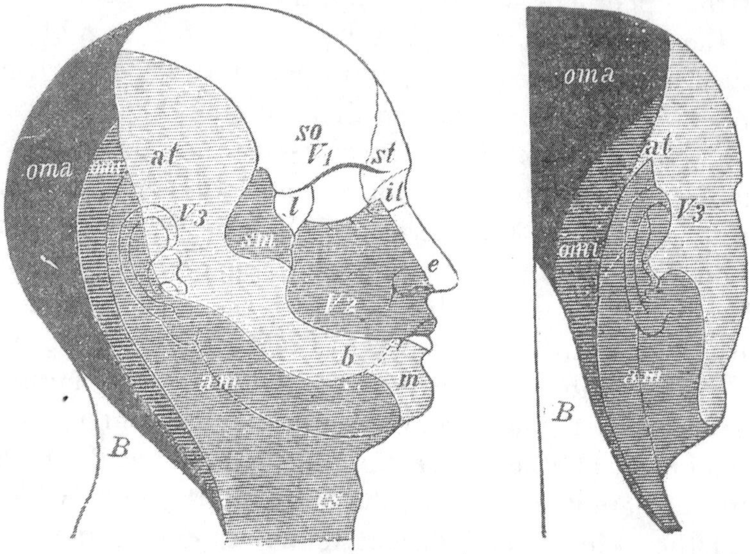

FIGS. 60, 61.—Distribution of the Cutaneous Sensitive Nerves upon the Head: *oma*, *omi*, the occipit. maj. and minor (from the N. cervical II. and III.); *am*, N. auricular magn. (from N. cervic. III.); *cs*, N. cervical superfic. (from N. cervic. III.); V_1, first branch of the fifth (*so*, N. supraorbit.; *st*, N. supratrochl.; *it*, N. infratrochl.; *e*, N. ethmoid.; *l*, N. lachrymal.); V_2, second branch of the fifth (*sm*, N. subcutan. malæ seu zygomaticus); V_3, third branch of fifth (*at*, N. auriculo-tempor.; *b*, N. buccinator; *m*, N. mental.); *B*, posterior branches of the cervical nerves.

hot irons to the skin without causing pain to the animal experimented upon.

Neuralgia of the face, headache, and toothache are all due to some interference with the normal functions of this nerve. It is not an uncommon thing to hear patients complain of headaches which seem to them to be in the brain itself. These deep-seated headaches may be due to affections of one or more of the recurrent branches which come off from the divisions of the nerve, and which are distributed to the dura mater and bones of the skull.

Lingual (*Gustatory*) *Nerve.*—This nerve is sometimes called the "lingual branch of the fifth nerve." It is the branch which is distributed to the mucous membrane of the mouth and the gums, and to the mucous membrane and papillæ of the tongue. It supplies the tongue with tactile sensibility, a quality of great advantage in enabling one to detect the physical properties of food, to recognize in it the presence of hard objects which it would be injurious to swallow, and to determine when it is ready for deglutition. Besides this tactile sensibility the lingual nerve supplies the anterior two-thirds of the tongue with the sense of taste, a special sense, and this power is lost when the fifth pair or the lingual branch is divided.

Mastication.—The muscles that have been mentioned as receiving branches of the inferior maxillary division are those concerned in the act of mastication. In this act the temporal and masseter close the mouth, the mylohyoid and digastric open it, while the pterygoids produce the lateral movement of the lower jaw. Division of the inferior maxillary paralyzes, therefore, all these muscles. If it be divided on one side, the muscles on the other side can still perform the act, but in an imperfect manner; if divided on both sides, all masticatory movements will be abolished.

Anastomosis of the Fifth Pair.—Besides the branches already mentioned, there are others which are termed *anastomotic branches.* Although the upper, middle, and lower parts of the face are supplied with sensation by the ophthalmic, superior maxillary, and inferior maxillary divisions respectively, still the boundaries of each are not absolute. Thus the skin of the nose is supplied by fibres from the ophthalmic and superior maxillary, and the skin of the temporal region is supplied from both the superior and inferior maxillary divisions. In addition to these branches, there are some which unite with other nerves and give a certain amount of sensibility to the parts to which these nerves are distributed. A striking instance of this is the branch which anastomoses with the facial nerve. This nerve is at its origin purely motor, and is distributed to the muscles of the face. These muscles are endowed with sensibility, but this is not due to fibres of the facial nerve, but to those of the fifth nerve, which anastomose with the facial and go with it to its termination in the muscles.

Connection of the Fifth Pair with the Special Senses.—After division of the fifth nerve the special senses of smell, sight, taste, and hearing are seriously affected. The Schneiderian membrane becomes swollen, and later assumes a fungous condition and bleeds readily when touched. There is also an accumulation of altered mucus in the nasal passages. The eye also undergoes marked changes: the conjunctiva becomes congested and the cornea opaque; later, most of the structures of the eye suffer from inflammatory changes to the degree of destruction. The sense of taste may likewise be lost, not only in the anterior two-thirds of the tongue, but also in the posterior third as well. Besides, the sense of hearing is also greatly impaired.

The explanation of these changes is not an easy one. Some authorities regard them as due to disturbance of trophic influences. The nerve-fibres which form the posterior or sensory root of the fifth pair in passing through the Gasserian ganglion are reinforced by fibres which have their origin in this collection of nerve-cells. Each of the three divisions of the trigeminus contains, therefore, fibres of the posterior root, and in addition fibres from the ganglion. The latter fibres are distributed to the structures to which the sensory fibres are distributed, and they are regarded as trophic nerves; that is, as nerves which regulate the nutrition of the parts to which they go. Among these parts are the mucous membrane of the nose, the cornea, the conjunctiva, and the mucous membrane of the tongue, and the loss of the special senses is believed to be due to altered nutrition of the affected parts. The sense of sight is resident in the retina and optic nerve, but it may be as perfectly abolished by rendering opaque the tissues through which light reaches these structures as by dividing the optic nerve. In like manner the olfactory nerves are the nerves of smell, but if the nasal mucous membrane be so affected in its nutrition as to render the functions of these nerves impossible, the sense of smell is as certainly abolished as if the olfactory bulb were broken up. This interference with the normal action of the nerves is seen in catarrhal affections of the nose, in which the sense of smell is much obtunded and sometimes even lost.

Some authorities, however, question the influence of so-called "trophic centres" except for nerves. They state that the inflammatory changes occurring in the eye, for instance, are due to the presence of foreign bodies lodging on the eyeball, which has lost its sensibility; that if the eye be so protected that irritating substances cannot injure it, the degenerative changes take place only after a considerable time; and that when they do occur it is probably even then due to injury, for it is a most difficult thing to protect the eye for a long time from all sources of irritation. Similar reasoning, it is claimed, excludes other so-called "trophic changes." It is, of course, a mooted question, but it seems to the writer that no explanation of the nutritive changes taking place after section of the trigeminus more satisfactorily accounts for them than that which regards the Gasserian ganglion as a trophic centre.

Ganglia of the Trigeminus.—Besides the Gasserian ganglion, there are, in connection with the fifth nerve, four ganglia which are by some writers described as a part of the sympathetic system. They are the ciliary or ophthalmic, the spheno-palatine or Meckel's, the otic or Arnold's, and the submaxillary.

The ciliary ganglion belongs, according to some authorities, to the third rather than to the fifth nerve. It is not larger than the head of an ordinary pin, and is situated in the orbit. The branches by which other nerves communicate with it are called its "roots;" of these there are three: the *sensory*, from the ophthalmic division of the fifth; the *motor*, from the motor oculi; and the *sympathetic*, from the cavernous plexus of the sympathetic. The nerves that go off from it are the short ciliary nerves, which, joining with the long ciliary nerves, form the nasal branch of the ophthalmic division, and together they are distributed to the ciliary muscles, the iris, and the cornea. These nerves supply motor influences to the sphincter and dilator pupillæ, sensibility to the iris, choroid, and sclerotic, and vaso-motor influences to the blood-vessels of the iris, choroid, and retina. If the trophic influence already spoken of exist, it must be conveyed to the eye through the ciliary nerves.

The Spheno-palatine or Meckel's ganglion, which is the largest of the four, is situated in the spheno-maxillary fossa. This ganglion also has three roots: the *sensory*, spheno-palatine, from the superior maxillary division of the fifth; the *motor*, large superficial petrosal nerve from the facial; and the *sympathetic*, large deep petrosal nerve from the carotid plexus of the sympathetic. The Vidian nerve is made by the union of these two latter nerves. The nerves from this ganglion are distributed to the posterior portion of the nasal passages and the hard and soft palate, giving them sensibility; to the levator palati and azygos uvulæ, giving them the power of motion; and to the blood-vessels of this region.

The Otic or Arnold's ganglion is situated on the inner side of the inferior maxillary division of the fifth, just below the foramen ovale. It likewise has three roots: the *sensory*, from the inferior maxillary and glosso-pharyngeal; the *motor*, from the facial and inferior maxillary; and the *sympathetic*, from the plexus around the middle meningeal artery. Its branches of distribution are to the tensor tympani, the tensor palati, and a small one to the chorda tympani. The mucous membrane of the tympanum and the Eustachian tube is also supplied by this ganglion.

The submaxillary ganglion, which is situated near the submaxillary gland, receives branches of communication from the lingual branch of the fifth, chorda tympani, and sympathetic plexus around the facial artery. Its branches of distribution are to the mucous membrane of the mouth and Wharton's duct, also to the submaxillary gland.

6. Abducens.—This nerve, which has its real origin in the floor of the fourth ventricle, escapes from the cranium by the sphenoidal fissure, being distributed to the external rectus muscle. It is purely a motor nerve, as is shown by the contraction of this muscle when the nerve is stimulated, and by its paralysis when the nerve is divided.

Paralysis of the Abducens.—When from any cause this nerve is so injured as to deprive it of its function, the internal rectus, having lost its antagonist the external rectus, turns the eye inward toward the nose, producing internal strabismus. There may also be some contraction of the pupil, because the radiating fibres of the iris, which cause dilatation of the pupil, are to a certain extent deprived of their innervation, this being supplied from the sympathetic, some of the nerves of which system run along with the abducens, and when this nerve is injured these sympathetic fibres may also be involved. It is said that this nerve is more frequently implicated in fractures at the base of the skull than any other cranial nerve.

7. Facial Nerve.—The facial nerve leaves the medulla oblongata at the groove between the olivary and restiform bodies. Its real origin is a nucleus on the floor of the fourth ventricle. It leaves the cranium by the internal auditory meatus, through which and the aqueduct of Fallopius it passes to emerge at the stylo-mastoid foramen. In the older nomenclature it was associated with the auditory nerve, in company with which it enters the auditory meatus, the facial, from its firm consistency, being called the portio dura, and the auditory, on account of its opposite quality, being called the portio mollis.

The facial has a very extensive distribution—the muscles of the face and external ear, the stylo-hyoid, posterior belly of the digastric, the platysma myoides, and the stapedius. It also gives off the chorda tympani, which is distributed to the submaxillary gland and ganglion, to the inferior lingualis muscle, and to the sublingual gland. Besides these it has most important branches of communication with the sympathetic system and with the glosso-pharyngeal, pneumogastric, and trigeminus nerves.

Physiological Properties of the Facial.—The facial is, originally, a purely motor nerve, and whatever sensibility is possessed by the parts to which it is distributed is not due to facial fibres, but to anastomotic fibres from other nerves, principally the fifth. The most pronounced function of the facial is its relation to expression. The so-called "expression" of the face is caused by different degrees of contraction of the facial muscles, and the different expressions, such as of fear, of anger, etc., are due to contraction of different muscles. The facial is therefore said to be the "nerve of expression," and when it is divided and the muscles paralyzed the reason for this title is readily understood.

Facial Paralysis.—When the facial nerve is divided or its functions otherwise abolished the following are the results:

(1) *Effect of Paralysis on Facial Expression.*—A complete loss of expression follows on the affected side; the wrinkles on that side are obliterated and the face is flattened out.

(2) *Effect of Facial Paralysis on the Eye.*—The muscle which closes the eye is the orbicularis palpebrarum: this muscle is innervated by the facial nerve, and in paralysis, therefore, the eye remains permanently open, the power to close it being lost. Inasmuch as the act of winking is but a rapid partial closing of the eye, this act is also abolished and the eyeball is liable to become dry. The act of winking spreads the tears which keep the eye moist. Unless provided against, this exposure of the eye may result in injury.

(3) *Effect of Facial Paralysis on the Mouth.*—The mouth is drawn by the unparalyzed muscles to the unaffected side. It is impossible to approximate the lips of the affected side to a glass; consequently, unless the head be thrown back, fluids will dribble from the corners of the mouth in drinking. The buccinator muscle being paralyzed, food finds its way into the space between the cheek and the gum, and mastication is seriously impeded. The lips being paralyzed, the consonants *b* and *p* cannot be pronounced distinctly.

(4) *Effect of Facial Paralysis on Taste.*—Accompanying facial paralysis may be impairment or abolition of the sense of taste. Authorities are not agreed as to the explanation of this result, but it is doubtless due to interference with the chorda tympani. Some attribute it to the influence which this nerve exercises over the circulation in the tongue and on the secretion of saliva: others regard the chorda tympani as the nerve of taste to the anterior two-thirds of the tongue, and as taking part in forming the gustatory nerve or lingual branch of the trigeminus. Indeed, there is a difference of opinion among anatomists as to the true source of the chorda tympani: some look upon it as a part of the fifth, some as a part of the seventh, and still others as a part of the ninth or glosso-pharyngeal, at least so far as concerns those fibres which are connected with the sense of taste.

8. Auditory.—The auditory nerve has its apparent origin from the lower border of the pons, in the groove between the olivary and restiform bodies. Its real origin is from the floor of the fourth ventricle. As already stated, the auditory nerve enters the internal auditory meatus with the facial nerve. It is distributed to the internal ear, and it is the special nerve of the sense of hearing. It will further be discussed in connection with that special sense.

9. Glosso-pharyngeal.—The superficial origin of the glosso-pharyngeal nerve is from the upper part of the medulla, in the groove between the olivary and restiform bodies. Its real origin is a nucleus in the lower part of the floor of the fourth ventricle. It escapes from the cranium through the jugular foramen, together with the pneumogastric and spinal accessory nerves. Its branches of communication are with the pneumogastric, facial, and sympathetic nerves. The glosso-pharyngeal gives off the tympanic branch, the nerve of Jacobson, which is distributed to the fenestra rotunda, the fenestra ovalis, and the lining membrane of the tympanum and Eustachian tube. As its name implies, the glosso-pharyngeal is distributed to the tongue and pharynx. The glossal portion supplies the posterior third of the tongue, the tonsils, and the mucous membrane of the pillars of the fauces and the soft palate, while the pharyngeal portion is distributed to the pharyngeal mucous membrane and to the muscles concerned in a part of the act of deglutition—namely, the styloglossus, digastric, and stylopharyngeus, and the superior and middle constrictors.

Physiological Properties.—The sensibility of the parts to which the glosso-pharyngeal nerve is distributed is due to this nerve. It is also a nerve of special sense, supplying the posterior third of the tongue and the palate with the sense of taste; and, finally, it is the motor nerve for the muscles enumerated which are concerned in passing the food from the back of the mouth into and through the pharynx to the œsophagus in the act of deglutition.

10. Pneumogastric.—This nerve is also called "ner-

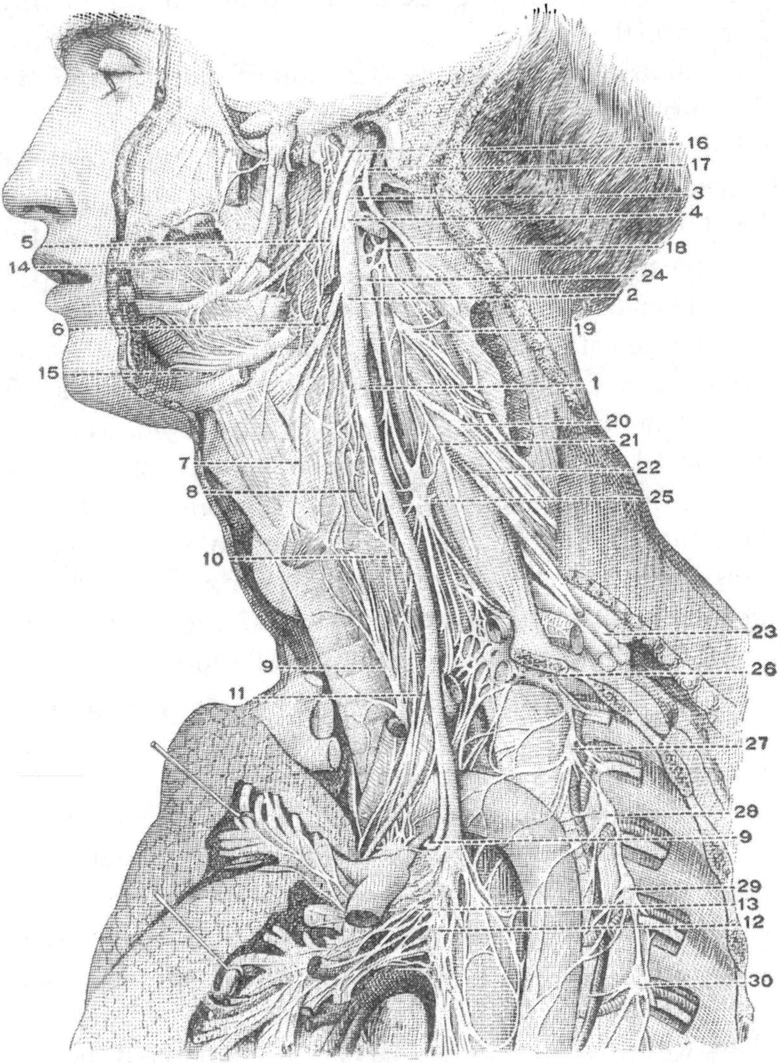

FIG. 62.—View of the Nerves of the Eighth Pair, their distribution and connections on the left side: 1, pneumogastric nerve in the neck; 2, ganglion of its trunk; 3, its union with the spinal accessory; 4, its union wlth the hypoglossal; 5, pharyngeal branch; 6, superior laryngeal nerve; 7, external laryngeal; 8 laryngeal plexus; 9, inferior or recurrent laryngeal; 10, superior cardiac branch; 11, middle cardiac; 12, plexiform part of the nerve in the thorax; 13, posterior pulmonary plexus; 14, lingual or gustatory nerve of the inferior maxillary; 15, hypoglossal, passing into the muscles of the tongue, giving its thyro-hyoid branch, and uniting with twigs of the

vus vagus" and "par vagum." Its common name is derived from two of the important organs, the lungs and stomach, to which it is distributed. Its apparent origin is by eight or ten filaments from the groove below the glosso-pharyngeal, while its deep origin is from a nucleus in the floor of the fourth ventricle, below and continuous with that of the same nerve.

At the jugular foramen, by which it escapes from the cranium, is found the ganglion of the pneumogastric or the jugular ganglion. The pneumogastric receives branches from the spinal accessory, facial, hypoglossal, and anterior branches of the first and second cervical nerves. It assists in forming the pharyngeal, laryngeal, pulmonary, and œsophageal plexuses. Among its important branches are the superior and inferior laryngeal nerves, the cardiac and the gastric branches. The pharyngeal branch is distributed to the mucous membrane and muscles of the pharynx and to the muscles of the soft palate. Its œsophageal branches supply the mucous membrane and muscular coat of the œsophagus, so that the act of deglutition, which begins in the mouth and is continued in the pharynx, is completed by the œsophagus. The superior laryngeal nerve is distributed to the crico-thyroid muscle and to the inferior constrictor, and it communicates with the superior cardiac nerve. Its further distribution is to the mucous membrane of the larynx and epiglottis as far as the vocal cords.

---

lingual; 16, glosso-pharyngeal nerve; 17, spinal accessory nerve, uniting by its inner branch with the pneumogastric, and by its outer passing into the sterno-mastoid muscle; 18, second cervical nerve; 19, third; 20, fourth; 21, origin of the phrenic nerve; 22, 23, fifth, sixth, seventh, and eighth cervical nerves, forming with the first dorsal the brachial plexus; 24, superior cervical ganglion of the sympathetic; 25, middle cervical ganglion; 26, inferior cervical ganglion united with the first dorsal ganglion; 27, 28, 29, 30, second, third, fourth, and fifth dorsal ganglia (from Sappey after Hirschfeld and Leveillé).

The superior laryngeal nerve is the sensitive nerve of the larynx. This sensibility is of great importance as a protection of the larynx and the respiratory organs below it from the entrance of foreign bodies, which would set up dangerous inflammatory processes. The instant such a substance touches the surfaces supplied by this nerve a violent expulsive cough occurs which ejects it. If the nerve be paralyzed, as it may be after diphtheria or in connection with brain disease, this protection is absent, and, owing to paralysis of the crico-thyroid, the ability to make tense the vocal cords is lost and the voice is hoarse.

The inferior or recurrent laryngeal nerve is distributed to all the muscles of the larynx except the crico-thyroid. It sends branches to the mucous membrane and muscular coat of the œsophagus, to similar structures of the trachea, and to the inferior constrictor. It is the motor nerve of the larynx. This nerve may be paralyzed under the same conditions as were mentioned in connection with the superior laryngeal, and all motion of the vocal cords is abolished. One nerve might be paralyzed, as when pressed upon by a tumor, when the corresponding vocal cord would alone be motionless.

The cardiac branches of the pneumogastric terminate in the superficial and deep cardiac plexuses. The pulmonary branches assist in forming the pulmonary plexuses whose branches are distributed to the lungs. The œsophageal branches form the œsophageal plexus or plexus gulæ. The gastric branches, which are the terminal filaments of the nerve, are distributed to the stomach and to the cœliac, splenic, and hepatic plexuses, the latter two supplying the liver and spleen.

In mentioning some of the branches of the pneumogastric their functions have also been referred to. In addition to these functions the movements of the stomach and the intestines are also performed under the influence of this nerve. It is through the cardiac branches that the inhibitory impulses from the medulla are sent to the heart. Through the pulmonary branches impulses reach the respiratory centre and influence respiration. Reference has previously been made to the depressor fibres, which run in the pneumogastric to the vasomotor centre, inhibiting its action and thus diminishing the work of the heart.

11. Spinal Accessory Nerve.—This nerve has two parts—one arising from a nucleus in the medulla below that of the pneumogastric, and the other from the intermedio-lateral tract of the cord. The former is the *accessory*, and the latter the *spinal*, portion. The accessory portion joins the pneumogastric, and it is distributed through the pharyngeal and superior laryngeal branches of that nerve. It is also probable that the fibres of the pharyngeal branch going to the muscles of the soft palate are fibres of this portion of the spinal accessory.

The inferior laryngeal nerve also contains fibres from this nerve, probably from the internal, anastomotic, or accessory portion, and experiments demonstrate that the power which the larynx possesses to produce vocal sounds is due to these fibres, for when the spinal accessory is torn out this power is lost. The other movements of the larynx, those which take place during respiration, are not interfered with under these circumstances, but only those of phonation. The inferior laryngeal nerve is, then, only partially made up of spinal accessory fibres: these fibres preside over phonation.

The other fibres, which are probably derived from the facial, hypoglossal, or cervical, or all of them, provide the nervous influence for the other movements. If the entire nerve be divided, movements both of phonation and of respiration will cease.

The spinal or external portion is distributed to the trapezius and sterno-mastoid muscles; it is therefore sometimes called the "muscular branch." This branch is believed to be brought into requisition when these muscles are needed for more than their ordinary activity, for the nervous force to supply the latter is furnished by cervical nerves. In unusual straining or in lifting or in the production of prolonged cries, these muscles are brought into requisition, and to supply the additional innervation which these acts seem to require is believed to be the office of the muscular branch of the eleventh nerve. The spinal accessory is, then, a motor nerve, although some writers regard a portion of the fibres of the accessory part as being sensory.

12. Hypoglossal.—The apparent origin of this nerve is by filaments, from ten to fifteen in number, from the groove between the pyramidal and olivary bodies: its real origin is in a nucleus in the floor of the fourth ventricle. It sends branches of communication to the pneumogastric, the sympathetic, the first and second cervical, and the gustatory. It is distributed to the sterno-hyoid, sterno-thyroid, omo-hyoid, thyro-hyoid, styloglossus, hyoglossus, genio-hyoid, and genio-hyoglossus muscles. It is a motor nerve to the tongue, so much so that it has been called the "motor linguæ." The movements over which it presides are those concerned in mastication and deglutition and in the production of articulate speech. When this nerve is paralyzed on one side, the tongue, when protruded, is directed toward the paralyzed side. When both nerves are involved in the paralysis, all motion of the tongue ceases.

2. The Senses.

It is by the senses that the individual is brought into relation with the world outside him. The senses are five in number: (1) General sensibility; (2) Smell; (3) Taste; (4) Sight; and (5) Hearing.

1. General Sensibility.—This kind of sensibility is so called because it is generally distributed over the entire body in the skin, and in those parts of mucous membrane adjacent to the skin. It is composed of a variety of sensations which are excited by a variety of stimuli, but it is still an unsettled question whether the nerves which conduct the impulses that excite these sensations are in all instances the ordinary sensory nerves of the skin, or whether there are special nerves, each one conducting only its own special stimulus. In treating of the subdivisions of general sensibility this question will again be referred to.

Sense of Touch.—The sense of touch, or tactile sensibility, gives knowledge of such qualities as hardness or softness, roughness or smoothness, sharpness or dulness, etc.; by it we become acquainted with the shape and consistency of objects, and are made aware of the presence or absence of irritating qualities in certain substances. The pungent vapors of some gases excite in the nose the ultimate fibres of distribution of the fifth pair of nerves, and not those of the first pair, and it is incorrect to describe this sensation as a smell. It is as truly a tactile sensibility as when a sharp-pointed instrument is brought in contact with the skin. The same is true of pungent liquids applied to the tongue, which are commonly, but erroneously, said to be tasted.

Tactile sensibility differs in different portions of the body. Its comparative delicacy is determined by applying the points of a pair of compasses to the surface of the body: the minimum distance at which they can be recognized as two points is the measure. At the tip of the tongue this distance is 1 mm. If the points be brought nearer together, they give the sensation of one point only. At the tips of the fingers it is 1.5 mm.; on the cheek it is 9.46 mm.; and in the middle of the back it is 50.43 mm.

Sense of Pressure.—When an object possessing considerable weight is laid upon the hand, there is a sensation produced which is that of "pressure." If an attempt be made to raise this object, there is a consciousness of the fact that to do this muscular power must be exerted, and this is called "muscular sense."

Sense of Temperature.—By this sense the difference in the temperature of bodies is recognized, and it is a well-known fact that the various portions of the body are endowed with different degrees of sensibility in this regard: the hand will bear a degree of heat which would cause great pain to some other parts of the body. The sense of temperature and that of touch are entirely distinct, and this fact may readily be demonstrated by pressing firmly on a sensitive nerve until the part to which it is distributed is almost devoid of the sense of touch, when it will be found that the sense of temperature is unaffected.

Sense of Pain.—When the stimuli that call out the sense of touch or of temperature are excessive, the sense of pain is produced, and when produced the other sensations are abolished; thus when a piece of iron very much heated burns the hand the sensation is the same as when the iron is very cold.

2. Sense of Smell.—The olfactory nerves are beyond all doubt the channels by which olfactory impressions reach the brain (Fig. 63.) They are nerves of the special

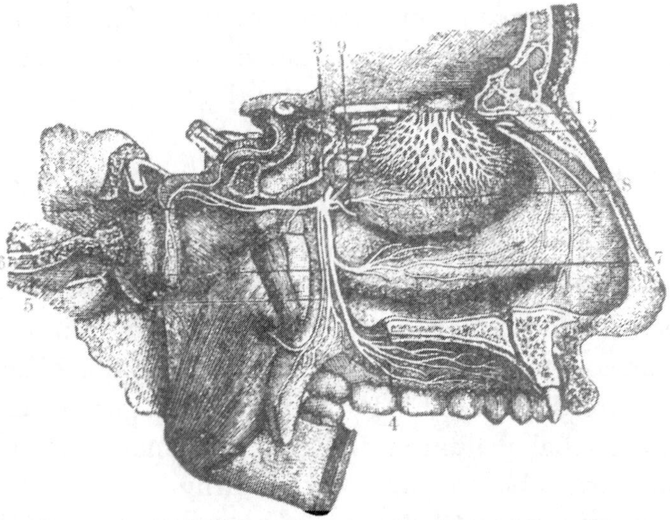

Fig. 63.—Nerves of the Outer Walls of the Nasal Fossæ: 1, network of the branches of the olfactory nerve, descending upon the region of the superior and middle turbinated bones; 2, external twig of the ethmoidal branch of the nasal nerves; 3, spheno-palatine ganglion; 4, ramification of the anterior palatine nerves; 5, posterior, and 6, middle, divisions of tbe palatine nerves; 7, branch to the region of the inferior turbinated bone; 8, branch to the region of the superior and middle turbinated bones; 9, naso-palatine branch to the septum cut short (from Sappey, after Hirschfeld and Leveillé).

sense of smell. The whole Schneiderian membrane is not supplied with olfactory fibres; hence only in that part where they are present, the olfactory membrane, does the sense of smell reside. The proof that the function of this nerve is that of smell is derived from experiments upon lower animals and from observations upon man. Animals whose sense of smell is very acute have the olfactory bulbs and tracts more highly developed—that is, the latter are larger—than in those animals in which the acuteness of the sense of smell is not marked. If the tracts be destroyed, the sense of smell is abolished. Although this experimental proof is not applicable in man, still there are cases on record in which an absence of the sense of smell during life has been found after death to accompany an absence of the olfactory tracts; and there are cases also of individuals whose sense of smell has been seriously impaired after injury to the tracts.

During ordinary respiration the inspired air does not pass over the olfactory membrane, but only over the lower part of the Schneiderian membrane, the respiratory portion. Hence if odors be faint, they are not detected, unless by a strong inspiration the air is carried up to and over that portion to which the olfactory nerves are distributed. If the nasal passages be closed by a catarrhal condition, the sense of smell is obtunded or may even be abolished temporarily.

It is important to distinguish between the sense of smell and general sensibility. The latter will hereafter be noticed at length, but for the present it will only be referred to. The mucous membrane of the nose has, in common with other mucous membranes and the skin, the power to recognize such physical properties in objects as consistency, temperature, etc. Thus if a sharp instrument were to be brought in contact with this membrane, it would be recognized as sharp, but this recognition is not due to the excitation of the olfactory nerves, but to the fibres of the trigeminus. The mucous membrane is therefore supplied by two nerves, the olfactory and the fifth. One is not liable to confound sharpness with odor, but the irritating effects of certain substances are often confounded with the sense of smell, when, as a matter of fact, it is not the olfactory, but the fifth pair, which is excited. Thus if acetic acid be brought in contact with the mucous membrane of the nose, it will excite the fibres of the fifth pair and will produce an irritating effect, but it would be incorrect to say that we smelled it. If, however, vinegar were substituted for the acetic acid, we should have the irritating effect of the acetic acid it contains, and in addition the olfactory nerves would be excited by the aromatic ingredients which with the acid form vinegar; and it would therefore be correct to say that we smelled the vinegar.

The acuteness of the sense of smell differs in different individuals, but in most it is well marked. It has been estimated that $\frac{1}{2000000}$ of a milligramme of musk may be detected by this sense. The emanations from objects which excite the sense of smell produce this effect by exciting the cells of Schultze, and the impulses are carried by the olfactory nerves to the brain.

3. Sense of Taste.—The sense of taste resides not only in the tongue, but also in the soft palate, the uvula, the pillars of the fauces, the tonsils, and the upper part of the pharynx. The nerve supplying the anterior two-thirds of the tongue with this sense is the lingual branch of the fifth pair, while the posterior portion depends for this power upon the glosso-pharyngeal. The relation which the corda tympani bears to the sense of taste has been discussed in connection with the facial nerve, of which it is a branch.

It is difficult to state exactly the difference in sensibility to sapid substances of the different portions of the tongue, but the most sensitive portions are the base, the tip, and the edges (Fig. 64): the middle portion is less sensitive, probably on account of the greater thickness of the epithelium, while the under surface is almost entirely insensitive.

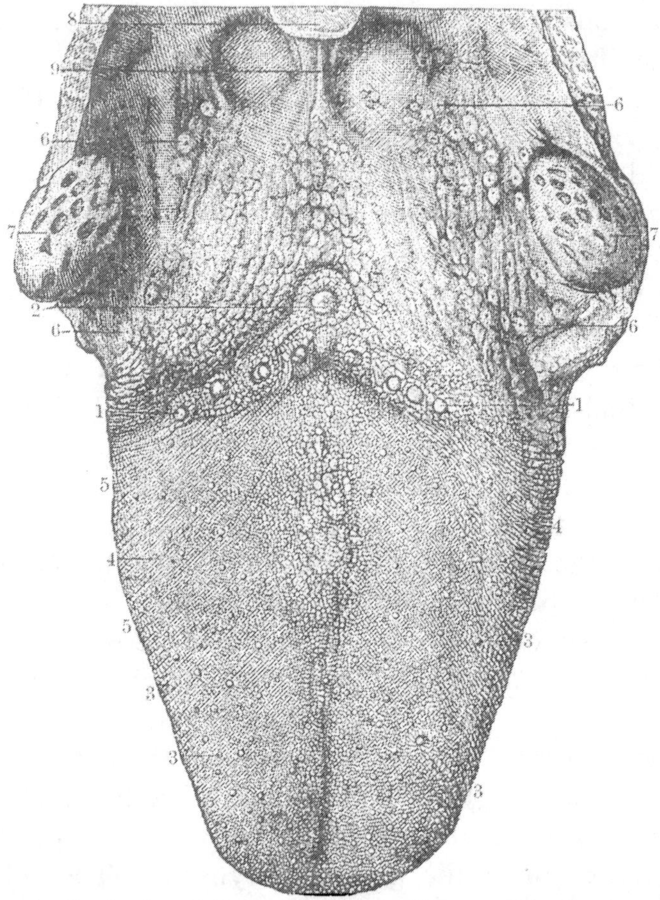

FIG. 64.—Papillar Surface of the Tongue, with the Fauces and Tonsils; 1, 1, circumvallate papillæ, in front of 2, the foramen cæcum; 3, fungiform papillæ; 4, filiform and corneal papillæ; 5, transverse and oblique rugæ; 6, mucous glands at the base of the tongue and in the fauces; 7, tonsils; 8, part of the epiglottis; 9, median glosso-epiglottidean fold (frænum epiglottidis) (from Sappey).

The mucous membrane of the tongue is covered with papillæ of three varieties—circumvallate, fungiform, and filiform. The *circumvallate papillæ*, eight or ten in number, form the boundary between the anterior two-thirds and the posterior third of the tongue. They are arranged in V-shape, the apex being backward. In these papillæ are the gustatory buds or "taste-goblets," which are believed to be connected with the sense of taste, although no connection of nerves with them has been traced. These bodies have also been found at the root of the tongue and on the posterior surface of the epiglottis. The *fungiform papillæ* are especially abundant at the sides and tip, and less so on the dorsum. The *filiform papillæ* are the most numerous of all the papillæ, and, though present on all portions of the mucous membrane of the tongue, are very abundant on the dorsum. The filiform papillæ are probably tactile organs, while the other two varieties are connected with the sense of taste.

The fact that the general sensibility of the tongue may be lost and the sense of taste remain would indicate that the channels for the transmission of these two sensations are different. It may be well to again call attention to the necessity for making a distinction between what may be tasted and what may be smelled, between savors and flavors. The sense of taste gives cognizance of the qualities sweet, sour, salty, etc., but to speak of an oily taste is incorrect: such a quality appeals to general sensibility only.

Conditions of the Sense of Taste.—That the sense of taste may be exercised requires the presence of certain conditions, one of which is that the substance must be in a state of solution or be soluble in the saliva. Insoluble substance are tasteless: for this reason calomel is especially suitable as a cathartic for children. Another condition is that the mucous membrane of the mouth must be moist. When the mouth is dry and substances

20

not already in a state of solution are taken in, there is no saliva present to dissolve them; consequently they are not tasted. This absence of taste is very marked in the parched condition of the mouth occurring during fevers.

To excite the sense of taste, sapid substances must pass by osmosis into the papillæ of the mucous membrane and there stimulate the terminal filaments of the nerves which preside over this sense. An important agent in causing this absorption is the movement of the tongue. It is a matter of common observation that if sapid substances be simply placed on the tongue, the sense of taste is not excited, but if the tongue be pressed against the roof of the mouth, absorption is promoted and the gustatory qualities are at once recognized.

It is to be noted also that a savor persists for a certain length of time, and that if it be desired to determine the comparative qualities of different substances by the sense of taste, there must either be intervals between the tests or something must be used to obliterate the taste of one of the articles before another is taken into the mouth. It is also noteworthy that some savors so powerfully impress the taste-organs that others fail to make any impression. This principle is made practical use of in rendering disagreeable medicines tasteless. Thus a few cloves eaten before taking a dose of castor oil will render the latter far less nauseous; a mouthful of brandy will have the same effect.

4. Sense of Sight.—The anatomy of the human eye (Fig. 65) is so complicated that only such points as are essential to an understanding of some of its more important functions will be referred to.

Sclerotic Coat.—The sclerotic coat is the outside and enclosing membrane of the eyeball, the anterior portion being the so-called "white of the eye." To it are attached the tendons of the muscles which move the eye-

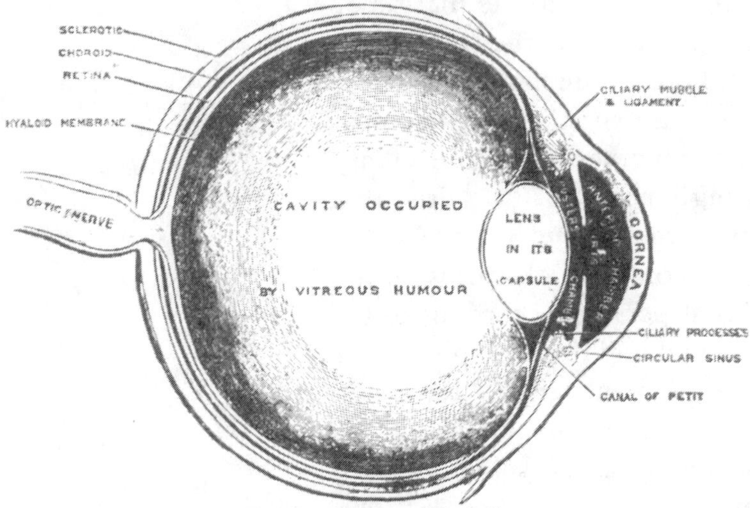

FIG. 65.—Section of Eyeball.

ball. In the anterior part the membrane is absent and its place is occupied by the cornea.

Cornea.—This structure is the most prominent portion of the eyeball, and by virtue of its transparency the iris can be seen through it.

Choroid.—Internal to the sclerotic is the choroid, a vascular membrane containing pigment. Its anterior portion is thickened, forming the ciliary body, the inner parts of which consist of folds, the ciliary processes.

Iris.—The iris is a muscular curtain behind the cornea, the fibres being both circular and radiating (Fig. 66). In the centre is an opening, the pupil, around which, on the posterior surface of the iris, are arranged the circular fibres forming the sphincter pupillæ, which receives its nervous supply from the motor oculi through the ciliary ganglion. The muscular fibres which form the dilator pupillæ are arranged in a radiating direction from the circumference to the margin of the pupil, where they blend with the fibres of the sphincter. These fibres are supplied with sympathetic nerves from the ciliary ganglion. It is the iris that gives to the eye its characteristic color, which varies in different persons according to the amount and the arrangement of the pigment, the latter being more abundant and more disseminated in dark than in light eyes.

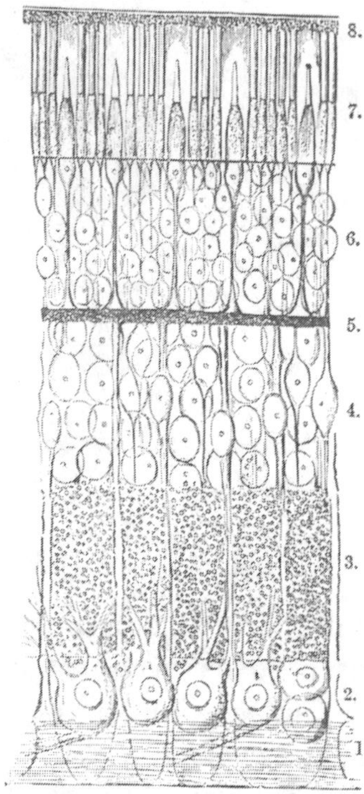

FIG. 67.—Diagrammatic Section of Retina, showing the relation of the different layers in the posterior part of the fundus (not the macula lutea) (Schultze): 1, nerve-fibre layer in which the retinal vessels run next to the vitreous humor; 2, layer of nerve-cells; 3, internal granular layer; 4, internal nuclear layer; 5, external granular layer; 6, external nuclear layer; 7, rods and cones with their extremities imbedded in the epithelial cells; 8, pigmented epithelium lying next to the choroid coat.

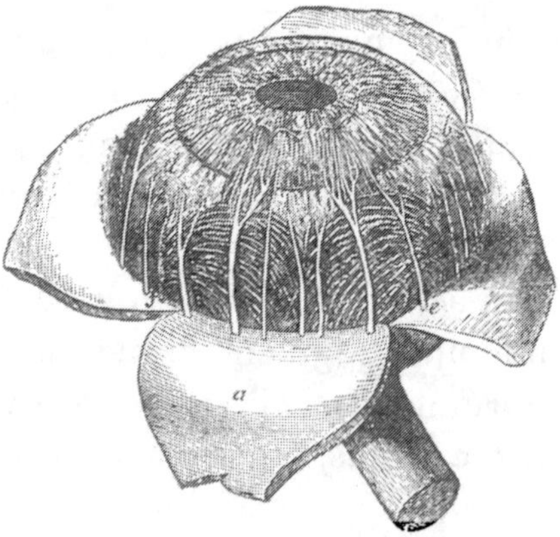

FIG. 66.—Choroid Membrane and Iris, exposed by the removal of the sclerotic and cornea: *a*, one of the segments of the sclerotic thrown back; *b*, ciliary muscle; *c*, iris; *e*, one of the ciliary nerves; *f*, one of the vasa vorticosa or choroidal veins (Quain).

Ciliary Muscle.—Between the sclerotic and choroid, anteriorly, is the ciliary muscle, a band about 3 mm.

broad, composed of radiating and circular unstriped fibres.

Retina.—The retina is the most internal of the tunics of the eye, and it is the portion which receives the rays of light. In the centre of the retina is the macula lutea, or yellow spot of Sömmering, and at its centre is a depression, the fovea centralis (Fig. 67). At a distance of about 2.5 mm. internal to the macula lutea is the optic disk, the entrance of the optic nerve. As at this point vision is absent, it is also called the "blind spot." Through its centre passes the central artery of the retina.

The structure of the retina is very complex, being made up of ten layers:

(1) *Membrana limitans interna*, the most internal layer.

(2) *Fibrous layer*, composed of nerve-fibres of the optic nerve.

(3) *Vesicular layer*, consisting of large ganglionic nerve-cells, one process from each of which passes into the fibrous layer, and which is regarded as connecting with a nerve-fibre, while from the other end of the cell goes off another process (in some more than one), which passes into the fourth layer.

(4) *Inner molecular or granular layer*, so called from its granular appearance, consists of minute fibres which are believed to connect with the adjoining layer.

(5) *Inner nuclear layer*, containing oval nuclei believed to be bipolar nerve-cells, one process of which passes into the inner molecular layer, and which is regarded by some as connecting, through this, with the ganglion-cells of the third layer: the other process passes into the sixth layer, and is believed to connect with the rods and cones. Besides the oval nuclei this layer contains other cells.

(6) *Outer molecular layer*, containing minute fibres and stellate cells, regarded as ganglion-cells.

(7) *Outer nuclear layer*, consisting of oval nucleated cells of two varieties; one variety, called "rod-granules," connects with the rods of the ninth layer, and the other, called "cone-granules," connects with the cones of that layer.

(8) *Membrana limitans externa* is the next layer.

(9) *Jacob's membrane, or layer of rods and cones*, is composed of rods and cones, the former solid bodies arranged perpendicularly to the surface, each of which is made up of an outer and an inner part joined together. The outer part presents a striated appearance, and is composed of disks, one upon another. The inner part connects with a rod-granule of the seventh layer. The cones, which are not so numerous as the rods, are conical in shape, their bases lying in the membrana limitans externa. They possess also an inner and an outer portion, the former being likewise striated, but the latter is more bulging.

(10) *Pigmentary layer*, consisting of a single layer of pigmented cells, was formerly regarded as belonging to the choroid.

The retina at the macula lutea differs in structure from that just described, inasmuch as the nerve-fibres of the second layer do not form a continuous layer; the third layer is composed of several strata of cells instead of one stratum; there are only cones, no rods, and in the seventh layer there are only cone-granules. At the fovea centralis are to be found only the cones, the outer nuclear layer, and a thin inner molecular layer.

Anterior and Posterior Chambers.—The anterior chamber is the space between the cornea and the iris, while the posterior chamber is the space between the peripheral part of the iris, the suspensory ligament, and the ciliary processes. The latter is very much smaller than it was formerly supposed to be; indeed, it hardly deserves the name of "chamber." Both these spaces are filled with aqueous humor, an alkaline fluid, 96.7 per cent. of which is water and 0.1 sodium chloride.

Vitreous Body.—This body is composed of transparent, jelly-like material, called also "vitreous humor," which is enclosed by the hyaloid membrane. In the

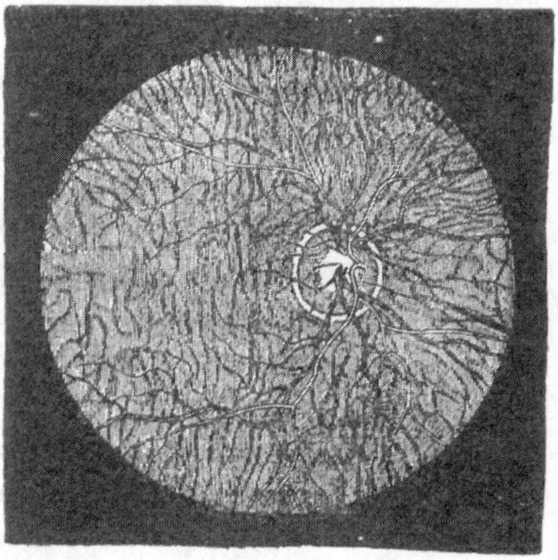

FIG. 68.—Fundus of an Eye containing little pigment, choroidal vessels visible (Wecker).

anterior portion, which is depressed, this membrane is wanting, and in the depression is the crystalline lens. The margin of the hyaloid membrane is attached to the margin of the lens, and it is called the "suspensory ligament."

Crystalline Lens.—The lens is transparent and doubly convex, being more convex on the posterior than on the anterior surface. It is situated behind the pupil, between the aqueous humor and the vitreous body, and is supported by these structures and the suspensory ligament. It is contained in its capsule, which is also transparent and highly elastic. The capsule is in contact with the border of the iris, but not with the rest of the structure, and the small space thus left is the posterior chamber.

Suspensory Ligament.—This ligament is a portion of the hyaloid membrane which encloses the vitreous body, and is situated between that body and the ciliary processes. It aids in supporting the lens.

Arterial Supply to the Eye.—The vessels which supply blood to the eye are the ciliary arteries and the arteria centralis retinæ (Figs. 68, 69). The nervous supply has already been considered.

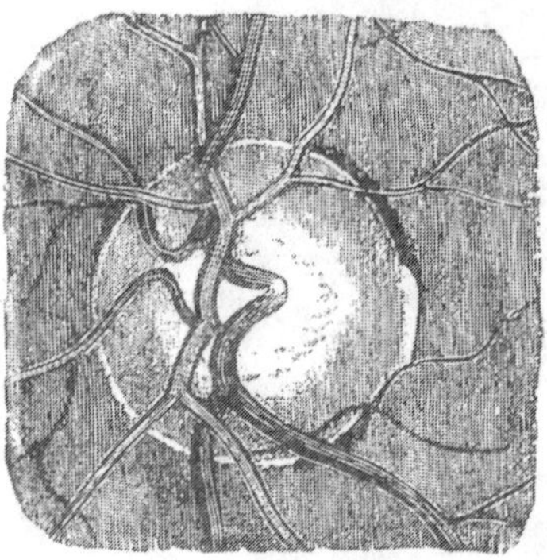

FIG. 69.—Normal Optic Disk of the Left Eye (after Jaeger).

Physiology of Vision.—The eye has very aptly been compared to a photographic camera, the transparent structure through which pass the rays of light representing the lenses, and the retina representing the sensitive plate on which the image is received, while the pigmented choroid coat is the representative of the lampblack with which the photographer darkens the interior of the camera-box to prevent any reflected light striking the plate and interfering with the sharpness of the picture. In the camera, in order to bring to a focus upon the plate the rays of light coming from objects at different distances, the photographer uses a focusing screw, by which the lens may be moved nearer to or farther from the object he wishes to photograph; and in order that clear images may be obtained by the eye it is necessary to accomplish the same result, for when the eye is focused for near objects those at a distance are blurred, and vice versâ. This fact may readily be demonstrated by looking through a piece of mosquito-netting at the windows of a house on the opposite side of a street. When the threads of the net can be seen distinctly the bars of the window will be indistinct, and when the bars of the window are clear and distinct, then the threads are blurred. In the optical apparatus of the eye there is no provision for altering the position of the lenses, but there is one which answers the same purpose, and which is called "accommodation." In connection with every camera there is an arrangement of openings or diaphragms by which a greater or lesser amount of light may be admitted according to circumstances. In the eye the iris serves a similar purpose. In many cameras it is necessary to have a number of such diaphragms, each having openings of different sizes, but some are provided with a single one, the size of whose opening can be altered; this is called an "iris diaphragm," and is a rude contrivance compared with the natural iris from which it derives its name, and which by means of its muscular fibres can alter in a moment the size of the pupil.

Rays of light coming from an object, in order to produce a distinct image of that object, must be brought to a focus upon the retina. If the media through which the light from an object passes to reach the retina were all of the same density as the air, and were also plane surfaces, an impression would be produced, but there would be no distinct image. Actually, before such rays do reach the retina, they must pass through certain media which, by reason of both density and shape,

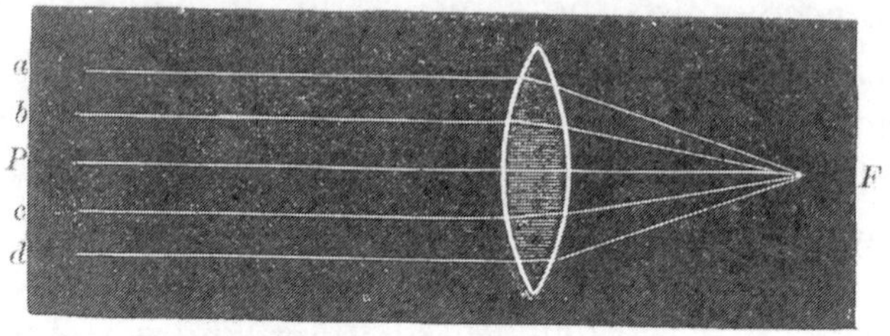

FIG. 70.—Principal Focus of a Convex Lens. The parallel rays, *a*, *b*, *c*, *d*, are refracted by the lens so as to unite at the point *F*, on the axis, *P*; the ray, *P*, undergoes no refraction. *F* is the principal focus.

refract them and bring them to a focus, thus producing a sharp and distinct image of the object looked at. These media are the cornea, the aqueous humor, the crystalline lens, and the vitreous body. The cornea by its density and convex shape refracts the rays falling upon it, but, as its anterior and posterior surfaces are parallel, the cornea and the aqueous humor may be considered together as one medium, the posterior surface of which, that of the aqueous humor covering the convex crystalline lens, is concave. The anterior convex surface of the cornea and the concave posterior surface of the aqueous humor act as a concavo-convex lens, so that there are in reality but three media: 1, cornea and aqueous humor; 2, crystalline lens; and 3, vitreous body. The optical axis of the eye passes through the centre of the cornea, directly backward through all these media until it terminates in the fovea centralis of the retina. Rays of light falling upon the cornea are refracted and made convergent, and this effect is increased by the lens, so that when the rays reach the retina they are brought to a focus. If the entire optical apparatus of the eye were rigid and immovable, it would be necessary, in order to obtain a clear image of an object, either for the individual to approach or to recede from the object, or to cause the object to do the same with reference to him, for only parallel rays—namely, rays coming from objects at a distance of 10 metres or more—are brought to a focus in the normal eye unless some change is brought about in the refractive media. If an object be within that distance, the rays of light coming from it are brought to a focus by altering the shape of the crystalline lens; this is accommodation.

Accommodation.—As already stated, the optical apparatus of the eye is in a state of rest when it is looking at objects more than 10 metres away; thus to see the stars, although millions of kilometres distant, no effort is

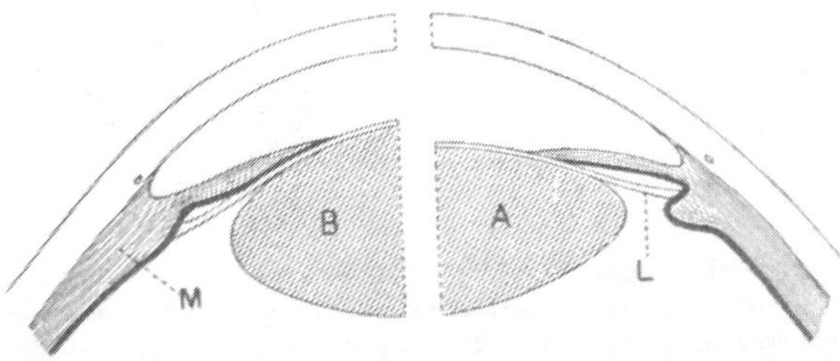

Fig. 71.—Diagram showing the Changes in the Lens during Accommodation. The ciliary muscle on the right is supposed to be passive, as in looking at distant objects: the suspensory ligament, *L*, is therefore tight, and compresses the anterior surface of the lens, *A*, so as to flatten it. On the left the ciliary muscle, *M*, is contracting, so as to relax the ligament, which allows the lens to become more convex. This contraction occurs when looking at near objects.

required; but if it be desired to see objects within that distance, there is a change in the refractive media until a point so close to the eye is reached that no amount of effort will enable them to be seen. The point at which objects cease to be seen distinctly is called the "near point," and it is, for a normal or emmetropic eye, about 12 cm., although it is not the same in all persons.

The accommodation of the eye is brought about especially by the change in the shape of the crystalline lens; thus in looking at near objects the eye becomes more convex. This accommodation is accomplished in the following manner: The lens is a very elastic structure, which is kept in a less convex condition when far

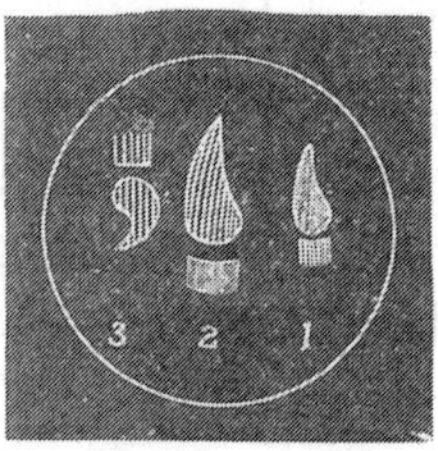

FIG. 72.

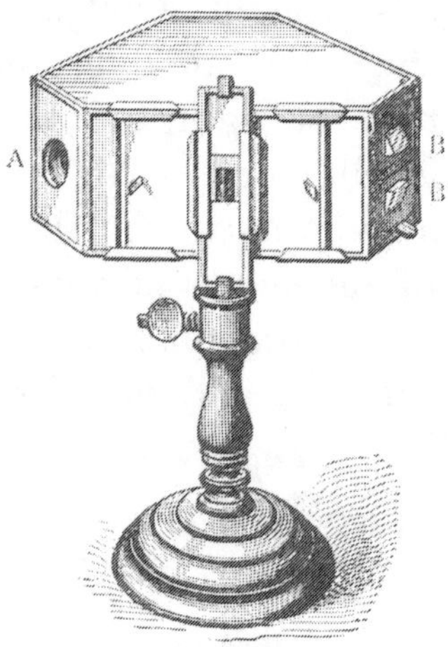

FIG. 73.

FIG. 72.—Diagram showing three reflections of a candle: 1, from the anterior surface of cornea; 2, from the anterior surface of lens; 3, from the posterior surface of lens. For further explanation see text. The experiment is best performed by employing an instrument invented by Helmholtz, termed a *phakoscope*.

FIG. 73.—Phakoscope of Helmholtz: at *B B'* are two prisms, by which the light of a candle is concentrated on the eye of the person experimented with; *A* is the aperture for the eye of the observer. The observer notices three double images, as in Fig. 72, reflected from the eye under examination when the eye is fixed upon a distant object; the position of the images having been noticed, the eye is then made to focus a near object, such as a reed pushed up; the images from the anterior surfaces of the lens will be observed to move toward each other, in consequence of the lens becoming more convex.

objects are looked at than its elasticity would cause it to assume were it allowed free play; but the lens is enclosed in a capsule to which the suspensory ligament is attached, and the tension of this ligament is such as to pull upon the anterior portion of the capsule and flatten it, at the same time flattening the anterior surface of the contained lens. But when a near object is to be looked at, the ciliary muscle contracts, and as its fixed point is at the junction of the cornea and sclerotic, this contraction draws the ciliary processes forward and relaxes the suspensory ligament, thus removing the influence which tends to flatten the lens and permits the latter by its elasticity to become more convex. The act is a voluntary one, the nervous supply for which is furnished to the ciliary muscle by the motor oculi through the ciliary nerves. At the same time that this muscular action is taking place the pupil becomes smaller and the eyes converge.

Phakoscope of Helmholtz.—The above explanation of the mechanism of accommodation is attributable to Helmholtz, who, to demonstrate it, has devised an apparatus called a "phakoscope" (Fig. 73), but it may also be demonstrated in the following manner: If a candle-flame be held at one side of the eye of a person who is looking at a distant object, and an observer look at the other side, he will see three images of the flame, the brightest and most distinct being an erect image which is formed by the anterior surface of the cornea. Besides this image there is a second image, which is also erect, but which is less distinct and larger; this image is formed at the anterior surface of the lens. A third image is also seen, which is inverted and also indistinct; this image is formed at the posterior surface of the lens, which, being concave forward, acts like a concave mirror and inverts the image. If the person then look at a near object, the second image becomes brighter and smaller, and at the same time approaches the first, while the first image undergoes no change, and the third a change so slight as not to be perceptible (Fig. 72). This proves that in accommodating the eye for near objects the change which takes place is an increase in the convexity of the anterior surface of the crystalline lens. The same may be shown by looking at the eye from the side, when in accommodation the iris may be seen to move forward, being pushed in that direction by the anterior surface of the lens with which it is in contact.

Emmetropia is a condition of the eye in which the principal focus falls exactly upon the layer of rods and cones of the retina when the accommodation is relaxed, or, as it is expressed, when the eye is in a state of accommodative rest. This is another way of saying that in this condition of the eye parallel rays are focused on the retina. An emmetropic eye is a normal eye.

Ametropia.—Whenever the permanent condition of an eye is not as described above it is one of ametropia. Of this condition there are several varieties.

Myopia.—A myopic eye is one that is abnormally elongated, and some authorities regard an increased convexity of the lens as constituting an essential part of this condition. The retina is so far from the lens that parallel rays are focused in front of it, and, crossing, do not form distinct images on the retina, the images being blurred. To correct this, concave glasses are used, which cause these rays to diverge as they enter the eye, and by adjusting the concavity to the amount of myopia parallel rays are thus brought to a focus on the retina as they are in the emmetropic eye without glasses. A myopic eye is commonly said to be a "near-sighted" one.

Hypermetropia.—In this condition the eye is shorter than normal, and the retina is too near the lens, so that parallel rays are brought to a focus behind the retina and indistinct vision is produced, as in the myopic eye. In the endeavor to overcome this defect the ciliary muscle is liable to overstrain in order to converge the rays to a focus upon the retina, and the constant effort is painful and injurious. The condition is corrected by the use of convex glasses.

Presbyopia, which is sometimes called "old sight," sometimes "long sight," is the condition of the eye seen in elderly people. In this condition it is difficult to see near objects, although the vision for those at a distance is unaffected. It is usually attributed to a lessened elasticity of the lens, though the ciliary muscle is also less strong, and some writers state that it depends on diminution of the convexity of the cornea. To aid in correcting it convex glasses are used.

Astigmatism.—In this condition the cornea is usually at fault, its curvature being greater in one meridian than in another, and consequently the rays of light from an object are not all brought to the same focus, and the image, therefore, is not distinct. For the correction of astigmatism glasses are worn which are segments of a cylinder—that is, curved in but one direction—and which are known as "cylindrical" glasses. The crystalline lens may also be at fault in astigmatism.

Functions of the Retina.—As odors excite the olfactory apparatus and savors excite the gustatory, so does light excite the retina. As neither odors nor savors reach the brain, where smell and taste are produced, but only the nerve-impulses which they excite and which the olfactory and gustatory nerves transmit, so when the light-waves fall upon the retina they go no farther; but the nerve-impulses which they there excite are carried to the brain by the optic nerve and produce the sensation called "light." Thus it is that a blow upon the eye or an injury to the optic nerve produces in the brain the impression of a flash of light, although the room in which the blow or injury was received may be absolutely dark.

That the optic nerve is itself insensitive to light is shown by the fact that at the point where it enters the eye, forming the optic disk, is the "blind spot," at which there is an entire absence of sight. This fact may be demonstrated in the following simple way: Look with the right eye at the round black spot here printed,

closing the left eye, and holding the book six inches from it. The spot and the cross can both be seen. Now carry the book away from the face farther and farther, still looking at the spot. A point will be reached where the cross will all at once disappear, and when this occurs the light from the cross falls upon the optic disk. If the book be carried still farther, the cross will again come in sight.

There is no doubt but that the portion of the retina which reacts to the stimulus of light is the layer of rods and cones, and of this layer the cones are especially sensitive. This is shown by the fact that the macula lutea (yellow spot) is the portion of the retina which is the most sensitive, and here there are no nerve-fibres, but rods and cones, and in the fovea centralis, which is the most sensitive portion of the macula, only cones are found. How the retina converts the impressions that light-waves produce upon it into nerve-impulses is still an unsettled question. One theory is that the light produces chemical changes in the retina, the result of which is to stimulate the nerve-fibres; another theory is that there are thermic influences produced by the light which have the same effect; while a third theory regards the pigment-cells of the retina as in some way connected with the phenomena.

Movements of the Eyeball.—The eyeball is moved by muscles which have already, to some extent, been considered in connection with the functions of the cranial nerves. The arrows in Fig. 74 indicate the direction in which the different muscles act. Thus it will be seen that the in-

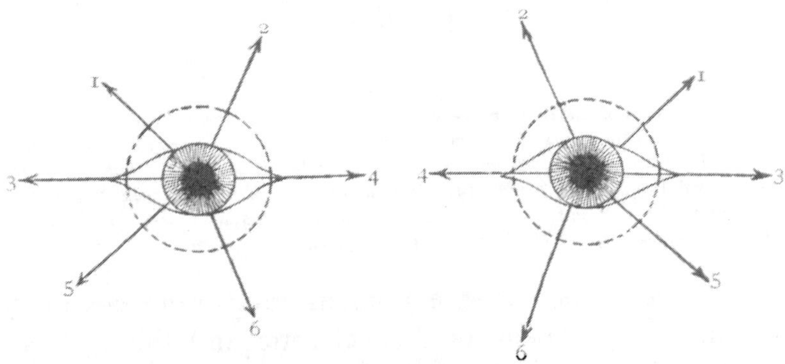

Fig. 74.—Movements of the Eyeballs: 1, inferior oblique; 2, superior rectus; 3, external rectus; 4, internal rectus; 5, superior oblique; 6, inferior rectus.

ternal rectus rotates the eye inward; the external rectus, outward; the superior rectus, upward and inward; the inferior rectus, downward and inward; the superior oblique, downward and outward; the inferior oblique, upward and outward. By a combination of two of these muscles various other movements are produced; thus the superior rectus and inferior oblique, acting together, rotate the eyeball vertically upward, while the inferior rectus and superior oblique jointly rotate it vertically downward.

Appendages of the Eye.—Lachrymal Apparatus.—To

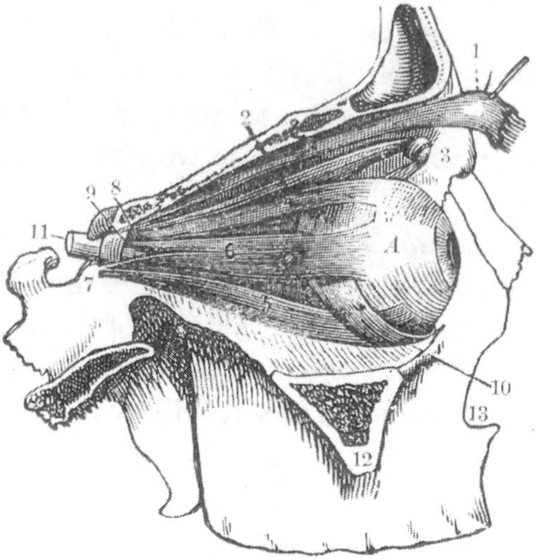

FIG. 75.—Muscles of the Eye: 1, the palpebral elevator; 2, the trochlear muscle; 3, the pulley through which the tendon of insertion plays; 4, superior rectus muscle; 5, inferior rectus muscle; 6, external rectus muscle; 7, 8, its two points of origin; 9, interval through which pass the oculo-motor and abducens nerves; 10, inferior oblique muscle; 11, optic nerve; 12, cut surface of the malar process of the superior maxillary bone; 13, the nasal notch; *A*, the eyeball.

keep the conjunctiva (the mucous membrane covering the anterior segment of the sclerotic and the cornea) moist and in normal condition is the function of the tears. They are secreted by the lachrymal gland, a compound racemose gland lodged in a depression at the upper and outer portion of the orbit (Fig. 76). Its ducts, about seven in number, open on the upper and outer half of the conjunctiva near its reflection on the eyeball. At the edge of the upper and lower eyelids, at their inner extremities, are openings (puncta lachrymalia)

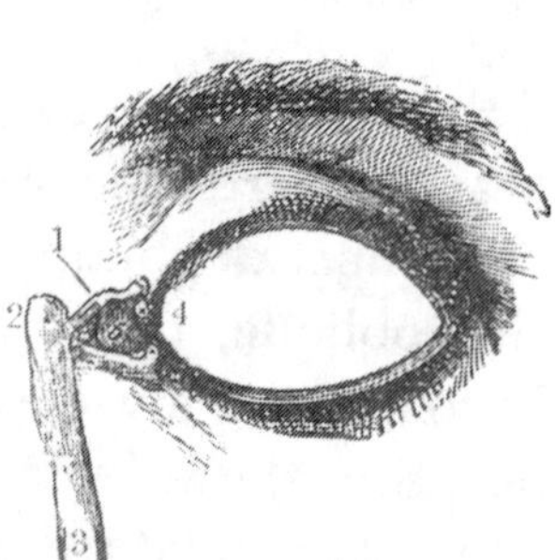

FIG. 76.—1, canaliculus; 2, lachrymal sac; 3, nasal duct; 4, plica semilunaris; 5, caruncula lachrymalis.

into which the tears pass after performing their function. These openings are the beginnings of the canaliculi, which open into the lachrymal sac, or the dilated upper extremity of the nasal duct, which discharges at the inferior meatus of the nose, the opening here being partially closed by a fold of mucous membrane, the valve of Hasner.

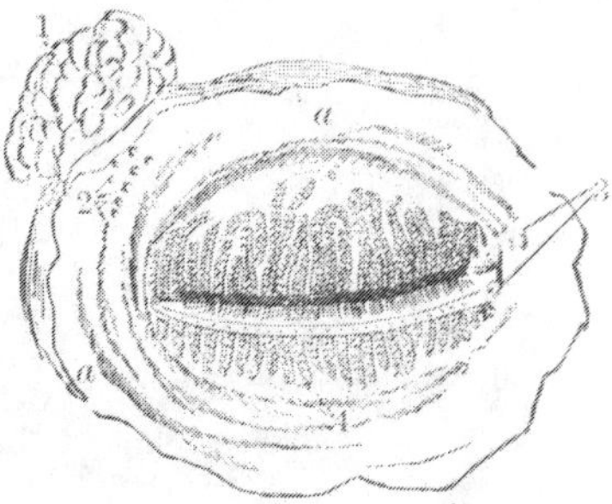

FIG. 77.—1, lachrymal gland; 2, its ducts; 3, punctum lachrymale; *a*, conjunctiva; 4, Meibomian glands.

Meibomian Glands.—On the posterior surface of the eyelids, beneath the conjunctiva, are the Meibomian glands (Fig. 77), thirty in number on the upper and fewer on the lower lid. Their ducts open on the edges of the lids, and their secretion prevents the adhesion of the lids and the tears from running over them on to the cheeks.

5. Sense of Hearing.—The ear, the organ of hearing, is divided into three parts, external, middle, and internal, the latter being essential, while the others are accessory (Fig. 78).

The external ear consists of the pinna or auricle and the external auditory canal or meatus. The office of the pinna is to collect the sound-waves and direct them to the canal, which they traverse to reach the membrana tympani. In some animals, such as the horse, the auricles are very important, enabling the animal to detect the direction from which sounds come, and they are capable of considerable movement; but in man they are not so important, although when the hearing is defective they are of assistance. That they are not essential to hearing is shown by the fact that when removed hearing is not affected, and also by the fact that in birds, where they are absent, the sense of hearing is well marked.

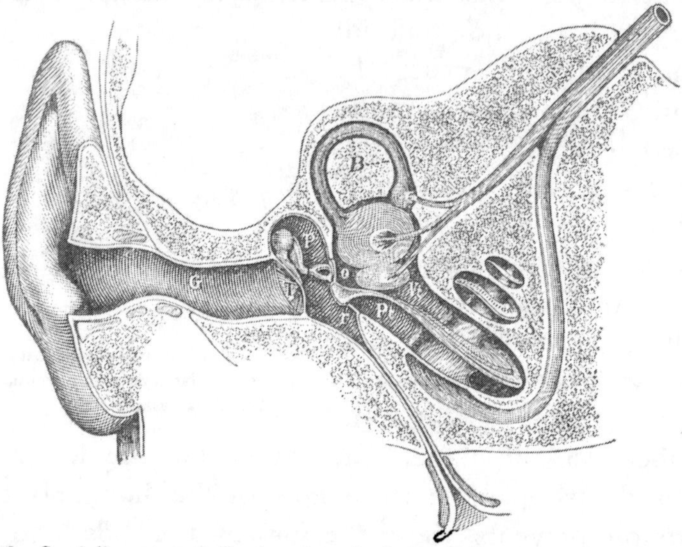

FIG. 78.—Semi-diagrammatic Section through the Right Ear (Czermak): *G*, external auditory meatus; *T*, membrana tympani; *P*, tympanic cavity: *o*, fenestra ovalis; *r*, fenestra rotunda; *B*, semicircular canal; *S*, cochlea; *Vt*, scala vestibuli; *Pt*, scala tympani.

The middle ear, *tympanum*, or tympanic cavity, is separated from the meatus by the membrana tympani. It is a cavity in the petrous portion of the temporal bone, is filled with air, and is in communication with the pharynx by means of the Eustachian tube. It is lined with mucous membrane covered with ciliated epithelium. In the tympanic cavity are the ossicles (Fig. 79), a chain of bones which con-

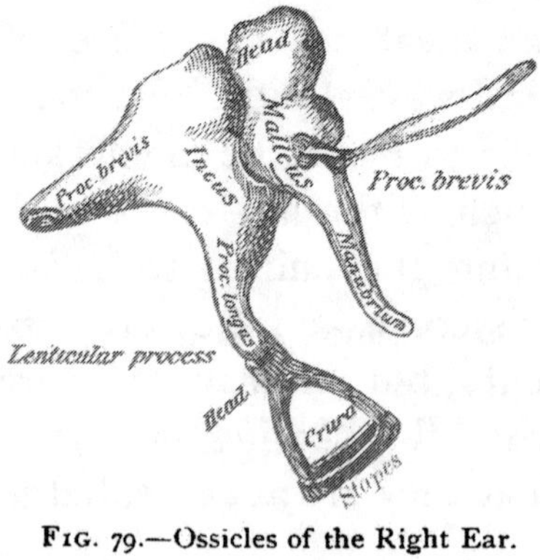

FIG. 79.—Ossicles of the Right Ear.

nect the membrana tympani with the labyrinth or internal ear. These bones are the malleus, the incus, and the stapes, otherwise known as the hammer, the anvil, and the stirrup, so called from their resemblance to these objects.

The internal ear, or labyrinth, consists of three parts, the vestibule, the semicircular canals, and the cochlea.

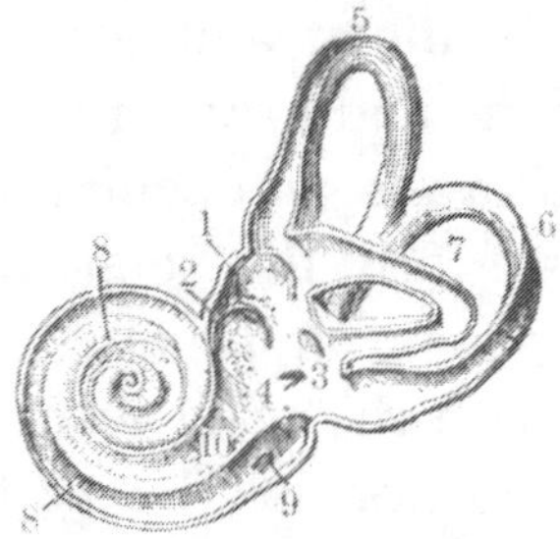

Fig. 80.—View of the Interior of the Left Labyrinth; the bony wall of the labyrinth is removed superiorly and externally: 1, fovea semielliptica; 2, fovea hemispherica; 3, common opening of the superior and posterior semicircular canals; 4, opening of the aqueduct of the vestibule; 5, the superior, 6, the posterior, and 7, the external, semicircular canals; 8, spiral tube of the cochlea (scala tympani); 9, opening of the aqueduct of the cochlea; 10, placed on the lamina spiralis in the scala vestibuli (Sömmering).

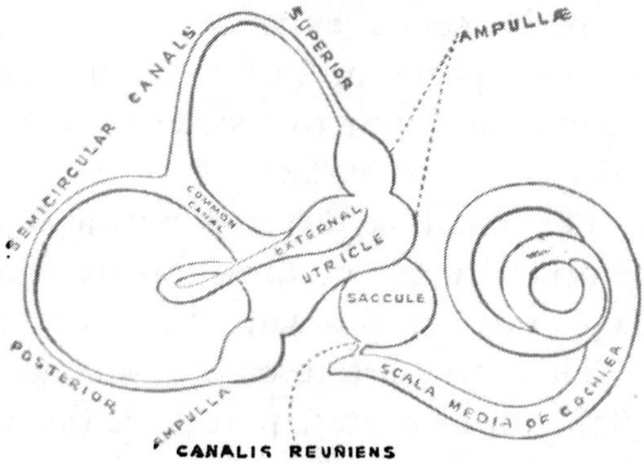

Fig. 81.—Diagram of the Membranous Labyrinth (Gray).

These are cavities in the temporal bone which communicate with the tympanum through the fenestra ovalis and fenestra rotunda, and with the internal auditory meatus, through which runs the auditory nerve, the nerve of hearing. These cavities form the osseous labyrinth. Within these is the membranous labyrinth, which contains the endolymph, while between the osseous and membranous labyrinths is a fluid, the perilymph.

Vestibule.—The vestibule is a common cavity with which all the other portions of the labyrinth are in communication. On its inner wall are openings through which filaments of the auditory nerve enter; on its outer wall is the fenestra ovalis, an opening closed by the base of the stapes; posteriorly the semicircular canals communicate by five openings, and anteriorly is the opening of communication with the scala vestibuli of the cochlea. The membranous portion of the vestibule consists of two sacs, the utricle and the saccule, in the walls of which nerve-filaments are distributed, and within are the otoliths, two small bodies consisting of grains of carbonate of lime.

Semicircular Canals.—These canals are three in number. The superior semicircular canal is vertical and at right angles to the posterior surface of the petrous portion of the temporal bone; the posterior is also vertical, but is parallel with the surface of the bone, while the external or horizontal is directed outward and backward. The arrangement of these canals is such that each one is at right angles with the other two.

Cochlea.—This structure resembles somewhat a snail-shell (Fig. 82). In its central portion is the axis, modiolus, or columella, around which winds a spiral canal divided into two parts by a partition partly bony and partly membranous. The bony portion is the lamina spiralis, and the membranous portion is the membrana basilaris, while the lower canal is the scala tympani.

The upper canal is subdivided by the membrane of Reissner, the larger part of the canal being the scala vestibuli, and the smaller the scala media, also called "canal of the cochlea." In the latter canal, covered over

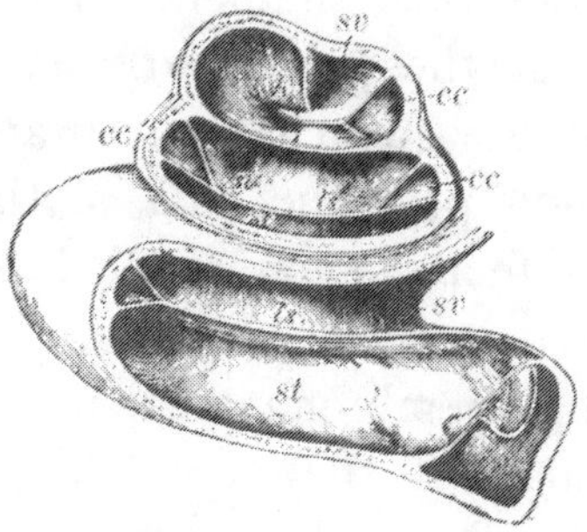

FIG. 82.—The Bony and Membranous Cochlea laid open: *st*, scala tympani; *sv*, scala vestibuli; *cc*, scala media or ductus cochlearis; *ls*, lamina spiralis ossea; *h*, helicotrema, or opening connecting the scalæ tympani and vestibuli.

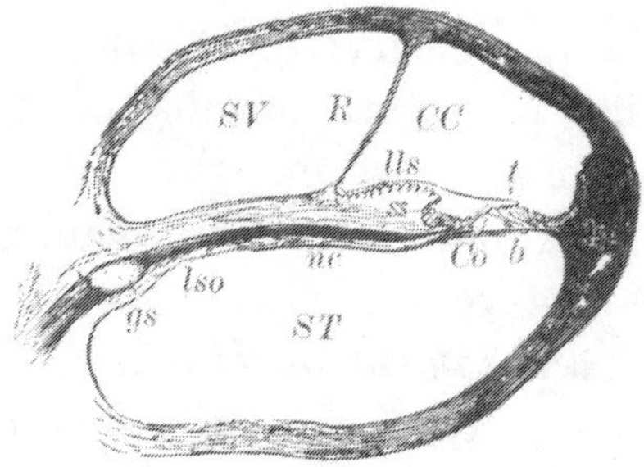

FIG. 83.—Section through one of the Coils of the Cochlea (diagrammatic): *ST*, scala tympani; *SV*, scala vestibuli; *CC*, canalis cochleæ or canalis membranaceus; *R*, membrane of Reissner; *lso*, lamina spiralis ossea; *lls*, limbus lamina spiralis; *ss*, sulcus spiralis; *nc*, cochlear nerve; *gs*, ganglion spirale; *t*, membrana tectoria (below the membrana tectoria is the lamina reticularis); *b*, membrana basilaris; *Co*, rods of Corti; *lsp*, ligamentum spirale (Quain).

by the membrana tectoria, is the organ of Corti, which is to the sense of hearing what the retina is to the sense of sight.

Organ of Corti.—This structure is located on the membrana basilaris, and extends throughout the length of the cochlea, winding with it. It is composed of cells whose arrangement has been likened to the keyboard of a piano. The two central cells, which are rod-like, are the inner and outer rods of Corti. They form an angle with each other, being separated at the base and meeting above, leaving a space between them, the zona arcuata. As there are rows of these rods, this space forms a tunnel extending the entire length of the cochlea. The number of the inner rods has been estimated at six thousand, and of the outer at four thousand five hundred. At the sides of these rods are rows of cells which are in communication with the terminal filaments of the auditory nerve. On the tops of these cells are hair-like processes, or cilia, covered by a delicate membrane with perforations, through which pass the cilia of the outer hair-cells. The membrana tectoria covers all these structures.

Mechanism of Hearing.—The membrana tympani is made to vibrate by the impulse of the sound-waves which reach it; through the ossicles these vibrations are communicated to the internal ear, the base of the stapes at its every movement sending a wave through the perilymph. This wave passes up the scala vestibuli from the fenestra ovalis, which the base of the stirrup closes, to the top of the cochlea, and comes down the scala tympani to the fenestra rotunda, in its course passing over and under the membranous labyrinth filled with endolymph, through which fluid the vibrations are communicated to the terminal filaments of the auditory nerve. It is supposed that these waves in the endolymph of the membranous vestibule cause the otoliths to come in contact with the nerve-filaments and to stimulate them. The nerves ending in the semicircular canals are believed to preside over the maintenance of the equilibrium of the body, and not to be connected with hearing. This will be referred to later. The cochlear division of the auditory nerve sends into the modiolus of the cochlea branches that pass in between the plates of the lamina spiralis, where they form a plexus in which are ganglion-cells, from which the nerve-filaments pass to the organ of Corti, terminating, it is believed, in the hair-cells.

The waves already referred to as being set in motion through the endolymph pass over and under these cells, with which the nerve-filaments are connected, and cause the basilar membrane on which they rest to vibrate. This motion is communicated to the outer rods of Corti, which in turn pass it to the hairs of the special auditory cells through the medium of the perforated membrane, and from there it passes to the nerves. Here it is converted into impulses which are transmitted to the brain, where sound is produced.

It has been supposed that the rods of Corti are so arranged as to vibrate with particular tones, one rod for each tone, but it is doubtful whether such a differentiation can be made out in the auditory apparatus. The rods are not present in the ears of birds, and there is no reason to believe that birds cannot appreciate musical tones. In the basilar membrane there are fibres enough to respond to all the notes that can be appreciated; that is, from thirty-three waves to thirty-eight thousand waves in a second. It is more probable that the rods simply act as levers to communicate the vibrations of the fibres of the basilar membrane to the terminal nerve-filaments in the auditory cells.

Just how one is able to distinguish the differences in the intensity (loudness), pitch, and quality of sounds is not understood. The explanation most generally accepted at the present time, as to pitch at least, is that as, when a tone is sung over the strings of a piano, certain strings are set in vibration sympathetically, so in the basilar membrane, where, as in the piano, there are fibres of different length, these respond to different tones, and that in connection with each tone there is a separate filament of the auditory nerve, so that if the note be a high one a certain fibre is set in vibration, and the nerve-filament in communication with it transmits an impulse to certain cells in the brain, which when excited give the impression of a high tone, and so with other tones and other nerve-cells.

The introduction of the telephone and a study of its mechanism have led some writers to question the explanations which are generally accepted of the mechanism of hearing, and to suggest that as the single telephone wire transmits the complex sounds produced by an orchestra to a distance where they are reproduced in all their variety of intensity, pitch, and quality, so "the cochlea does not act on the principle of sympathetic vibration, but that the hairs of all its auditory cells vibrate to every tone, just as the drum of the ear does; that there is no analysis of complex vibration in the cochlea or elsewhere in the peripheral mechanism of the ear; that the hair-cells transform sound-vibrations into nerve-vibrations similar in frequency and amplitude to the sound-vibrations; that simple and complex vibrations of nerve-molecules arrive in the sensory cells of the brain, and there produce, not sound again of course, but the sensations of sound, the nature of which depends not upon the stimulation of different sensory cells, but on the frequency, the amplitude, and the form of the vibrations coming into the cells, probably through all the fibres of the auditory nerve." This explanation has been put forth by Prof. William Rutherford under the title of the "Telephone Theory of the Sense of Hearing."

Although sound-waves for the most part are transmitted to the internal ear through the tympanum, they may also be transmitted through the bones of the head. Thus vibrating bodies—a tuning-fork, for example—may be placed on the top of the head and the sound will be heard, or it may be held between the teeth with the same result. This fact is made use of in the audiphone, a fan-like device held in the teeth by the deaf. If the essential portions of the auditory apparatus be so diseased as to cause deafness, no such device as the audiphone will be of any use.

Eustachian Tube.—To permit the membrana tympani to respond properly to the sound-waves that reach it, the pressure of the atmosphere must be the same on both sides, and as the external pressure is subject to constant changes, a provision for a similar change on the tympanic side is essential. This is accomplished by the Eustachian tube, the channel of connection between the tympanic cavity and the pharynx. The pharyngeal orifice of this tube is closed except during swallowing, at which time it is opened. If it were always open the sound of one's own voice would be so loud as to be extremely disagreeable.

Semicircular Canals.—These structures have probably no connection with hearing, nor are they designed to distinguish the direction from which sound-waves come, as when diseased the hearing is in no wise affected, but under these circumstances there is a feeling of giddiness and the movements of the body are uncertain. If one of them be cut, the head of the animal experimented upon is violently moved to and fro in the plane of the canal which was divided, and it walks in an unsteady manner. The canals are therefore regarded as being connected with the maintenance of equilibrium.

Sympathetic Nervous System.—The sympathetic ner-

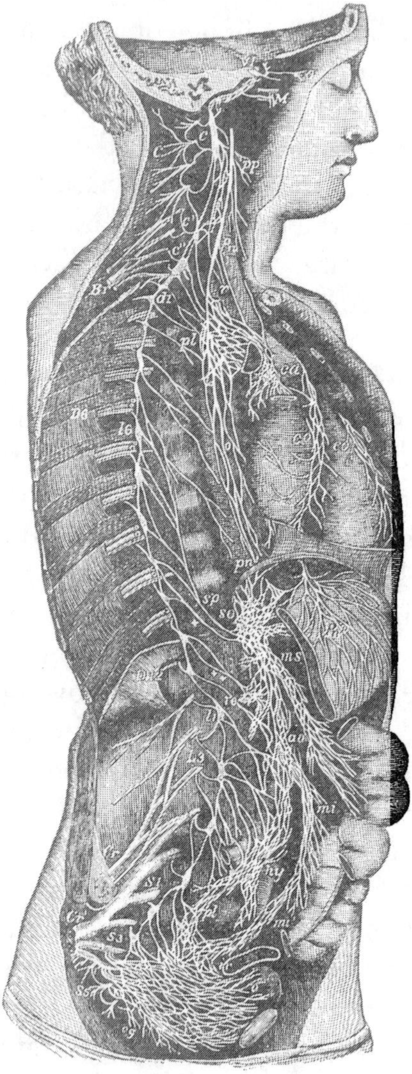

FIG. 84.—Diagrammatic view of the Sympathetic Cord of the Right Side, showing its connections with the principal cerebro-spinal nerves and the main præaortic plexuses. (Reduced from Quain's Anatomy.)

Cerebro-spinal Nerves.—VI., a portion of the sixth cranial as it passes through the cavernous sinus, receiving two twigs from the carotid plexus of the sympathetic nerve; O, ophthalmic ganglion connected by a twig with the carotid plexus; M, connection of the spheno-palatine ganglion by the Vidian nerve with the carotid plexus; C, cervical plexus; Br, brachial plexus; D 6, sixth intercostal nerve; D 12, twelfth; L 3, third lumbar nerve; S 1, first sacral nerve; S 3, third; S 5, fifth; Cr, anterior crural nerve; Cr, great sciatic; *pn*, vagus in the lower part of the neck; *r*, recurrent nerve winding round the subclavian artery.

Sympathetic Cord.—*c*, superior cervical ganglion; *c'*, second, or middle; *c''*, inferior; from each of these ganglia cardiac nerves (all deep on this side) are seen descending to the cardiac plexus; *d* 1, placed immediately below the first dorsal sympathetic ganglion; *d* 6, is opposite the sixth; *l* 1, first lumbar ganglion; *c g*, the terminal or coccygeal ganglion.

Præaortic and Visceral Plexuses.—*pp*, pharyngeal, and, lower down, laryngeal plexus; *pl*, post. pulmonary plexus spreading from the vagus on the back of the right bronchus; *ca*, on the aorta, the cardiac plexus, toward which, in addition to the cardiac nerve from the three cervical sympathetic ganglia, other branches are seen descending from the vagus and recurrent nerves; *co*, right or posterior and *co'*, left or anterior coronary plexus; *o*, œsophageal plexus in long meshes on the gullet; *sp*, great splanchnic nerve formed by branches from the fifth, sixth, seventh, eighth, and ninth dorsal ganglia; +, small splanchnic from the ninth and tenth; + +, smallest or third splanchnic from the eleventh; the first and second of these are shown joining the solar plexus, *so*; the third descending to the renal plexus, *re*; connecting branches between the solar plexus and the vagi are also represented; *pn'*, above the place where the right vagus passes to the lower or posterior surface of the stomach; *pn''*, the left distributed on the anterior or upper surface of the cardiac portion of the organ: from the solar vous system consists of ganglia and nerves (Fig. 84). The four ganglia which some writers describe as sympathetic ganglia of the head have been described in connection with the trigeminus.

Sympathetic Ganglia and Nerves.—From the base of the skull to the end of the spinal column there is on each side of the latter a chain of ganglia (twenty-four in number) which are connected in a series by nervous matter, each being spoken of as a ganglionic cord. At the coccyx these cords unite in one ganglion, the ganglion impar, and they are called "lateral," "vertebral," or "vaso-motor" ganglia. Besides these ganglia there are three gangliated plexuses—the *cardiac* in the thoracic cavity, the *solar* in the abdominal, and the *hypogastric* in the pelvic cavity. These are spoken of as "collateral" ganglia. There are besides ganglia in the viscera, as, for instance, in the heart; these are terminal ganglia. The ganglia on the posterior roots of spinal nerves are also regarded as belonging to the sympathetic system.

The sympathetic ganglia differ in no important particular from the ganglia already described. The nerve-cells are small, and are to a considerable extent unipolar. The nervous matter which connects the ganglia consists of both white and gray nerve-fibres. The ganglia are

---

plexus large branches are seen surrounding the arteries of the cœliac axis, and descending to *ms*, the sup. mesenteric plexus; opposite to this is an indication of the supra-renal plexus; below *re* (the renal plexus), the spermatic plexus is also indicated; *ao*, on the front of the aorta, marks the aortic plexus, formed by nerves descending from the solar and sup. mesenteric plexuses and from the lumbar ganglia; *mi*, the inf. mesenteric plexus surrounding the corresponding artery; *hy*, hypogastric plexus placed between the common iliac vessels, connected above with the aortic plexus, receiving nerves from the lower lumbar ganglia, and dividing below into the right and left pelvic or inf. hypogastric plexuses; *pl*, the right pelvic plexus; from this the nerves descending are joined by those from the plexus on the sup. hemorrhoidal vessels, *mi'*, by nerves from the sacral ganglia, and by visceral nerves from the third and fourth sacral spinal nerves, and there are thus formed the rectal, vesical, and other plexuses, which ramify upon the viscera, as toward *ir*, and *v*, the rectum and bladder.

also intimately connected with the cerebro-spinal nerves by both white and gray fibres. The white fibres which pass from the spinal nerves to the ganglia are continuous with the white fibres just described in the branches of communication between the ganglia. The gray fibres pass from the ganglia to the spinal nerves.

The most recent writers are inclined to regard the cerebro-spinal and sympathetic systems not as distinct, but as parts of one great whole, and the intimate relationship between the two is strongly confirmatory of this view. The history of the development of both is the same: the vaso-motor nerves, which are called "sympathetic," have their real origin in the cord and medulla, and, so far as known, the ganglia of the sympathetic do not respond reflexly to stimuli, as they would be expected to do if they were independent centres.

Functions of the Sympathetic.—The efferent fibres of the sympathetic are distributed to the muscles of the vascular system as vaso-motor fibres; that is, vaso-constrictor and cardio-accelerator, and vaso-dilator and cardio-inhibitory. The vaso-constrictor and cardio-inhibitory nerves pass out from the spinal cord by the anterior roots of the spinal nerves from the second dorsal to the second lumbar, and pass to the lateral ganglia of the sympathetic. They are at this time medullated fibres, but in the ganglia they become non-medullated, and also increase in number, and go to their various points of distribution. The cardio-accelerator fibres pass into the stellate inferior cervical ganglion, where they lose their medullary sheath, and leave it as non-medullated fibres, to be distributed to the heart. The vaso-dilator or vaso-inhibitory nerves are doubtless as numerous as the vaso-constrictor, but far less is known of them. The nervi erigentes which pass to the hypogastric plexus, the chorda tympani, and the small petrosal nerve are illustrations of this class of inhibitory fibres, as is also the cardio-vagus, the inhibitory nerve of the heart. These nerve-fibres have no connection with the lateral ganglia, but they pass on to the collateral or terminal ganglia.

The sympathetic efferent fibres are also distributed to the muscles of the viscera, and are viscero-motor and viscero-inhibitory. The fibres which supply innervation to the muscles of the lower portion of the œsophagus, the stomach, and the intestines, by virtue of which they perform their peristaltic movements, are of this character. The viscero-inhibitory are but little understood. In addition to these there are also glandular nerves which are distributed to secreting organs: of these little is known except as to the parotid, submaxillary, and lachrymal glands.

The functions of the sympathetic ganglia are, so far as known, threefold: 1, to change the medullated into non-medullated fibres; 2, to divide the fibres into a large number of filaments; and 3, to exercise a trophic or nutritive influence on the distal portions of the nerves, and possibly on the structures to which they are distributed. The centres in the cord with which the sympathetic nerves are connected are Clark's vesicular column, Stilling's sacral nucleus, which is in that part of the cord corresponding to the second and third segments of the sacrum, and a third in the neighborhood of the vagal nucleus, that is, the portion of the medulla in which the vagus nerve has its origin.

IV. REPRODUCTIVE FUNCTIONS.

THE reproductive functions are those concerned in the perpetuation of the species. In the lower forms of animal life, where the individual consists of a single cell, this process of reproduction is very simple, consisting of the division of the cell into two, each of which has the same power of dividing to form new individuals in the same manner as itself was formed. This is *asexual* reproduction. In the higher animals the reproduction is *sexual;* that is, it requires the union of two elements produced in the organs of two individuals, the male and the female, neither of which can accomplish the process alone.

1. REPRODUCTIVE ORGANS.

These organs, which are also called the genital or generative organs, are in the male the testes, each with its duct, the vas deferens, and the reservoir, the vesicula seminalis, and the penis; and in the female, the ovaries, Fallopian tubes, uterus, and vagina.

Genital Organs of the Male.—*Testes.*—The testes, or testicles (Fig. 85), two in number, are situated in the scrotum. They are composed of lobules, the number of which in each testis is variously estimated at from two hundred and fifty to four hundred. In each lobule are convoluted seminiferous tubules, tubuli seminiferi, varying in number from one to three.

Spermatozoa.—In the interior of the testes are several layers of epithelial cells which, from the fact that they form the essential part of the semen, are called "seminal cells." At the time of puberty some of these cells, mother-cells, undergo division, producing thereby a

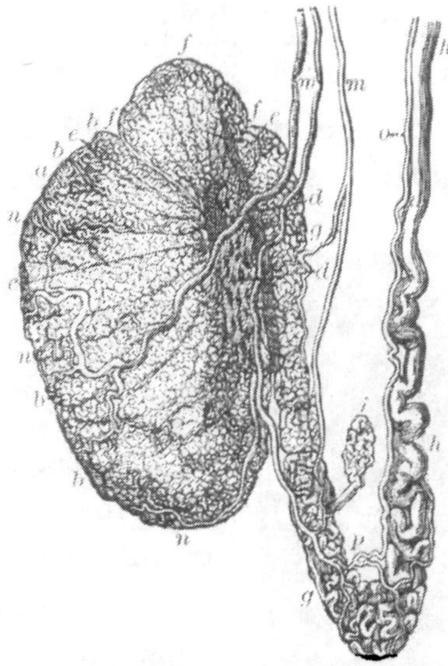

FIG. 85.—Testicle and Epididymis of the Human Subject: *a*, testicle; *b*, lobules of the testicle; *c*, vasa recta; *d*, rete testis; *e*, vasa efferentia; *f*, cones of the globus major of the epididymis; *g*, epididymis; *h*, vas deferens; *i*, vas aberrans; *m*, branches of the spermatic artery to the testicle and epididymis; *n*, ramification of the artery upon the testicle and epididymis; *o*, deferential artery; *p*, anastomosis of the deferential with the spermatic artery (Kölliker).

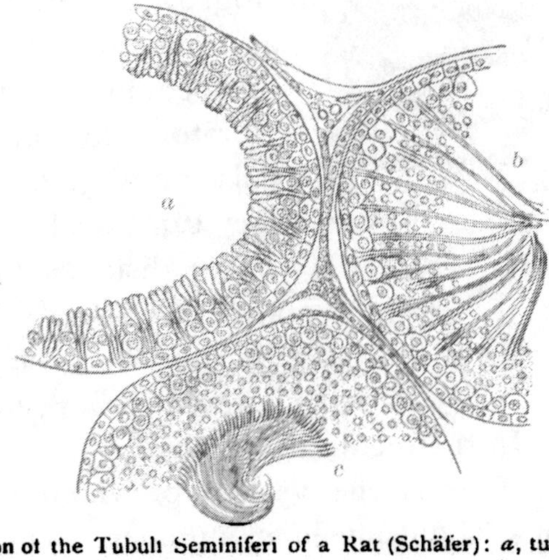

FIG. 86.—Section of the Tubuli Seminiferi of a Rat (Schäfer): *a*, tubuli in which the spermatozoa are not fully developed; *b*, spermatozoa more developed; *c*, spermatozoa still more developed.

22

number of smaller cells. These daughter-cells are called "spermatoblasts," and it is these cells that are changed into the spermatozoa which are the fecundating elements of the semen. Each spermatozoon consists of a head, a body, and a tail. These terms do not indicate any special organization, but are used simply for purposes of description, as we speak of the head of an arrow. The spermatozoa of different animals vary in size, although their general appearance is much the same. The human spermatozoon is about 0.055 mm. long (Fig. 87, *a*), while that of menobranchus is 0.57 mm. (Fig. 87, *c*). These structures are endowed with the power of locomotion, due to the vibratory motion of their tails or *flagella*, by which they can travel for a considerable distance in the generative passages of the female.

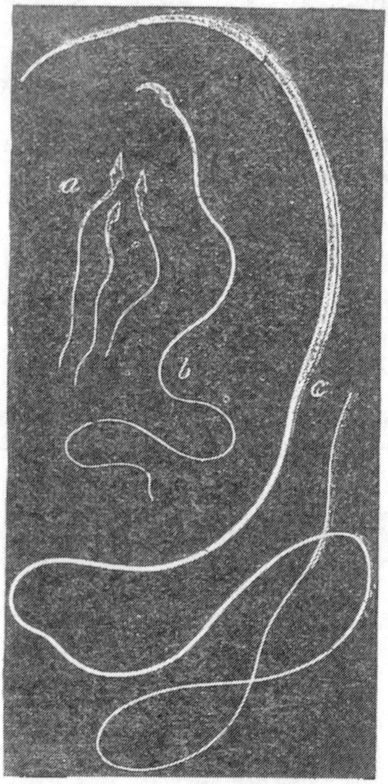

FIG. 87.—Spermatozoa: *a*, human; *b*, of the rat; *c*, of menobranchus (magnified 480 times).

The seminiferous tubules terminate at the apices of the lobules in the vasa recta (straight tubes), about thirty in number. In the mediastinum these tubes form a network, the rete testis, the vessels of which end in the vasa efferentia, about fifteen in number. These vessels connect the testicles with the epididymis, the continuation of which is the vas deferens.

Vas Deferens and Vesicula Seminalis.—The vas deferens may be regarded as the excretory duct of the testis (Fig. 88). It terminates at the base of the bladder, where it unites with the duct of the vesicula seminalis to form the ejaculatory duct, which discharges into the prostatic portion of the urethra.

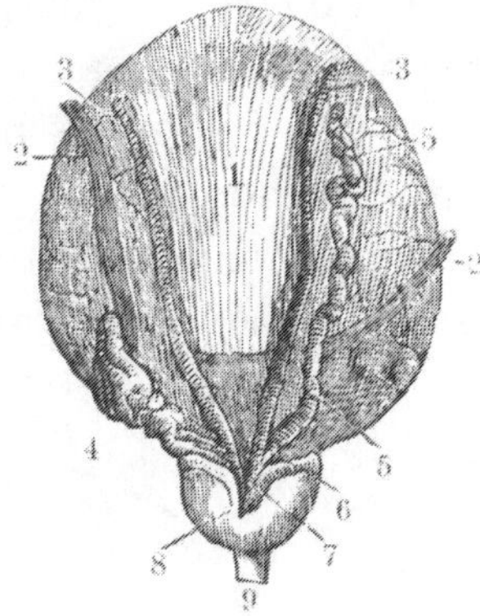

Fig. 88.—Posterior View of the Fundus of the Bladder: 1, peritoneum extending as far down as the transverse line; 2, ureters; 3, deferent canals; 4, seminal vesicle of the left side; 5, right seminal vesicle dissected so as to show its tubular character; 6, duct of the seminal vesicle, joining the deferent canal to form, 7, the ejaculatory duct; 8, prostate; 9, membranous portion of the urethra.

The spermatozoa traverse the following vessels after leaving the seminiferous tubules: vasa recta, rete testis, epididymis, and vas deferens. The mucous membrane lining each of these channels adds its secretion as the spermatozoa pass along, until the vesicula seminalis is reached, which acts as a reservoir for the semen. The lining of the vasa recta and the rete testis is a single layer of flattened epithelium; that of the vasa efferentia, the epididymis, and the vas deferens is columnar and ciliated. The spermatozoa, up to the time that they reach the seminal vesicles, display but little of their characteristic motion. This is probably due to the fact that they are more or less agglutinated, but in these reservoirs there is formed a considerable quantity of secretion which dilutes the semen, and at this time the oscillatory motions of the spermatozoa become very marked.

Genital Organs of the Female.—*Ovary.*—The ovaries (Figs. 89, 90, 91), two in number, are analogues of the testicles. They are situated in the posterior part of the broad ligament, one on each side of the uterus. The human ovary weighs about 8 grammes, and consists of stroma and Graafian vesicles or follicles. The stroma is made up of spindle-shaped cells, which are regarded by some authorities as non-striated muscle-cells, and by others as connective-tissue cells, together with connective tissue. The outer layer of the ovary, formerly called

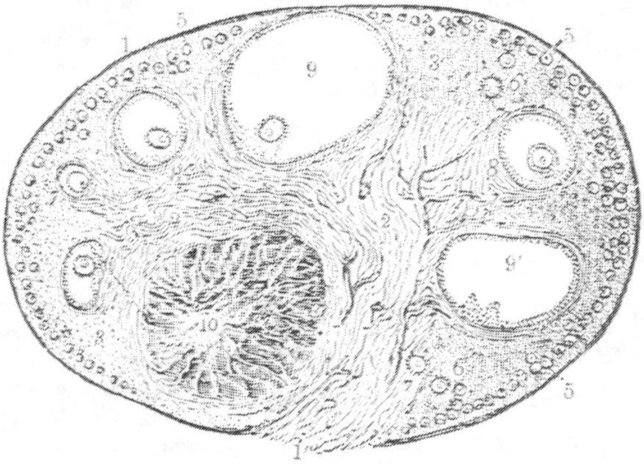

FIG. 89.—Section of the Ovary of a Cat, enlarged six times (Schrön): 1, outer covering and free border of the ovary (epithelium and albuginea); 1′, attached border; 2, vascular zone, or medullary substance; 3, parenchymatous zone, or cortical substance; 4, blood-vessels; 5, Graafian follicles in their earliest stages, lying near the surface; 6, 7, 8, more advanced follicles, imbedded more deeply in the stroma; 9, an almost mature follicle, containing the ovum in its deepest part; 9′, a follicle from which the ovum has accidentally escaped; 10, corpus luteum.

"tunica albuginea," is now regarded as condensed stroma. The covering of the ovary is a single layer of columnar cells, the germinal epithelium of Waldeyer. This is quite different in appearance and structure from the peritoneum, which is covered by flattened endothelium.

The Graafian vesicles are sacs in the ovarian stroma varying in size according to the period of their development. The wall of a vesicle is called the "membrana propria," and is made up of two layers—an external layer of capillary blood-vessels, the tunica vasculosa, and an internal or fibrous layer, the tunica fibrosa. The latter is lined with granular cells arranged somewhat in the form of a membrane, making the membrana or tunica granulosa. At one part of this membrane the cells are accumulated, forming the discus or cumulus proligerus,

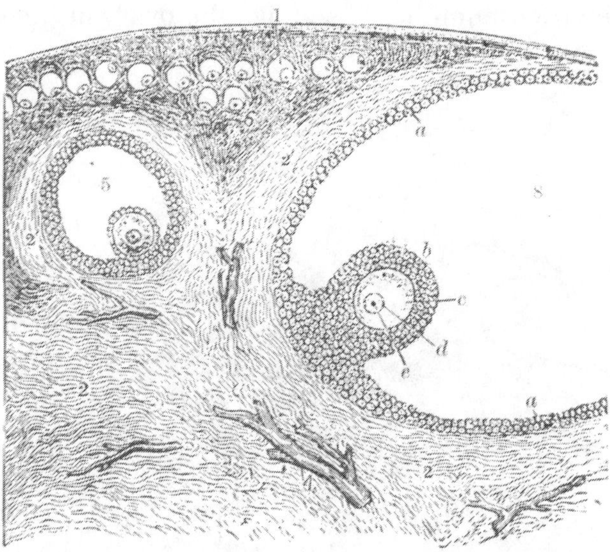

Fig. 90.—Part of the same section as represented in Fig. 89, more highly enlarged (Schrön): 1, small Graafian follicles near the surface; 2, fibrous stroma; 3, 3′, less fibrous, more superficial stroma; 4, blood-vessels; 5, a follicle still further advanced; 6, one or two more deeply placed; 7, one further developed, enclosed by a prolongation of the fibrous stroma; 8, part of the largest follicle; *a*, membrana granulosa; *b*, discus proligerus; *c*, ovum; *d*, germinal vesicle; *e*, germinal spot.

in the midst of which an ovum is imbedded. Between the discus proligerus and the membrana granulosa, except where the two are united, is a fluid, the liquor folliculi.

When during fœtal life the ovary is formed, some of these cells, which have been mentioned above as composing the germinal epithelium of Waldeyer, come to be situated in the stroma, and by a growth of the latter they are cut off from the surface. Around them the ovicapsule forms, and the included cells, with one exception, become the cells of the membrana granulosa. The one cell referred to becomes the *ovum*.

Parovarium.—The parovarium (Fig. 91), also called the "organ of Rosenmüller," is above the ovary in the broad

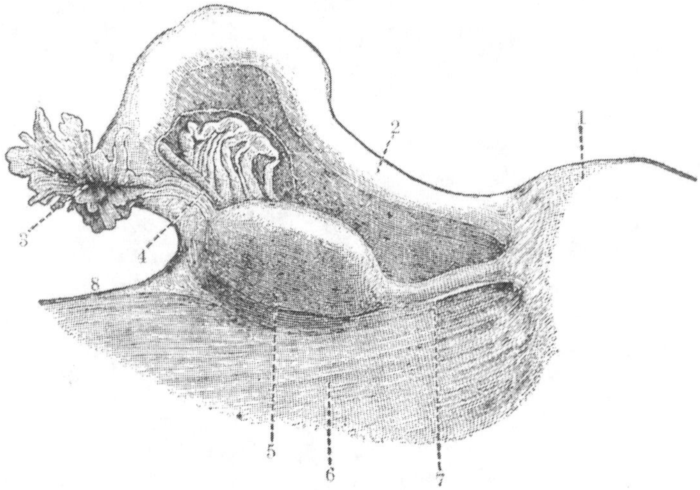

Fig. 91.—Posterior View of Left Uterine Appendages (Henle): 1, uterus; 2, Fallopian tubes; 3, fimbriated extremity and opening of the Fallopian tube; 4, parovarium; 5, ovary; 6, broad ligament; 7, ovarian ligament; 8, infundibulo-pelvic ligament.

ligament, between the latter and the Fallopian tube. It is the remains of the Wolffian body, a fœtal organ.

Ovum.—The human ovum, which is on an average 0.25 mm. in diameter, is composed of an external enveloping membrane, the vitelline membrane or zona pellucida, within which is an albuminous material, the vitellus, in the midst of which is the germinal vesicle with its contained germinal spot.

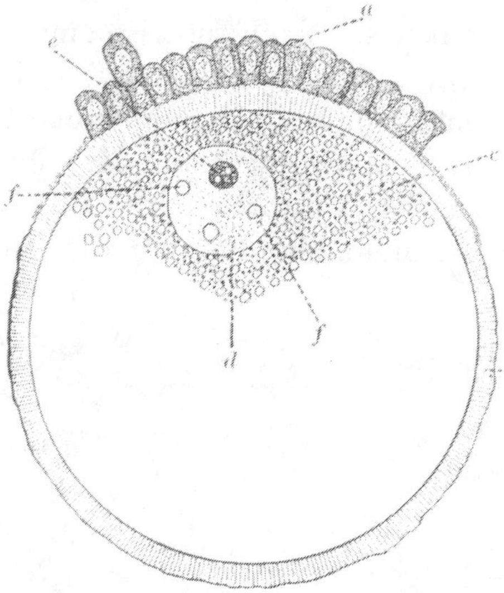

FIG. 92.—Mature Ovum of Rabbit (Waldeyer): *a*, cells from the discus proligerus (epithelium of ovum); *b*, zona pellucida; *c*, vitellus; *d*, germinal vesicle; *e*, germinal spot; *f*, large globules with dull lustre in the germinal vesicle.

Fallopian Tubes.—The Fallopian tubes are each about 10 cm. long, and extend from the angles of the uterus to

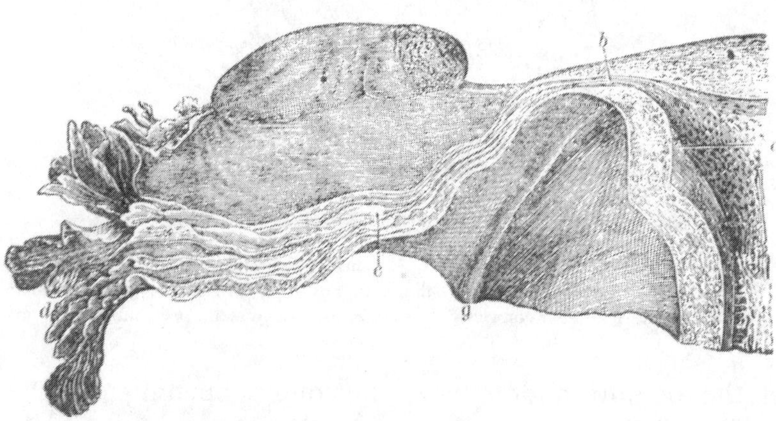

FIG. 93.—Fallopian Tube laid open (from Playfair, source unknown): *a*, *b*, uterine portion of tube; *c*, *d*, folds of mucous membrane; *e*, tubo-ovarian ligament, or fimbria ovarica; *f*, ovary; *g*, round ligament.

the sides of the pelvis. Each tube is composed of three coats—serous, muscular, and mucous. The muscular coat contains both longitudinal and circular fibres. The mucous coat is covered by columnar ciliated epithelium, and it consists of three parts, the isthmus, the ampulla, and the infundibulum. In this latter portion

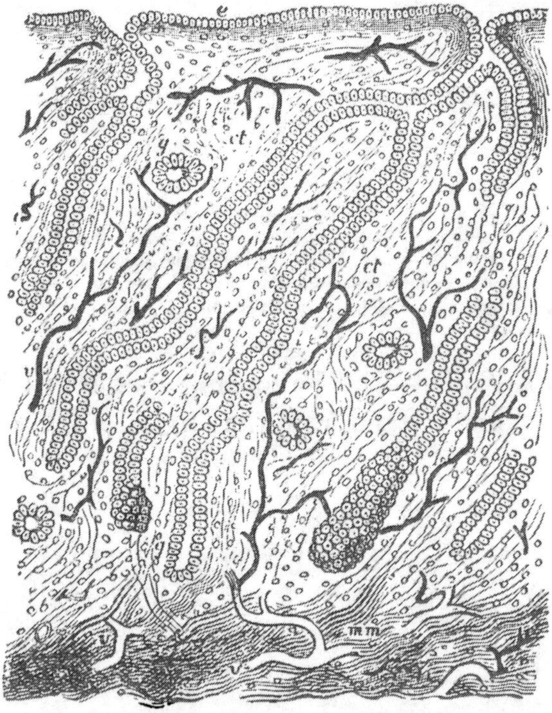

Fig. 94.—Vertical Section through the Mucous Membrane of the Human Uterus (Turner): *e*, columnar epithelium—the cilia are not represented; *g*, *g*, utricular glands; *ct*, interglandular connective tissue; *v*, *v*, blood-vessels: *mm*, muscular layer.

is the ostium abdominale, the outer opening of the tube, which is surrounded by the fimbriæ, one of which, the fimbria ovarica, is attached to the ovary. The fimbriæ are also lined by ciliated epithelium. The canal of the tube is, at its junction with the uterus, very narrow, scarcely admitting a bristle; in the other portion it is larger.

Uterus.—The uterus is about 7.5 cm. long, 5 cm. broad, and 2.5 cm. thick, and weighs about 32 grammes. It is divided into body and neck—corpus and cervix—and consists of three coats—serous, muscular, and mucous. The mucous coat is covered by columnar ciliated epithelium, except at the lower third of the cervix, where the cilia are absent, and the epithelium gradually changes until at the external os it is squamous. In the mucous membrane of the body are the uterine glands.

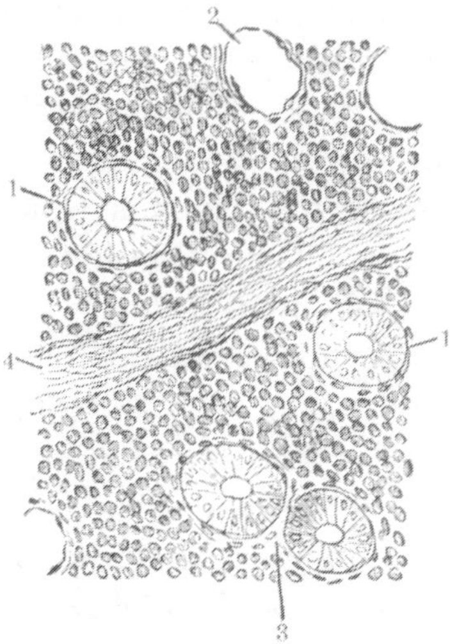

FIG. 95.—Section of the Mucous Membrane of the Uterus, parallel to the surface (Henle): 1, 2, 3, glands (the epithelium has fallen out from 2); 4, blood-vessel.

2. OVULATION.

At undetermined periods the liquor folliculi of the Graafian vesicles increases, and as a result the membrana propria becomes distended until the distention reaches such a degree that this membrane bursts and the contents, including the ovum, are discharged. The ripening and discharge of ova constitute *ovulation*, which is believed by many authorities to occur at regular intervals of about four weeks. Others think that this process does not take place so frequently, and that the intervals are very irregular and unknown. J. Bland Sutton, in his *Surgical Diseases of the Ovaries and Fallopian Tubes*, says: "In the ovary of the human fœtus ova ripen, form follicles, and undergo suppression during the last month of intra-uterine life. The life of the human ovary may be divided into the following periods of activity and repose: The first period extends from the seventh month of intra-uterine life to the end of the first year. Ova ripen in such abundance that in some cases a marked diminution in the number of the ova is appreciable at the second year after birth. To this succeeds a period of comparative repose, terminating at the tenth or twelfth year; then the ripening of ova is again easily detected, and goes on independently of menstruation, even after the accession of the climacteric."

In an uncertain proportion of instances the ova find their way into the Fallopian tube. The mechanism by which this is accomplished is still a matter of doubt. One theory maintains that the fimbriated extremity is so approximated to the ovary as to bring the ostium abdominale against the part at which the Graafian vesicle is about to rupture, and that the escaping ovum thus enters the tube. Tait has found in certain cases upon which he has operated the tube grasping the ovary, and he attributes this action to muscular fibres which develop at the period of puberty and which atrophy at the menopause, so that ova can enter the tube only during the active life of these fibres, and then, and then only, can pregnancy take place, though both before puberty and after the menopause ovulation may occur, the ova under these circumstances falling into the abdominal cavity, where they disintegrate. According to this theory, if ovulation takes place and the tube does not grasp the ovary, the ovum when discharged would not enter the tube, but would fall into the abdominal cavity.

The second theory is, that this grasping of the ovary by the tube does not occur, but that the ovum is carried into the ostium abdominale by the current created by the ciliated epithelium lining the tube and the fimbriæ. The fimbria ovarica, which is attached to the ovary, forms a little groove leading to the ostium, and if an ovum should find its way into it the ciliated epithelium would doubtless carry it to the opening of the tube.

While neither of these theories has been demonstrated as the sole explanation of the cause of the passage of the ovum into the tube, it is possible that both are in a measure correct. If the actual grasping of the ovary by the tube does not, as a rule, occur, there may still be a partial approximation and the current may complete the process. It is to be remembered that the ovum is but 0.25 mm. in diameter, and there seems no reason to question the power of the current to draw so small a body into the tube. Once in the tube, it is carried on to the uterus by the ciliated epithelium.

3. Menstruation.

At about the age of fourteen years a bloody discharge takes place from the vagina at intervals of about four weeks. This is the *menses*, and the process is *menstruation.* It should be noted that the period of life at which menstruation appears is by no means uniform in all individuals.

Prof. Skene lays down the following rules in his *Diseases of Women:*

1. Menstruation should begin at puberty; that is,

when the woman is maturely developed, no matter what the age may be.

2. It should recur at regular intervals; about every twenty-eight days is the average time. A regular periodicity is normal, but the duration of the periods often differs in different persons.

3. The discharge should always be fluid in consistence and sanguineous in color.

4. The flow should continue a definite length of time, the duration depending upon the habit of each case; at least there should not be any great deviation from this rule. The duration is usually from three to five days, and the total amount is about four or five ounces.

At about the age of forty-five years menstruation ceases: this is the *menopause*, or climacteric, or change of life. The cessation is not abrupt, but gradual. The menstruation becomes irregular, and finally ceases altogether.

Composition of Menses.—The menstrual flow is composed of blood from the uterine blood-vessels. Some authorities think some of the blood is from the Fallopian tubes. Whether there is also present the broken-down mucous membrane of the uterus or simply exfoliated epithelium is still a mooted question.

The changes which take place in the mucous membrane of the body of the uterus during menstruation are not agreed upon by authorities. Some hold to the view that the entire membrane, down to the muscular coat, is thrown off; others that only the epithelial layer is cast off; while still others think that even this slight amount of destruction is absent. J. Bland Sutton maintains that there is no discharge of mucous membrane, basing his opinion upon observations he made on the macaque monkey, in which animal there seems to be a true menstruation. The evidence seems to support the theory that the extent to which tissue is destroyed is no greater than involves the epithelium.

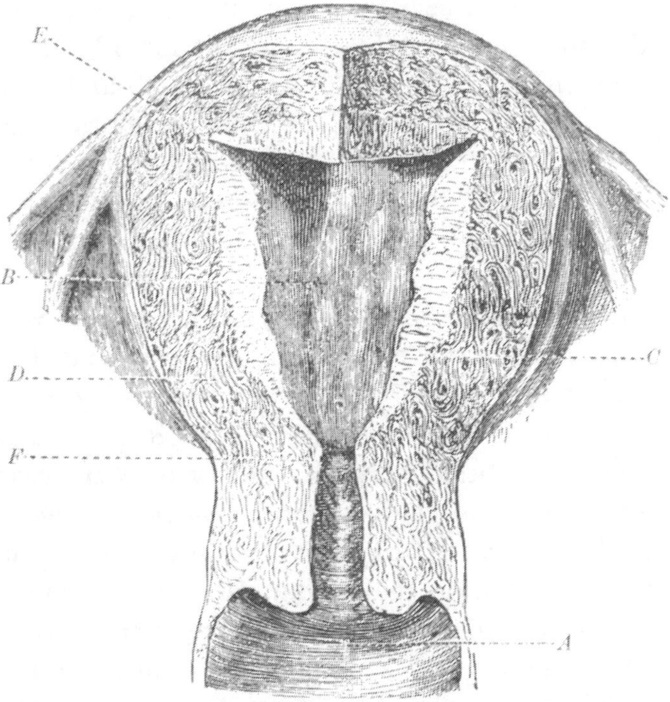

FIG. 96.—Uterus during Menstruation (Courty), cut open to show the swelling of the whole organ, and particularly the mucous membrane: *A*, mucous membrane of cervix; *B*, *C*, mucous membrane of corpus, much thickened; *D*, muscular layer; *E*, uterine opening of tube; *F*, os internum (the mucous membrane tapers down to these openings).

Cause of Menstruation.—The cause of menstruation is still undetermined. Some writers regard it as dependent on a special nerve-centre. It is claimed that in the removal of the ovaries and tubes to produce a premature menopause, as is done by surgeons for certain diseased conditions, this is more certainly accomplished if a large nerve-trunk which lies in the angle between the round ligament and the tube is included in the ligature, so as to destroy its function; but the evidence on this point is not convincing.

Relation between Ovulation and Menstruation.—The relation between these two processes is as yet undetermined, although physiologists in the main hold that at the time of the discharge of an ovum from the ovary there is such a condition of the uterus as brings about its increased vascularity and the oozing from its vessels of the menstrual blood. They believe that at each menstruation there is discharge of an ovum. Other writers—and these are principally surgeons who have devoted much time to the study of diseases of women, and who have large experience in operations for the removal of the ovaries—differ very materially from the physiologists. One of the number (A. Reeves Jackson, in an article entitled "Ovular Theory of Menstruation: Will it Stand?" in the *American Journal of Obstetrics*) says: "Menstruation may occur without accompanying ovulation; ovulation may occur without accompanying menstruation; and ovulation is the irregular but constant function of the ovaries, while menstruation is the regular rhythmical function of the uterus." Lawson Tait, the celebrated surgeon, says that "ovulation and menstruation are not only not concurrent, but ovulation is much less frequent than menstruation." J. Bland Sutton, already referred to, says: "It is very difficult to uproot ancient tradition, especially one so ancient as the belief in the intimate association of ovulation and menstruation, but evidence is rapidly accumulating which will show that the two processes are not so intimately connected as was formerly supposed."

PLATE IV.

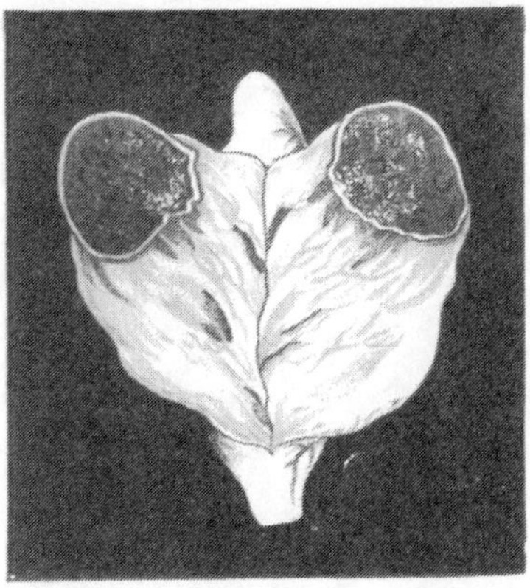

1

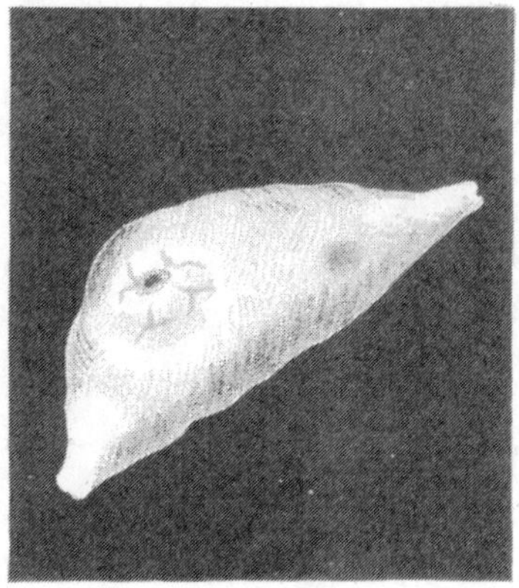

2

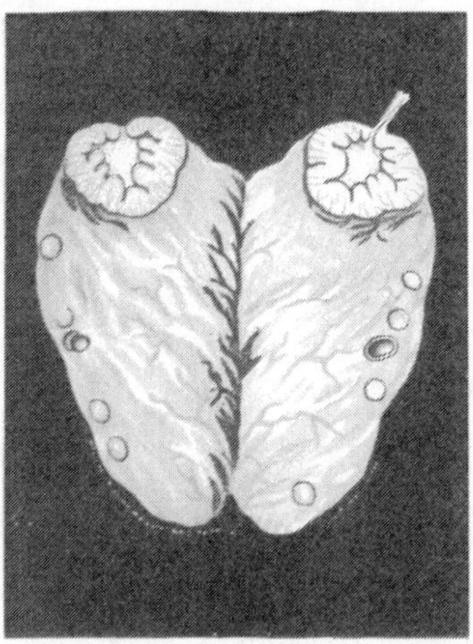

3

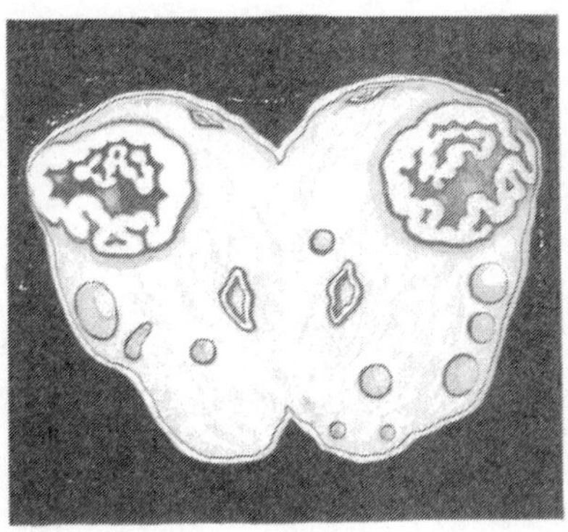

4

FIG. 1.—Ovary of Woman two days after Menstruation, showing earliest stages of transformation of a ruptured and bloody Graafian follicle into a corpus luteum.

FIG. 2.—Ovary of Woman nine days after Menstruation: The dark spot is the cicatrice; the surrounding yellow circle is the corpus luteum shining through the transparent tissue.

FIG. 3.—Ovary of Woman at term of Pregnancy, showing corpus luteum with firm white central clot.

FIG. 4.—Ovary of Woman twenty days after Menstruation: Besides large fresh corpus luteum are seen two smaller old ones, and Graafian follicles of different sizes (*Dalton*).

It would appear, then, that the relation existing between ovulation and menstruation is not definitely determined, but that they are in some manner associated cannot be questioned, for the removal of the ovaries, as a rule, is followed by a discontinuance of menstruation.

Formation of Corpus Luteum (Pl. 4).—After an ovum is discharged from a Graafian vesicle certain changes take place in the latter structure, which changes result in the formation of a corpus luteum. The cavity of the vessel is filled with blood which, like blood elsewhere, coagulates. The serum becomes expressed from the clot, and is absorbed, and later the clot, which at first was red, becomes decolorized. The membrana propria becomes thickened and convoluted, especially opposite the point at which the ovum escaped, and subsequently becomes of a yellow color; whence its name. This body becomes smaller and smaller and finally disappears. As a corpus luteum forms whenever a vesicle ruptures, it is no evidence of pregnancy. If impregnation take place, the corpus luteum becomes larger and remains for a longer time than when pregnancy does not occur. The length of time required for the descent of the ovum to the uterus is unknown, but is believed to be about seven days. During the passage it receives a covering of albuminous material from the mucous membrane of the tube.

Maturation of the Ovum.—The changes which take place in the ovum itself during the descent have been studied in lower animals, and it is inferred that the same changes occur in the human ovum; they constitute the maturation of the ovum. To understand these changes thoroughly it is necessary to be familiar with karyokinesis, the process of indirect division of the nuclei of cells. The ovum is a cell whose nucleus is the germinal vesicle, and the nucleolus is the germinal spot. The germinal vesicle has its enclosing membrane, the nuclear membrane, and the protoplasm of the vesicle is

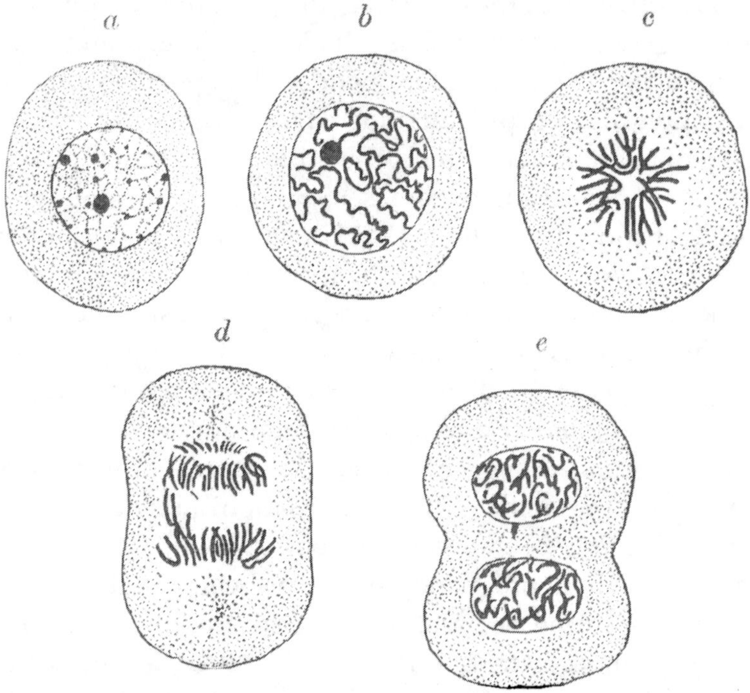

FIG. 97.—Karyokinesis, or Indirect Cell-division: *a*, cell with nucleus in quiescent state (the nucleus contains nucleoli and a network of threads); *b*, formation of coarse chromatin threads in nucleus; *c*, disappearance of nucleolus and membrane of nucleus; arrangement of threads in loops, forming the "rosette;" *d*, angles of loops directed toward the poles of the cell, which are formed of achromatic threads; *e*, beginning division of the cell; this is followed by a gradual return of the nucleus to the quiescent state (*a*).

reticulated. This vesicle approaches the surface of the ovum, and as a result of several changes that take place in it a polar globule is formed, and later a second one. These globules have no further office, but what remains of the vesicle after their separation returns to the centre of the ovum, and now receives the name of "female pronucleus." It is to be understood that the changes in the ovum which have been described occur entirely independently of impregnation; indeed, it is questionable whether an ovum can be considered as mature until the stage has been reached in which the female pronucleus has been formed.

Impregnation.—During coitus, or sexual intercourse, the seminal fluid is forcibly thrown into the vagina, and by virtue of their vibratile movements the spermatozoa enter the canal of the cervix uteri and pass through the canal of the body into the Fallopian tube, in which it is believed that they meet the ovum in its descent, probably in the upper portion. Here fecundation or impregnation occurs.

It was formerly held that the spermatozoa might fertilize the ovum while the latter was still in the ovary, and that its development there, more or less complete, constitutes *ovarian pregnancy*, and also that in some instances the ovum so impregnated, instead of going through with development in the ovary, might drop into the abdominal cavity, and there develop, constituting *abdominal pregnancy*; but the present view is that ovarian pregnancy rarely occurs, if ever, and that abdominal pregnancy results from the rupture of a Fallopian tube in which an impregnated ovum has previously lodged and developed. If this view be correct, every extra-uterine pregnancy resolves itself originally into a tubal pregnancy, and fertilization of the ovum always takes place in the tube, probably in the upper portion, for it is probable that the layer of albuminous material added to the exterior of the ovum by the mucous membrane of the Fallopian tube in the lower part of the canal would serve as an obstacle to the entrance of the spermatozoa.

Method of Fertilization.—In the vitelline membrane of the ova of some animals there is a minute opening called the "micropyle," by which a spermatozoon gains access to the interior. Such an opening does not exist in the

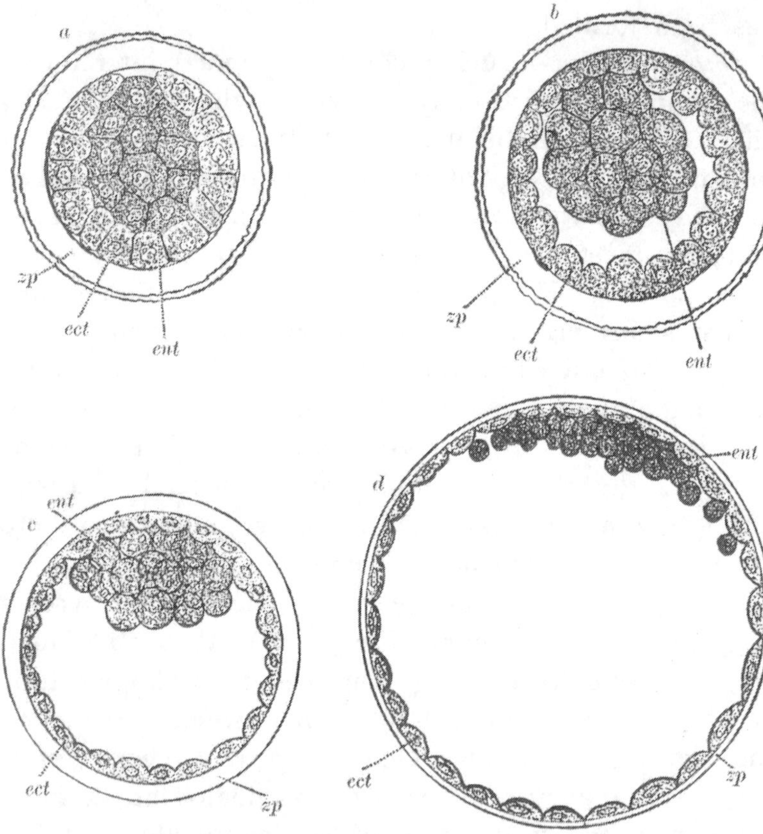

FIG. 98.—Sections of the Ovum of a Rabbit, showing the formation of the blastodermic vesicle (E. Van Beneden): *a*, *b*, *c*, *d*, are ova in successive stages of development; *zp*, zona pellucida; *ect*, ectomeres, or outer cells; *ent*, entomeres, or inner cells.

human ovum. Some histologists have described the vitelline membrane as possessing a porous structure, and it has been suggested that through one of these pores a spermatozoon might pass. It is by no means established that such pores exist. However, in some way the spermatozoon passes through the membrane into the protoplasm; here its tail disappears and the head assumes a spherical form, and to it the name of "male pronucleus" is given. The male and female pronuclei then unite to produce the "fecundation nucleus." After this occurs the ovum consists of a mass of protoplasm with a nucleus, and is spoken of as the "segmentation sphere," because it undergoes segmentation.

Segmentation.—This consists in the production of two segments by the same process of indirect division which took place in the germinal vesicle; these again divide, forming four, and, the same process continuing, the entire ovum is broken up into a mass of spherical cells which, from the resemblance to a mulberry, is named "morula." These cells separate into two layers with fluid between them, except at one place where the two layers are in contact. The blastodermic vesicle is now formed. It is probable that development has reached this stage at about the tenth day, by which time the ovum has entered the uterus. The albuminous secretion of the Fallopian tube serves as pabulum or food to the cells in this process.

Formation of Embryo.—The next change which takes place is the formation of three layers from the two just described. They are termed the *epiblast*, the *mesoblast*, and the *hypoblast;* together they form the *blastoderm.* The epiblast is most external, in contact with the vitelline membrane, which takes no part in the changes thus far described.

It would perhaps be too much to say that the embryo is now formed, yet the subsequent changes are but the modification and differentiation of the cells which compose these three layers. The epiblast forms the brain and spinal cord, portions of the organs of special sense, and the epidermis, and also takes part in the formation of the chorion and amnion. The mesoblast forms the vascular, osseous, and muscular systems and the endothelium which lines the serous cavities. The hypoblast forms the lungs, the epithelium of the alimentary canal and of the glands which are offshoots from this canal. The membrane which lines the allantois and the yolk-sac are also formed from the hypoblast.

The segmentation just described is such as takes place in the human ovum and that of other mammalia. It is a process in which the entire mass of protoplasm undergoes division: such ova are said to be "holoblastic." In the ova of birds and of reptiles only a portion undergoes this segmentation, the rest serving as food. Such ova are "mesoblastic." As an illustration of the latter may be mentioned the fowl's egg, in which the processes of development have most thoroughly been studied. In this egg only a minute portion, the cicatricula, becomes converted into the chick, while the great body of material nourishes the growing embryo until it leaves the shell and is able to gain its own livelihood. As such an embryo is never attached to the parent, it must have within itself all the material necessary for its development and maintenance until freed from its enclosing shell, hence the large size of the ovum; while in the mammal this supply is not necessary, for the attachment to the maternal structures is made at an early period of its history, and from the parent all necessary sustenance is obtained.

Inasmuch as development has been so much more thoroughly studied in the hen's egg than in any other, and inasmuch as the processes are in many respects probably the same as in the human ovum, the development of the chick will be described, referring to the principal points of difference as they are reached in the description, giving, however, only a general view of the subject, which is much too extensive and complicated to discuss in any other manner in this connection.

Development of Chick.—If the shell of a hen's egg be broken during the first day of its incubation and the blastoderm be examined, it will be seen that there is a clear central portion, the area pellucida, and a portion outside of this, the area opaca, which is much less clear. The embryo forms in the area pellucida, and the membranes and structures which are to nourish it form in the area opaca. On the second day, the area opaca having meanwhile extended, within it are formed red blood-corpuscles and vessels, and during the same time in the area pellucida the heart is formed. These structures arise, as has been stated, from the cells of the mesoblast.

At one extremity of the area pellucida a fold forms in the blastoderm, and, as this is the anterior end, it is called the "cephalic fold." A similar fold, the tail fold, forms at the other extremity of the area pellucida. In the same manner lateral folds form on the sides. All these folds, which include the three layers of the blastoderm, approach one another below, and by so doing form a canal, the embryonal sac. This sac is bounded above by the blastoderm, anteriorly by the cephalic fold, posteriorly by the tail fold, and laterally by the lateral folds, while below it is in communication with the vitellus. This embryonal sac subsequently becomes divided into two, one division forming the alimentary tract and the other the body-walls, the umbilicus being the point at which the folds all unite. These folds just described are to be carefully distinguished from the membranes, the amnion, the chorion, etc. The folds, as stated, involve the epiblast, the mesoblast, and the hypoblast, while in the formation of the membranes the various layers play different parts.

Membranes of the Embryo.—Amnion.—The mesoblast about the embryo splits into two laminæ, the parietal and the visceral. The parietal (external) joins with the epiblast to form the *somatopleure*, from which the amnion and the body-walls are developed, while the visceral lamina unites with the hypoblast to form the *splanchnopleure.* From this structure are developed the walls of the *allantois*, the yolk-sac, and the alimentary canal. Between the somatopleure and the splanchnopleure is the pleuro-

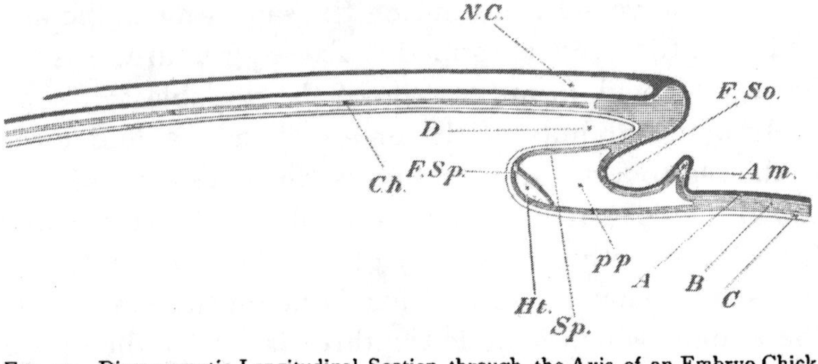

FIG. 99.—Diagrammatic Longitudinal Section through the Axis of an Embryo Chick (Foster and Balfour): *N. C*, neural canal; *Ch*, notochord; D, foregut; *F. So*, somatopleure; *F. Sp*, splanchnopleure; *Sp*, splanchnopleure forming the lower wall of the foregut; *Ht.* heart; *pp*, pleuroperitoneal cavity; *Am*, amniotic fold; *A*, epiblast; *B*, mesoblast; *C*, hypoblast.

peritoneal cavity, which later is divided by partitions into pericardial, pleural, and peritoneal cavities. From the somatopleure folds form which rise above the embryo on all sides, meeting over its back and fusing together. These are the amniotic folds. As each fold is double, when they unite two membranes result: the inner, next the embryo, is the amnion, and the outer, toward the vitelline membrane, is the false amnion (Fig. 100). The amnion and the vitelline membrane fuse to-

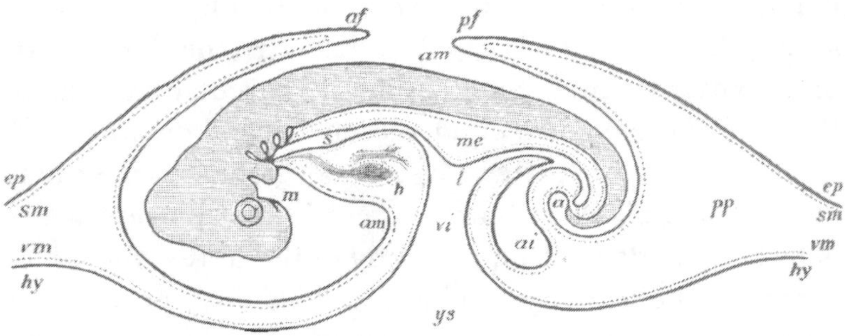

FIG. 100.—Diagrammatic Longitudinal Section of a Chick on the Fourth Day (Allen Thomson): *ep*, epiblast; *hy*, hypoblast; *sm*, somatopleure; *vm*, splanchnopleure; *af*, *pf*, folds of the amnion; *pp*, pleuro-peritoneal cavity; *am*, cavity of amnion; *ai*, allantois; *a*, position of the future anus; *h*, heart; *i*, intestine; *vi*, vitelline duct; *ys*, yolk; *s*, foregut; *m*, position of the mouth; *me*, the mesentery.

gether, forming the chorion. The true amnion has epiblast for its inner and mesoblast for its outer layer, and the space between it and the embryo is the amniotic cavity, in which the liquor amnii accumulates.

Yolk-sac.—The yolk-sac is a very important structure in the fowl and in birds generally, as it is upon the yolk that the nutrition of the embryo depends; but in mammals it is of little importance, as the nutritive material in the vitellus is insignificant in amount.

Allantois.—The allantois is a projection of the splanchnopleure into the pleuro-peritoneal cavity. It subsequently communicates with the posterior portion of the intestinal canal, and its lining is hypoblast. This structure projects more and more into the pleuro-peritoneal cavity, following up the folds that have been described as forming the true and the false amnion. The allantois at last comes in contact with the chorion, which, it will be remembered, was formed by the fusion of the false amnion with the vitelline membrane, and into the villi of that structure it sends processes. It is especially developed in the part corresponding to the attachment of the ovum to the uterine wall. The allantois has two layers, a mesoblastic and a hypoblastic. In the former are blood-vessels which come from the vascular system of the embryo, the connecting vessels becoming the umbilical arteries. At a later stage of development the cavity of the allantois disappears, except in that portion which is to be included within the body of the fœtus, and which becomes the urinary bladder, and in that portion between the bladder and the umbilicus, which becomes the urachus.

Chorion.—This membrane, as already stated, is formed by the union of the vitelline membrane and the false amnion. When first formed, it is smooth, but becomes shaggy by the growth from it of processes called "villi." These villi are at first scattered over the whole exterior of the ovum, but later they are found only at the point of attachment of the ovum to the uterus, where the placenta is to be formed. In these villi are blood-vessels from the fœtal vascular system.

Placenta.—When the impregnated ovum reaches the cavity of the uterus the mucous membrane of that organ is prepared to receive it, and it finds a lodgement there. Under the stimulus of impregnation the whole mucous membrane becomes thickened, and at the termination of utero-gestation the entire mucous membrane of the body is cast off; it is called the "decidua vera." Especially marked is this thickening at the point of attachment of the ovum, and to this part the name "decidua serotina" is applied (Fig. 101). As a result of this stimulus the mucous membrane increases around the ovum, finally completely enclosing it. This new formation is the "decidua reflexa."

The villi of the chorion find their way into the depressions of the decidua serotina, and their walls become atrophied, being finally represented only by epithelial cells covering the capillary blood-vessels which have come from the allantois. The blood-vessels in the decidua serotina become converted into blood-spaces, sinuses, to which the uterine arteries carry blood, and from which the uterine veins carry the blood away. It will be seen, therefore, that the fœtal blood-vessels are surrounded by the maternal blood in the uterine sinuses, the two fluids being separated only by the thin wall of the fœtal capillaries, through which the interchanges of oxygen and carbon dioxide take place, and also the passage of the nutritious material to supply the growing fœtus, and in the reverse direction pass the effete products to be eliminated. The structure which performs all these important offices is the *placenta*, made up of both maternal and fœtal tissues. It seems hardly necessary to say that the blood of the mother and that of the child

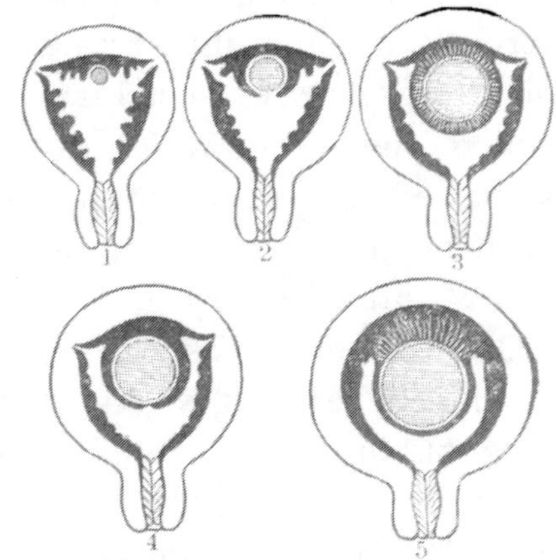

FIG. 101.—Series of Diagrams representing the Relationship of the Decidua to the Ovum at Different Periods. The decidua are colored black, and the ovum is shaded transversely. In 4 and 5 the vascular processes of the chorion are figured. (*Copied from Dalton.*) 1, ovum entering the congested mucous membrane of the fundus—decidua serotina; 2, decidua reflexa growing around the ovum; 3, completion of the decidua around the ovum; 4, general growth of villi of the chorion; 5, special growth of villi at placental attachment, and atrophy of the rest.

never come in contact, but are always separated by the walls of the fœtal capillaries.

At birth the placenta is cast off, and in the contraction of the uterine muscular tissue the mouths of the maternal blood-vessels are closed, and thus hemorrhage is prevented. The blood which escapes during a normal labor is that which was in the sinuses. The functions of the placenta are thus seen to be threefold—nutritive, respiratory, and excretory.

Circulation in the Embryo.—*Vitelline Circulation.*—During the earliest weeks of human fœtal life the contents of the ovum supply the growing embryo with nutrition. This is done by means of vessels which compose the vitelline circulation, but, important as this circulation is in the fowl's egg, it is of very brief duration in the human subject, for the supply of nutritious material is soon exhausted, probably at the sixth week.

Placental or Fœtal Circulation.—By the sixth week the placenta is formed and the connection has been made by which the embryo receives its nourishment from the maternal blood. From this time until birth the fœtus depends upon the placental or fœtal circulation for its nourishment and maintenance.

The blood of the fœtus is freed from much of its impurities in the placenta, and there likewise it receives oxygen and nutritive materials. It returns to the fœtus through the umbilical vein, passing to the liver. In this organ the current is divided: the greater part joins with the venous blood of the portal vein; a second portion goes directly into the hepatic circulation; while a third part goes through the ductus venosus into the ascending vena cava without passing through the liver. The currents all meet again in the ascending vena cava, here mixing with the blood returning from the lower extremities. The ascending vena cava discharges its

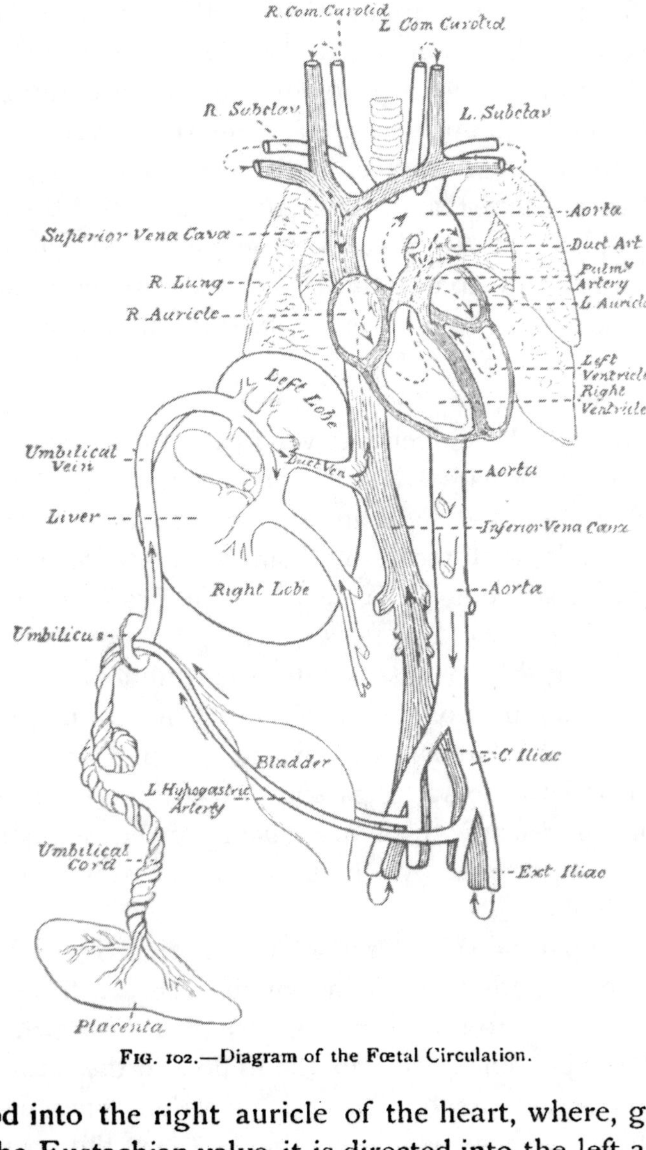

FIG. 102.—Diagram of the Fœtal Circulation.

blood into the right auricle of the heart, where, guided by the Eustachian valve, it is directed into the left auricle through the foramen ovale. From this cavity it passes into the left ventricle, thence into the aorta, which distributes it to the head and upper extremities. It will be seen from this description that to these three portions of the body the blood from the placenta is distributed. This blood is not very pure, for it has been deteriorated by the impure blood returning from the lower extremities, with which it mixes in the ascending vena cava; but it is the purest and most nutritious blood the fœtus receives, and this accounts for the greater development of the upper portion of the body as compared with the lower, which is so striking a feature in the new-born babe.

The blood returns from the head and upper extremities through the descending vena cava to the right auricle, and thence passes into the right ventricle. There is probably always a slight mixing of the currents in the right auricle, that returning from the placenta and that from the descending vena cava, but at first this is very slight; later it is doubtless greater. From the right ventricle the blood passes into the pulmonary artery, a very small portion going through the capillaries of the lungs, the larger part passing through the ductus arteriosus into the aorta, passing down this vessel to the internal iliac, from which are given off the hypogastric or umbilical arteries by which the blood is conveyed to the placenta.

By comparing this description with that of the circulation in the adult the points of difference will be seen. It may be well to note here that there are six principal points of difference between the fœtal and the adult circulatory apparatus, besides less important ones of size and shape. These points of difference are the presence in the fœtal heart of the Eustachian valve and the foramen ovale, in the venous system of the umbilical vein and the ductus venosus, and in the arterial system of the umbilical arteries and the ductus arteriosus.

Changes in the Circulation at Birth.—During intra-uterine life the respiratory centre in the medulla is supplied with blood containing sufficient oxygen to prevent any inspiratory impulse, and there is therefore during this period no attempt at respiration on the part of the fœtus. (See Resistance Theory of Respiration, p. 251.) As soon, however, as the connection between the parent and the child is severed, whether by separation of the placenta or by tying of the umbilical cord, the respiratory centre, being no longer supplied with oxygen, sends out impulses to the respiratory muscles, and respiration begins. This may be hastened or assisted by slapping the skin or dashing water upon it, but under ordinary circumstances these measures are not called for. The fact that respiration will take place while the fœtus is still enclosed in its membranes, without the reflex influence of exposure to the air, shows that this is not the essential, but only a contributing, cause. It is the stoppage of the placental circulation which starts the respiratory movements.

Although during fœtal life some blood flows through the pulmonary capillaries, still the amount is small, and, there being no air in the pulmonary alveoli, the lungs will sink if placed in water. The first respiratory movement causes an enlargement of the thoracic cavity and a consequent distention of the lungs, the air passing into the alveoli, and the blood, which is at the same time in the pulmonary capillaries, becomes oxygenated and returns to the left auricle as arterial blood. The expansion of the thorax reduces the resistance to the flow of the blood through the pulmonary circulation, and as a result a large amount of blood goes to the lungs; this means a lessened amount through the ductus arteriosus, and, following the law that a diminution of function is followed by atrophy, this vessel begins to diminish in size, and becomes closed between the fourth and tenth days, and in later life is to be found as a fibrous cord between the left pulmonary artery and the aorta.

With the termination of the placental circulation the flow through the ductus venosus ceases, and within a few days this vessel closes, and remains only as a fibrous cord in the fissure of the same name in the liver: that portion of the umbilical vein which is within the body of the child becomes the round ligament of the liver. The blood flowing into the right auricle from the inferior vena cava finds it easier to pass into the right ventricle than into the left auricle, which is now filled with blood from the lungs, and hence takes this course, while the blood cannot flow into the right auricle through the foramen ovale by reason of the valve which has been forming in the left auricle during the latter part of intra-uterine life to close this opening. The opening is not permanently closed for a considerable time after birth, in some cases a year, and sometimes not at all. As a result of these various changes the fœtal circulation becomes converted into that of the adult.

INDEX.

E.

F.

G.

N.

O.

P.

V.

W.

Y.

Z.